PHYSICAL ACTIVITY IN
REHABILITATION AND RECOVERY

PHYSICAL ACTIVITY IN REHABILITATION AND RECOVERY

HOLLY BLAKE

EDITOR

Nova Science Publishers, Inc.

New York

NOTICE TO THE READER
The Publisher has taken reasonable care in the preparation of this book, but makes no expressed or implied warranty of any kind and assumes no responsibility for any errors or omissions. No liability is assumed for incidental or consequential damages in connection with or arising out of information contained in this book. The Publisher shall not be liable for any special, consequential, or exemplary damages resulting, in whole or in part, from the readers' use of, or reliance upon, this material.

Independent verification should be sought for any data, advice or recommendations contained in this book. In addition, no responsibility is assumed by the publisher for any injury and/or damage to persons or property arising from any methods, products, instructions, ideas or otherwise contained in this publication.

1006935389

This publication is designed to provide accurate and authoritative information with regard to the subject matter covered herein. It is sold with the clear understanding that the Publisher is not engaged in rendering legal or any other professional services. If legal or any other expert assistance is required, the services of a competent person should be sought. FROM A DECLARATION OF PARTICIPANTS JOINTLY ADOPTED BY A COMMITTEE OF THE AMERICAN BAR ASSOCIATION AND A COMMITTEE OF PUBLISHERS.

LIBRARY OF CONGRESS CATALOGING-IN-PUBLICATION DATA
Physical activity in rehabilitation and recovery / editor, Holly Blake.
     p. ; cm.
Includes bibliographical references and index.
ISBN 978-1-60876-400-6 (hardcover)
1. Exercise therapy. 2. Medical rehabilitation. I. Blake, Holly, 1975-
[DNLM: 1. Exercise Therapy--methods. 2. Exercise--physiology. 3. Physical Exertion--physiology. 4. Rehabilitation--methods. WB 541 P5785 2009]
RM725.P49 2009
615.8'2--dc22
                          2009039007

Published by Nova Science Publishers, Inc. ✛ *New York*

CONTENTS

Preface   **vii**

Editorial: Exercise in Rehabilitation: Towards a Population-Based
                  Promotion of Physical Activity   **1**
                  Holly Blake

Chapter 1   Physical Activity for Health: Adult Recommendations,
                  Interventions and Evaluation   **5**
                  Charlotte Emma Hilton

Chapter 2   Physical Activity and Long-Term Conditions   **17**
                  Holly Blake

Chapter 3   Exercise Promotion and Rehabilitation of Neurological
                  Conditions   **51**
                  Helen Dawes

Chapter 4   The Role of Exercise in the Management of Long
                  Term Pain: A Biopsychosocial Approach   **101**
                  Paula Banbury, Caroline Neal and Elizabeth Johnson

Chapter 5   Physical Activity in Traumatic Brain Injury Rehabilitation   **131**
                  Holly Blake

Chapter 6   Aerobic and Resistance Exercise in Patients with Congestive
                  Heart Failure   **155**
                  Pamela Bartlo

Chapter 7   Exercise Based Cardiac Rehabilitation   **183**
                  Frances Wise

Chapter 8   "Within You and without You": Internal and External
                 Factors in the Realisation of Exercise Principles   **211**
                 Alison Mckeown

Chapter 9   Representation and Perceptions of Injury in Sport
                 and Exercise: The 'Common Sense' Model   **229**
                 Martin S. Hagger

Chapter 10   The Role of Physical Exercise in Occupational
                 Rehabilitation   **261**
                 Amanda Griffiths and Alec Knight

Chapter 11   Exercise Interventions in the Treatment of Depression   **279**
                 Sumaira Malik, Phoenix Kit Han Mo and Holly Blake

Chapter 12   Psychological Outcome Measures to Evaluate Exercise
                 Interventions   **313**
                 Shirley A. Thomas and Roshan das Nair

Author Biographies   **341**

Index   **349**

PREFACE

Increasing physical activity at a population level is an important public health priority. Exercise is increasingly recognised as an essential lifestyle behaviour in maintaining health, preventing disease and rehabilitating a broad range of conditions. This book compiles research evidence and clinical perspectives on the benefits and pitfalls of exercise in rehabilitation and recovery from illness or injury. The content focuses on the growing and important concept of increasing physical activity in people with long-term health conditions, maintaining active lifestyles for physical health and wellbeing, prevention of secondary illness and recovery from injury. In an eclectic collection of chapters, readers are provided with an outline of population trends in physical activity, presenting the international focus on increasing population-level physical activity through a range of approaches. The importance of physical activity for those with 'chronic' health conditions is discussed using examples from UK strategy for the management of long-term conditions. Several chapters present the nature and outcomes of exercise prescription and consider the implications of exercise promotion or intervention in musculoskeletal disorders (e.g. chronic back pain, arthritis), neurological conditions (e.g. stroke, TIA, Parkinson's, Multiple Sclerosis, Traumatic Brain Injury), cardiorespiratory illnesses (e.g. coronary heart disease, heart failure) and other common health conditions (e.g. COPD, cancer, obesity and diabetes). Both the physical and psychological outcomes of exercise are considered and several clinical case studies are presented. The implications of exercise in mental health are discussed (e.g. in the treatment of depression) and the relevance of cognitive representations of illness and coping strategies in rehabilitation are discussed in relation to musculoskeletal injury. Motivational factors and barriers to exercise in rehabilitation are discussed in the context of exercise programme design. A range of common outcome measures used for the psychological evaluation of exercise interventions are reviewed. The evidence relating to physical activity for occupational rehabilitation and work capability of absent employees is also presented together with organizational case studies. Chapters are compiled by academics and health professionals providing a combination of theory, current research evidence, and examples from practice.

Chapter 1 - This chapter aims to review the current recommendations for physical activity for adults and the initiatives that have been developed to assist individuals in meeting them. The challenges of evaluating physical activity and exercise initiatives are discussed with considerations for the future development of exercise interventions, their evaluation and recommendations for practitioners.

Chapter 2 - This chapter describes the prevalence of ill health in our society and the associated burden on health and social care services, using examples of long-term conditions management strategies within the UK. An argument is presented that in those with long term conditions, maintaining a physically active lifestyle is important in helping to reduce further disability, increasing independence, improving prognosis and psychosocial outcomes and to help prevent the onset of secondary disease. Rehabilitation may include structured exercise intervention targeted at specific functional improvements, general physical conditioning, or recommendations to increase lifestyle physical activity, with exercise interventions tailored to the specific needs of individuals. This chapter presents an overview of the benefits of physical activity for health and quality of life in a diversity of health conditions.

Chapter 3 - This chapter explores the effect of an active lifestyle on the general health, well being and role in prevention of the primary disease and occurrence of secondary diseases for selected conditions affecting the central nervous system. It will give an initial overview of neurological conditions, consider the barriers and facilitators for engagement and long term maintenance of physical activity, and finally explore physical activity levels and interventions in people with stroke, Parkinson's disease (PD) and Multiple Sclerosis (MS). The aim is not to cover detailed discussion of exercise prescription for attainment of specific functional recovery within rehabilitation, but rather to scrutinise exercise prescription for health and wellbeing in primary and secondary prevention.

Chapter 4 - The benefits of exercise and activity in the management of long term pain are well documented. A wealth of information exists about the most effective treatments for this complaint. It is generally accepted that the evolution of a new model for understanding the complex phenomenon of persistent pain has been more useful to patients and professionals working in this clinical area. The limitations of a purely medical approach have been acknowledged and a biopsychosocial model is proposed, applying principles of cognitive behavioural therapy to achieve more effective results for patients. Exercise has always been considered a pivotal feature of pain management programmes but evidence for which type or style has varied, and researchers continue to debate this issue. However a body of evidence has been building to explore the involvement of beliefs, thoughts and feelings in influencing prognosis for patients with long term pain. This is reflected in this chapter and it is acknowledged that a biopsychosocial approach should be employed when treating people with long term pain who present with barriers to increasing their activity levels.

Chapter 5 - Traumatic brain injury (TBI) can result in a range of physical, cognitive, emotional and behavioural problems. Exercise is increasingly advocated in brain injury rehabilitation since individuals with long-term conditions are at particular risk of deconditioning and secondary disease or impairment as a result of inactivity. Maintaining an active lifestyle can help brain injured individuals to regain confidence and independence, and further, exercise has been associated with reductions in physical and cognitive impairments, fatigue and depression, which often accompany TBI. This chapter identifies some key arguments for promoting exercise in TBI, and provides an overview of the research evidence evaluating exercise intervention in this population identifies some major limitations of existing work in this field and provides suggestions for further investigation. A case study is presented which shows the introduction of an alternative form of exercise intervention into the community day centre setting.

Chapter 6 - Congestive heart failure (CHF) is a common disease that leads to multiple body system changes. People with CHF experience difficulties with left ventricular function and heart rate control. They also sustain changes at the skeletal muscles that lead to inefficiencies in muscle function. These central and peripheral changes lead to multiple symptoms, the most common of which are decreased exercise tolerance and dyspnoea. Research has focused on exercise for people with CHF and has shown promising results. Both aerobic and resistance exercise have been shown to have positive effects on the cardiovascular system and several peripheral systems. Exercise has been shown to be safe and able to improve the quality of life for people with CHF. Recommendations for exercise prescription, based on the literature, are outlined in this chapter.

Chapter 7 - Cardiovascular disease is the leading cause of death in developed nations, and there is a clear link with physical inactivity. The benefits of exercise, both aerobic and resistance training, in patients with Coronary Heart Disease are well documented. Both modalities are important components of cardiac rehabilitation and can contribute to secondary prevention of heart disease with corresponding improvements in patient survival. This chapter describes the benefits of exercise for cardiac patients, details how exercise is prescribed in this group, and considers safety and contra-indications.

Chapter 8 - The main aim of this chapter is to explore internal and external motivational factors in relation to exercise and physical activity undertaken for preventative or rehabilitative reasons. A brief social context is provided and evidence for the benefits of engaging in structured exercise as part of rehabilitation and condition management programmes is discussed. Barriers to exercise are presented and the increased effect they have in the rehabilitative context. The chapter concludes with an evaluation in favour of the health benefits.

Chapter 9 - The common-sense model of illness perceptions suggests that people's lay representations of illness assist them in coping with health threats by guiding their coping responses to produce adaptive illness outcomes. The present theoretical and empirical chapter reviews the literature with respect to the common-sense model and reports an empirical study that sought to examine relations among lay perceptions of sport-related musculoskeletal injuries, generalized coping strategies to deal with injury, and important functional and emotional outcomes in injured sports participants and athletes. Specifically, the cross-lagged effects between injury perception and coping procedures were tested among sport injured athletes (N = 126, 81 men, 45 women, mean age = 21.46, SD = 6.42) over a period of four weeks. Confirmatory factor analyses supported the construct validity of self-report measures of injury perception dimensions (identity, serious consequences, time, personal control, and treatment control), coping dimensions (active and planning coping and venting emotions), and the emotional (anxiety, depression) and functional (sport functioning, physical functioning) outcomes. Autoregressive path analyses revealed a moderate degree of stability in the illness perception constructs over a 4-week period. There was only one cross-lagged relationship with personal control (time1) predicting active coping (time 2) and vice-versa. Personal control was the most prominent predictor of both functioning and emotional outcomes. In addition, planning coping was negatively related to emotional outcomes, while injury identity was important in predicting physical functioning and both emotional outcomes. Importantly, few of the injury perceptions at time 1 predicted outcomes at time 2, indicating that immediate beliefs about the injury and coping styles are most relevant. Results are discussed with respect to the common-sense model and practical recommendations to change cognitive perceptions of injury such as personal control and emotional representations that impact upon anxiety and depression. It is proposed that practitioners adopt planning and active coping strategies to improve injury outcomes.

Chapter 10 - Given the accepted role of physical exercise in rehabilitation in healthcare settings, it is surprising that exercise has been subject to little research in occupational environments. Employers, on the other hand, are beginning to credit exercise with some potential significance. This chapter presents the scientific evidence to date, and using the UK as an example, explores the disconnect between academic considerations, policy-level and employer-led imperatives. It focuses on three areas of concern to employers: (a) common mental health issues, (b) musculoskeletal disorders, and (c) cardiovascular conditions and respiratory disorders. Reviewers of the scientific literature have frequently commented upon the lack of methodological rigour in relation to the extant evidence. However, such criticisms should be tempered by a realistic appreciation of the nigh-impossibility of conducting experimental or quasi-experimental investigations in the turbulent world of real organisations. The authors conclude that although evidence remains mixed at present, the role of physical exercise in occupational rehabilitation looks promising.

Chapter 11 - Depression is a common psychiatric problem affecting millions of people worldwide. Whilst conventional treatments for depression have involved the use of antidepressant medications or 'talking' therapies, in recent years the concept of exercise therapy has received increasing attention as a potential alternative or supplementary treatment for depression. Research suggests that exercise interventions can be beneficial for alleviating depressive symptoms in individuals with a diagnosis of depression. Furthermore, it appears that exercise may be equally as effective as the use of antidepressant medications or psychotherapy. However, there are methodological shortcomings in much of the published literature, which may limit the generalisability of findings. There is a need for further well-designed research to clarify the role of exercise in the treatment of depression. Recommendations for future research and practice are outlined in this chapter.

Chapter 12 - Psychological outcome measures are becoming more commonplace in the evaluation of exercise interventions. This chapter provides guidance on what factors should be considered when selecting an outcome measure. It is important to evaluate the psychometric properties of the measure, how the measure is going to be completed and who you are completing it with, in order to select the appropriate measure and increase the validity of the findings. In addition, it is necessary to pre-define the primary end-point and to agree what magnitude of different on the outcome measure is clinically meaningful. This chapter includes an overview of outcome measures that have been commonly used to assess quality of life and mood in the evaluation of exercise interventions.

In: Physical Activity in Rehabilitation and Recovery   ISBN: 978-1-60876-400-6
Editor: Holly Blake   © 2010 Nova Science Publishers, Inc.

EDITORIAL: EXERCISE IN REHABILITATION: TOWARDS A POPULATION-BASED PROMOTION OF PHYSICAL ACTIVITY

Holly Blake

It is universally accepted that physical activity is essential for health and wellbeing. Sedentary lifestyles are associated with a range of non-communicable diseases, many of which are associated with an increased risk of morbidity and mortality, and are increasing in prevalence at alarming and often 'epidemic' rates in the Western world. For our society, this results in considerable economic burden as health and social care systems struggle to cope with the increasing demands of preventable disease caused by sedentary lifestyles. From the individual's perspective, there is no longer any doubt that inactivity has devastating effects on physical and psychological health, and that physical activity exerts a profound effect on both short and long-term health and quality of life for people with chronic health problems.

Population-based policies and strategies for promoting physical activity are in place and being implemented widely in our institutions, schools, colleges, workplaces, prisons and in community settings. Yet there is a growing recognition that the benefits of physical activity extend from the general population to particular groups, such as those living with long-term conditions or those who have sustained injury. There have been notable advances in the promotion of exercise in these populations due to the increased risk of secondary disease as a result of inactivity. Exercise is therefore rapidly becoming a cornerstone of rehabilitation programmes, delivered in both acute and community settings for injured individuals or those with chronic disease. Nonetheless, long-term behavioural change is also essential to help people to develop effective strategies for incorporating physical activity into their daily lives and taking responsibility for their own health. Adoption of healthy lifestyle behaviours is becoming a key focus within both primary and secondary prevention settings.

Rehabilitation programmes for a diversity of health conditions commonly include structured, supervised exercise interventions and recommendations for increasing lifestyle physical activities. Assimilating the available evidence into current practice however, can be challenging on many levels. Measuring quality in healthcare needs to be explicit, and although quality measurement is becoming widespread, the use of different assessments or outcome measures often makes research study outcomes difficult to compare. Also, whilst a diverse range of measures exist, we are still lacking a generic, simple tool which can be used in clinical practice to evaluate the level of physical activity participation, or rather, extent of sedentary behaviour on which personalised medical advice can be based. The measure closest to achieving this is the short-form International Physical Activity Questionnaire (IPAQ) although various other self-report questionnaire tools have been adopted for use in different clinical populations. Similarly, the availability of accurate biological markers of activity levels would allow for greater objectivity and scientific quality amongst physical activity research studies since the majority of studies rely heavily on self-reported outcomes. Heart rate monitors and motion sensors (pedometers and accelerometers) are increasingly used in physical activity research although their use can be expensive in clinical practice and problematic in certain populations.

There is no longer any doubt that physical activity is essential in the prevention of chronic disease and premature death, and physical activity is certainly both inversely and linearly associated with mortality. Nevertheless, for many health conditions we await further research to inform us about the optimal frequency, duration and intensity of exercise required for health benefit, for effective rehabilitation or for recovery. In some instances, firm conclusions as to the effectiveness of exercise intervention cannot be drawn from the current evidence base. However, we cannot say that physical activity is *not* beneficial in these cases, but rather that there is not yet enough quality research evidence to support it. This highlights the lack of scientifically rigorous research studies within the research literature. It seems that physical activity now plays a fundamental role in rehabilitation and many simple, or complex, interventions with or without supervision have demonstrated positive health outcomes in a range of settings. However, studies promoting physical activity, particularly amongst the sedentary, are plagued with high drop-out rates and poor adherence to exercise regimes. Unfortunately, however, it is likely that the individuals in most need of exercise intervention are the ones who are least compliant in exercise programmes. Despite the known benefits of a physically active lifestyle, and the increasing prevalence of interventions to encourage physical activity, only a small proportion of the general population meet internationally recognised guidelines for physical activity which suggests that there are barriers to exercise for all of us. Furthermore, many individuals with long term health conditions do not exercise regularly, and report specific barriers and determinants to exercise participation which need to be addressed. Services targeting certain population groups therefore need to be easy to access, readily available and provide supportive environments for lifestyle change.

Exercise is a normal human function, which can be undertaken by most people with a high level of safety. However, physical exercise is not without its risks, and as is the case for the general population, the hazards of exercise for people with long-terms conditions are likely to include unexpected cardiac events, or musculoskeletal injury (a chapter which follows presents a discussion of cognitive perceptions of injury and coping strategies). Exercise in those with long-term conditions is therefore based on the premise that the benefits outweigh any potential risks, and intervention design will undoubtedly need to take into account the severity of the condition and accompanying symptoms or clinical deficits, potential complications and any other co-existing conditions, as well as secondary factors such as patient mood, familial support, social integration and cultural issues. Some individuals will need to be medically supervised during exercise participation, and exercise prescription should always be evidence-based and tailored to the specific needs of the individual.

This book compiles research evidence and clinical perspectives on the benefits and pitfalls of exercise in rehabilitation and recovery from illness or injury. The content focuses on the growing and important concept of increasing physical activity in people with long-term health conditions, maintaining active lifestyles for physical health and wellbeing, prevention of secondary illness and recovery from injury. The eclectic collection of chapters that follows begins with an outline of population trends in physical activity, presenting the international focus on increasing population-level physical activity through a range of approaches. The importance of physical activity for those with 'chronic' health conditions is discussed using examples from UK strategy for the management of long-term conditions. Several chapters present the nature and outcomes of exercise prescription and consider the implications of exercise promotion or intervention in musculoskeletal disorders (e.g. chronic back pain, arthritis), neurological conditions (e.g. stroke, TIA, Parkinson's, Multiple Sclerosis,

Traumatic Brain Injury), cardiorespiratory illnesses (e.g. coronary heart disease, heart failure) and other common health conditions (e.g. COPD, cancer, obesity and diabetes). Both the physical and psychological outcomes of exercise are considered and several clinical case studies are presented. The implications of exercise in mental health are discussed (e.g. in the treatment of depression) and the relevance of cognitive representations of illness and coping strategies in rehabilitation are discussed in relation to musculoskeletal injury. Motivational factors and barriers to exercise in rehabilitation are discussed in the context of exercise programme design. A range of common outcome measures used for the psychological evaluation of exercise interventions are reviewed. The evidence relating to physical activity for occupational rehabilitation and work capability of absent employees is also presented together with organizational case studies.

The information presented in several of the chapters that follow sheds light on the effectiveness of exercise interventions for individuals with chronic conditions who may be defined as 'high risk'. Whilst this is imperative information in the light of rehabilitation and recovery from illness or injury, a key concept remains. It is not unreasonable to assume that *all* individuals would benefit from an increase in physical activity level, particularly those individuals who were previously sedentary. Whilst we know that exercise can help aid recovery from many illnesses and injuries, maintaining a physically active lifestyle is vital in the prevention of a wide range of life-threatening diseases. Therefore, encouragement of exercise participation and the integration of physical activity within the daily routine seems an appropriate strategy for all of us. That is, the importance of physical activity in rehabilitation, recovery and secondary prevention, cannot be divorced from the necessity for a population-based strategy of *preventative* medicine, thus focusing on increasing energy expenditure in the *whole* population, promoting activity from an early age, and making a resolute difference to population health in future generations.

In: Physical Activity in Rehabilitation and Recovery   ISBN: 978-1-60876-400-6
Editor: Holly Blake   © 2010 Nova Science Publishers, Inc.

Chapter 1

PHYSICAL ACTIVITY FOR HEALTH: ADULT RECOMMENDATIONS, INTERVENTIONS AND EVALUATION

*Charlotte Emma Hilton**

School of Science and Technology, Nottingham Trent University, UK.

ABSTRACT

This chapter aims to review the current recommendations for physical activity for adults and the initiatives that have been developed to assist individuals in meeting them. The challenges of evaluating physical activity and exercise initiatives are discussed with considerations for the future development of exercise interventions, their evaluation and recommendations for practitioners.

INTRODUCTION

The diverse health benefits of physical activity are well documented and the importance of a physically active lifestyle for people with long-term conditions is addressed more specifically in the chapter that follows. A UK report from the Chief Medical Officer (Department of Health (DH), 2004) communicates that adults should be accumulating 30 minutes of at least moderate intensity physical

---

* Tel: +44115 8486601; Email: charlotte.hilton@ntu.ac.uk

activity on five or more days a week in order to maintain good general health (5 x 30 moderate). This amount is also reported as sufficient enough to improve psychological well-being although 45-60 minutes of moderate intensity physical activity daily is recommended for the prevention of obesity.

The report acknowledges the significant role physical activity has in the prevention and management of up to 20 chronic diseases and the consequent financial burden physical inactivity has on the economy. In England, the cost of physical inactivity to the economy is estimated to be around £8.2 billion with an additional cost of £2.5 billion for the cost of obesity alone (DH, 2004). The role of physical activity in terms of disease prevention, management, improved mental well-being and the potential economic savings result in physical inactivity being considered as a major public health issue. In the UK, a health survey for England data indicated that in 2003, only 37% of men and 24% of women met the current physical activity guidelines suggested by the Government (DH, 2005). In 2004, it was estimated that 60% of men and 70% of women were not sufficiently active enough to benefit their health (DH, 2004). More recent health survey data for England identified that 40% of men and 28% of women met the current physical activity guidelines (DH, 2006).

In 2002, the Government proposed to increase the proportion of the English adult population who participate in 30 minutes of moderate physical activity five or more times a week to 70% by the year 2020. This would require participation levels in England to double in just over 15 years. As a result, physical activity is increasingly being considered the best investment in health and has been included into recent UK public health policy (DH, 2004a; DH, 2004b; DH 2005; National Institute for Health & Clinical Excellence (NICE), 2006a).

Initiatives to increase the levels of physical activity worldwide are two-fold and include a) self-directed attempts made by the public, usually in response to advice from a clinician and/or b) formal referrals made by clinicians that aim to assist individuals with long-term disease management such as diabetes or hypertension, for example.

INITIATIVES TO INCREASE PHYSICAL ACTIVITY IN THE GENERAL POPULATION

A recent review of initiatives to increase physical activity in the UK identified four main methods to increase physical activity, namely a) brief interventions in primary care, b) exercise referral schemes, c) pedometers and d) community based programmes for walking and cycling (NICE, 2006a). The use of brief interventions in primary care received a favourable response and NICE recommended that this method of increasing physical activity should be implemented wherever possible. However, because of the varied evidence base for the efficacy of exercise referral schemes, pedometers and walking and cycling programmes, NICE recommended that these methods only be endorsed by those funding the initiative when part of a properly designed and controlled research study to determine effectiveness.

BRIEF INTERVENTIONS IN PRIMARY CARE

Historically, brief interventions have been developed to facilitate behaviour change for those with addictive behaviour problems such as drug or alcohol dependence. Brief interventions are often designed to target both cognitions (the level at which an individual identifies with the severity of the problem behaviour) and the behaviour itself (the manner in which an individual responds to the problem-behaviour). The aim is for a skilful practitioner to help an individual identify the nature and severity of a problem-behaviour and support them in developing the necessary skills to reduce this behaviour and make lifestyle changes.

In the context of physical activity behaviour change, the UK NICE guidance (NICE, 2006a) encourages public health practitioners to take the opportunity whenever possible to identify inactive adults and advise them to aim for the physical activity recommendation. However, a consensus on exactly *how* this advice should be delivered is still lacking and implementation advice provided by NICE in the same year only stipulates that practitioners should be provided with training that equips practitioners with *techniques* for delivering brief advice and follow-up procedures (NICE, 2006b). There is little evidence that simply advising someone to take more exercise is effective (e.g. Hillsdon, Thorogood, & Foster, 2002). Therefore, more is needed regarding appropriate consultation methods that aim to facilitate behaviour change. One such method that is growing in the design and delivery of exercise initiatives including brief interventions is motivational interviewing (MI). This directive, client-centred style of counselling has been described as a method that helps clients to explore and resolve their ambivalence about changing behaviour (Rollnick & Miller, 1995). In the context of brief interventions within primary care, practitioners have incorporated adaptations of MI (AMI) into consultations that draw upon the fundamental principles, methods and communication style of MI in order to facilitate behaviour change in consultations where time may be restricted.

EXERCISE REFERRAL SCHEMES

Perhaps the most common method of increasing physical activity, particularly for clinical populations is via an exercise referral scheme. Indeed, the exercise referral scheme has been deemed as the most prolific initiative developed (Crone, Johnston & Grant, 2004). The design of a typical exercise referral scheme includes a 'patient pathway' that allows for health professionals (usually General Practitioners and Practice Nurses) working within primary care to refer patients for programmes of structured exercise. Each scheme will have a specific set of medical inclusion criteria, usually based around particular levels of Body Mass Index (BMI) or Blood Pressure (BP), for example. The referring health practitioner has the ability to signpost eligible patients to a scheme whereby it is commonplace for a scheme coordinator to identify appropriate opportunities for physical activity based upon medical history, disease profile and patient choice. For those that are signposted to structured exercise within a gym setting, instructors supporting these individuals should hold a qualification to work with special populations. Exercise referral schemes are typically designed to offer a programme of exercise for around 12 weeks and in the UK, guidelines have been published to assist organisations with scheme design and evaluation (DH, 2002).

The efficacy of exercise referral schemes in terms of increasing physical activity levels, particularly in the longer-term is poor (NICE, 2006c). Although only four randomised controlled trials of exercise referral schemes were included in a review by NICE, it was deemed that such schemes should only be considered beneficial in increasing physical activity levels in the short-term (6-12 weeks) and that in the longer term (over 12 weeks) and very long-term (over one year) schemes are ineffective. However, it is important to be mindful that current measures of physical activity are not designed to detect change over time which is problematic when attempting to quantify this measure without the use of tools such as accelerometers for example, or when those responsible for assessing patient outcomes are reliant upon self-reported physical activity level. In practice, those responsible for the evaluation of exercise referral schemes do not have access to objective yet expensive measures of physical activity as an academic institution would. Moreover, the evaluation guidelines provided by the National Quality Assurance Framework (NQAF) (DH, 2002) are limited (Dugdill, Graham, & McNair, 2005) and as a consequence, practitioners often struggle to select the most appropriate outcome measures to detect the diverse outcomes of a referral into exercise. Consequently, an increasing number of schemes seek to collaborate with local universities in an attempt to improve evaluation procedures and the quality of data collected. This may also contribute to fulfilling the evaluation recommendations communicated by NICE (2006) that stipulate an exercise referral scheme should only be endorsed by practitioners, policy makers and commissioners when part of a properly designed and controlled research study to determine effectiveness (NICE, 2006a).

PEDOMETERS

Pedometers are a tool designed to measure the total number of steps accumulated in a day. The instrument measures step-count via the detection of hip motion and as such is intended to measure step count exclusively, as opposed to other modes of activity that may contribute to daily physical activity total. The accuracy of pedometers has been the subject of much debate both in terms of the precision of total daily step measurement, and also the manner in which the device is used. In a recent study in America, the notion of reactivity (i.e. a change in behaviour due to the awareness of being monitored) has been addressed. The randomized controlled crossover study subjected 28 healthy white male (n = 12) and female (n = 16) adults to two conditions. Half the group wore sealed pedometers for one week whereby the total number of daily steps could not be seen and these step counts were recorded by a researcher. Following a two-week break when no pedometer was worn or recording taken, the same participants wore an unsealed pedometer whereby total step count could be seen and these were recorded by the participants. The other half of the experimental group completed this protocol in reverse order. There was no significant difference in sealed vs. unsealed pedometers in daily step total leading the authors to propose that reactivity does not challenge the validity of pedometer self-monitoring in healthy adults (Matevey, Rogers, & Dawson, 2006).

Despite debate regarding measurement accuracy, it is generally agreed that the pedometer provides a useful tool for both patient and practitioner to gain baseline data regarding physical activity levels prior to any intervention. Subsequently, the pedometer may be used to set appropriate goals in terms of increases in total daily steps. A recent UK study concluded that the use of pedometers should be encouraged for those whom are overweight or obese especially given the prevalence of obesity in the UK (Clemes, Hamilton, & Lindley, 2008). Historically, the public health message of ten thousand daily steps has been used to set long-term goals for pedometer users and, although still considered beneficial, in practice, this is being reduced in favour of communicating the 5 x 30 moderate guidelines.

COMMUNITY BASED PROGRAMMES FOR WALKING AND CYCLING

The use of walking and or cycling to increase physical activity levels is twofold. One method involves the organisation of structured groups who meet to purposefully walk or cycle. The other is the promotion of walking and cycling into everyday lifestyle as a means of active travel. In the UK an organisation dedicated to supporting organised led health walks – The Walking the way to Health Initiative (WHI) reports favourable physical activity levels for those attending health walks in England and Scotland. Survey data from 750 participants attending health walks revealed that 65% of individuals met the current recommended levels of physical activity just from walking alone (WHI, 2006).

Overall, the potential for such interventions to impact upon health outcomes is positive. Rather than encourage those that require an increase in physical activity for health to engage in structured exercise as per an exercise referral scheme, active travel via walking, cycling, the use of public transport or a combination is considered a valuable intervention. Support for a plausible link between active travel and the management of overweight and obesity has been offered from a recent Australian study where causal relationships for the management of weight and active travel were noted for men in particular (Wen & Rissel, 2008). A recent one-year intervention delivered in Belgium reported a positive influence on blood parameters, blood pressure, mental health and quality of life for middle-aged healthy adults who had cycled to work at least three times a week as part of the one-year controlled study (Geus, Hoof, Aerts, & Meeusen, 2008).

When considering if the key to better health lies within an increase in walking or cycling, it is best to adopt a person-centred approach and to assume that the likelihood of maintaining health behaviour change is increased if the choice regarding mode of activity resides with the person undertaking the health behaviour change. That said, interventions should always be matched to the physical capabilities, desired health outcomes, disease profile and age of the person undertaking exercise behaviour change. Shephard (2008) has suggested that cycling should be preferable for young commuters, while walking should be considered for older persons. As with all the interventions described, the most challenging component of increasing physical activity both at the individual and population level is the perceptions of those who need to be targeted most. The public knowledge base of the benefits of physical activity for health rarely stretch beyond that of weight management and body image for most, which may impact upon motivation for engagement in active travel and other forms of opportunity for physical activity. In addition, it is common for people to report perceived barriers to physical activity. New Zealand survey data (N = 7894) revealed that only a small percentage of people (21%) perceived that they could replace car journeys on at least two days of the week with transport-related physical activity. Furthermore, respondents who reported higher activity levels were more likely to strongly agree with replacing car journeys than those who were sedentary (Badland & Schofield, 2006). Nevertheless, supporting active travel remains a feasible consideration for improving national health profiles and contributing to the prevention and management of chronic disease.

THE EVALUATION OF EXERCISE INITIATIVES AND RECOMMENDATIONS FOR PRACTITIONERS

Prior to the publication of the NICE guidelines (NICE, 2006a) the evaluation of exercise initiatives was infrequent and sporadic. Pedometer and walking schemes tend to focus on rates of attendance to demonstrate at least a need for the service to be delivered. Indeed, some schemes adopt an attendance monitoring approach to infer that attendance and participating in a walking scheme, for example automatically demonstrates that attendees will be in receipt of the benefits of exercise.

Brief interventions in primary care are commonplace for specific long-term conditions. However, their application for the promotion of physical activity is a relatively new concept and one of the most challenging issues is determining some amount of standardisation as to the method of delivery (i.e., the manner in which consistent conversations about physical activity are delivered). A feasibility trial of a care pathway designed to support and signpost patients to opportunities for physical activity received a favourable response from those primary health care practitioners responsible for the delivery of the initial design. In particular, focus group interviews with the practitioners who were trained to incorporate MI methods into primary care consultations revealed that MI was considered as particularly valuable in helping patients change exercise behaviour (Hilton, Milton, & Bull, 2009). Incorporating MI methods into the design and delivery of exercise referral initiatives has been recommended previously (Dugdill, et al., 2005) which may indicate moves towards more specific guidelines regarding the delivery method of schemes in the future.

It is the efficacy of exercise referral schemes that has been given considerable attention in the literature (e.g. Dugdill, Graham, & McNair, 2005; Harrison, Roberts & Elton, 2004; Morgan, 2004 & Riddoch, Puig-Ribera, & Cooper, 1998) and is the source of much debate. Primarily perhaps because exercise referral schemes may be more successful in some areas than others. For example, exercise referral schemes may impact upon a person's attitudes and beliefs regarding exercise more significantly than measurable physiological change. It is safe to assume that the least likely impact of such a short 12-week referral for exercise would be physiological outcomes, and yet this is the most frequently measured outcome. Relevant psychological and environmental parameters tend to be ignored (Dugdill et al., 2005) despite these parameters also being some of the most likely outcomes for those referred (DH, 2002). For these reasons, attempting to summarise the generic efficacy of exercise referral becomes challenging.

Qualitative methodology is often utilised to gain a greater understanding of the 'how' and 'why' of exercise referral and assist statistically in an environment where scheme participant sample sizes may be small. More importantly, these types of studies can recognise the value of person-centred methods of healthcare practice, and focus on the person with the disease rather than the course of the disease itself (Bauman, Fardy, & Harris, 2003). However, communicating qualitative data to those who fund schemes is difficult in terms of a historical favour of quantitative data within healthcare systems and concerns regarding generalizability of results.

The tools with which to capture such diverse responses to, and outcomes of exercise for those who had previously been sedentary are poor in terms of their transferability from research to practice. For example, current measures of physical activity level are unable to detect change over time and therefore the validity of data collected via questionnaires in this way is debatable. Measures that seek to determine psycho-social outcomes of exercise interventions (typically generic quality of life measures) are not specific to those items of importance for exercise referral populations. Such measures have usually been developed for research purposes and the transferability of their use in practice is sometimes difficult (the psychological outcomes measures commonly used in exercise interventions will be addressed in more detail further in this book).

CONCLUSION

In short, the literature has a lot to offer in terms of furthering our understanding about not only the benefits of physical activity for the general population and those with long-term conditions but also with regard to the efficacy of those initiatives that have been designed to increase physical activity and perhaps more importantly, those attributes that may play a key role in determining if an individual will attempt to engage in physical activity or not. The long-term focus of any intervention designed to increase physical activity should be behaviour change. Any intervention designed to help people change their physical activity behaviour should a) ensure that the intervention has procedures in place for addressing behavioural change, including resources such as behaviour change counselling training for those whom are to deliver the intervention at patient level (e.g. motivational interviewing), b) ensure that the aims and objectives of the intervention match the evaluation methods used to collect evidence of patient outcomes (i.e. an intervention designed to assess the impact of exercise upon psychological outcomes should not consider physiological assessments such as weight loss as a primary measure of efficacy), c) ensure that, wherever possible links with local academic institutions are made in order to assist with the management and analysis of large and complicated programme evaluation data sets and d) ensure that the intervention is person-centred and that the motivation for change alongside choice of physical activity is initiated by the patient and not the practitioner. It is probable that this will enhance the likelihood of an individual starting a programme of exercise and also long-term behaviour change.

At a more global level, we have seen how the Government, communities and individuals have responded to the high levels of physical inactivity and the physical activity related health profile of the UK and internationally. In order to make a real impact at the population level, multidisciplinary engagement from those responsible for transport, leisure services, urban planning and public health messages is required. The related ill-health consequences of a sedentary lifestyle are an urgent worldwide consideration and the subtleties of poor participation levels lie deeply rooted within the complexities of attitudes, beliefs and perceived motivation. Physical inactivity is a complex problem to which there is no simple solution. However, designing the right transport systems, ensuring adequate opportunities to leisure services and designing an environment that aims to facilitate active lifestyles, all have a role to play in tackling disease prevention and management, increasing physical activity, improving health inequalities and enhancing quality of life.

REFERENCES

Badland, H., & Schofield, G. (2008). Perceptions of Replacing Car Journeys with Non Motorized Travel: exploring Relationships in a Cross-Sectional Adult Population Sample. *Preventative Medicine, 43,* 222-225.

Bauman, A. E., Fardy, J.H., & Harris, P.G. (2003). Getting it Right: Why Bother with Patient-Centred Care? *The Medical Journal of Australia, 179,* 253-256.

Clemes, S.A., Hamilton, S.L., & Lindley, M.R. (2008). Four-Week Pedometer Determined Activity in Normal Weight, Overweight and Obese Adults. *Preventative Medicine,* 325-330.

Crone, D., Johnston, L., & Grant, T. (2004). Maintaining quality in exercise referral schemes: A case study of professional practice. *Primary Health Care Research & Development, 5,* 96-103

Department of Health. (2002). Exercise Referral Systems: A National Quality Assurance Framework. London: HSMO.

Department of Health. (2004a). *Choosing Health. Making Healthy Choices Easier.* London: HMSO.

Department of Health. (2004b). *At Least 5 a Week. Evidence of the Impact of Physical Activity and its Relationship to Health. A Report from the Chief Medical Officer.* London: HMSO.

Department of Health. (2005). *Choosing Activity. A Physical Activity Action Plan.* London: HMSO.

Department of Health. (2005). *Health Survey for England.* London: The Stationary Office.

Department of Health (2006). *Health Survey for England: Updating of Trend Tables to Include 2005 Data.* London: Information Centre.

Dugdill, L., Graham, R. C., & McNair, F. (2005). Exercise referral: The public health panacea for physical activity promotion? A critical perspective of exercise referral schemes; their development and evaluation. *Ergonomics, 48,* 1390-1410.

Geus, B.D., Hoof, E.V., Aerts, I., & Meeusen, R. (2008). Cycling to Work. Influences on Indexes of Health in Untrained on Untrained Men and Women in Flanders. Coronary Heart Disease and Quality of Life. *Scandinavian Journal of Medicine and Science in Sports, 18,* 498-510.

Harrison, R.A., Roberts, C., & Elton, P.J. (2004). Does Primary Care Referral to an Exercise Programme Increase Physical Activity 1 Year Later? A Randomized Control Trial. *Journal of Public Health, 27,* 25-32.

Hillsdon, M., Thorogood, M., & Foster, C. (2002). Advising people to take more exercise is ineffective: A randomised control trial of physical activity promotion in primary care. *International Journal of Epidemiology, 31,* 808-815.

Hilton, C.E., Milton, K. & Bull, F.C. (2009).Lets Get Moving: A Feasibility Trial of a 'Physical Activity Care Pathway' in Primary Care Settings. *Journal of Sport and Exercise Sciences, 26* (S2) S1-S143.

Matevey, C., Rogers, L.Q., & Dawson, E (2006). Lack of Reactivity during Pedometer Self-Monitoring in Adults. *Measurement in Physical Education and Exercise Science 10,* 1-11.

Morgan, O. (2004). Approaches to Increase Physical Activity: reviewing the Evidence for Exercise referral Schemes. *Journal of the Royal Institute for Public Health, 119,* 361-370.

National Institute for Health and Clinical Excellence. (2006a). *Four Commonly used Methods to Increase Physical Activity: Brief Interventions in Primary Care, Exercise Referral Schemes, Pedometers and Community-based Exercise Programmes for Walking and Cycling.* London: UK.

National Institute for Health and Clinical Excellence. (2006b). *Implementation Advice: Four Commonly used Methods to Increase Physical Activity.* London: UK.

National Institute for Health and Clinical Excellence. (2006c). *A Rapid Review of the Effectiveness of Exercise Referral Schemes to Promote Physical Activity in Adults.* London: UK.

Rollnick, S., & Miller, W.R., (1995). What is Motivational Interviewing? *Behavioural and Cognitive Psychotherapy, 23,* 325-334.

Riddoch, C., Puig-Ribera, A., & Cooper, A. (1998). *Effectiveness of Physical Activity Schemes in Primary Care: A Review.* London: Health Education Authority.

Shephard, R.J. (2008). Is Active Commuting the Answer to Population health? *Sports Medicine, 38,* 751-758.

Walking the Way to Health Initiative. (2006). *Walking the Way to Health Initiative 2000-2005. National Evaluation of Health Walk Schemes.* The Countryside Agency.

Wen, L.M., & Rissel, C. (2008). Inverse Associations between Cycling to Work, Public Transport, and Overweight and Obesity: Findings from a Population based Study in Australia. *Preventative Medicine, 46,* 29-32.

In: Physical Activity in Rehabilitation and Recovery   ISBN: 978-1-60876-400-6
Editor: Holly Blake   © 2010 Nova Science Publishers, Inc.

Chapter 2

PHYSICAL ACTIVITY AND LONG-TERM CONDITIONS

*Holly Blake**

Faculty of Medicine and Health Sciences, University of Nottingham, UK.

ABSTRACT

This chapter describes the prevalence of ill health in our society and the associated burden on health and social care services, using examples of long-term conditions management strategies within the UK. An argument is presented that in those with long term conditions, maintaining a physically active lifestyle is important in helping to reduce further disability, increasing independence, improving prognosis and psychosocial outcomes and to help prevent the onset of secondary disease. Rehabilitation may include structured exercise intervention targeted at specific functional improvements, general physical conditioning, or recommendations to increase lifestyle physical activity, with exercise interventions tailored to the specific needs of individuals. This chapter presents an overview of the benefits of physical activity for health and quality of life in a diversity of health conditions.

* Tel: +44 (0)115 8231049; Fax: +44 (0)115 8230999; Email: Holly.Blake@nottingham.ac.uk

LONG-TERM CONDITIONS: PREVALENCE AND SERVICE USE

Long-term conditions (LTC) are health conditions of a prolonged duration, generally longer than a year, that may affect any aspect of a persons' life. Symptoms may be transient or permanent, and often these conditions have no cure but individuals may be able to adjust their lifestyle in order to manage their symptoms, reduce the risk of secondary consequences, and maintain or improve their quality of life. The World Health Organisation (WHO) defines long term conditions, also called 'chronic' conditions, as health problems that require ongoing management over a period of years or decades. This includes a wide range of health conditions including non-communicable diseases (e.g. cancer and cardiovascular disease), communicable diseases (e.g. HIV/AIDS), certain mental disorders (e.g. schizophrenia, depression), and ongoing impairments in structure (e.g. blindness, joint disorders) (Department of Health, 2005c).

Long-term conditions are prevalent in today's society and are a major cause of disability both in the UK and internationally. Some of the most common LTCs include hypertension, chronic heart disease, asthma, diabetes, cancer, neurological disorders and severe mental health conditions. In Engand, the General Household Survey (2005) revealed that 15.4 million people have a LTC and this figure predicted to increase to 18 million by 2025, with this increase concomitant with changing population demographics and an ageing population, and also the increasing incidence of preventable disease which is often associated with poor lifestyle choices. UK prevalence rates for long-term conditions are available from a range of sources including the General Medical Services (GMS) Quality and Outcomes Framework (QOF) (BMA/NHS Convention, 2003). The QOF is an annual reward and incentive programme detailing general practitioner practice achievement results, an important part of which is achievement points for general practices for the management of common LTCs. However, whilst these figures provide a general picture of the prevalence of long-term conditions the figures do not distinguish between those suffering from single or multiple conditions.

In the UK, it is estimated that the most common conditions include (in order of highest prevalence): hypertension (almost 7 million), obesity, asthma, diabetes, coronary heart disease, stroke and transient ischaemic attack, chronic obstructive pulmonary disease, heart failure, cancer, severe mental health conditions and epilepsy (>300,000). What our national figures do show is that ill health in our population is rising, and this places significant burden on health and social care services which must become responsive to meet this increase in demand.

With advances in medicine meaning a reduction in the prevalence of communicable disease, the predominant disease pattern in England, and also other developed countries, is now one of chronic illness rather than acute disease. In fact, recent UK figures show that more than 30% of the population suffer from a LTC, and this has significant cost implications since this group are intensive users of primary and secondary care services, taking more than half of all general practitioner appointments, two-thirds of hospital outpatient appointments and nearly three-quarters of all inpatient bed days (Department of Health, 2007a). A handful of conditions, associated by common risk factors and underlying determinants, are responsible for a large part of the disease burden, with just seven risk factors accounting for 60% of disease burden in Europe: high blood pressure (12.8%); tobacco (12.3%), alcohol (10.1%), high blood cholesterol (8.7%), overweight (7.8%); low fruit and vegetable intake (4.4%) and physical inactivity (3.5%) (World Health Organisation, 2006). These risk factors frequently cluster in individuals and interact to impact further on disease outcome.

MANAGING PEOPLE WITH LONG-TERM CONDITIONS: THE UK SELF-CARE AGENDA

It has been estimated that 69% of the total health and social care spend in England and 78% of healthcare spending in the US is accounted for by the treatment and care of people with LTCs. There are clear messages in UK policy about the health benefits and financial benefits that can be made through investment in the management of LTCs, and one of the key high-level outcomes identified in UK policy is to ensure that people have 'improved quality of life, health and wellbeing' which will enable them to be more independent (Department of Health, 2007b). As well as improvements in clinical care, support for patient *self-care* is now significant in UK government agenda, and this is intended to reduce the proportion of our health and social care services used by people with LTCs.

Self-care is all about individuals taking responsibility for their own health and wellbeing, although we still have some way to go in promoting good health and providing individuals with the knowledge and tools they need to manage their condition and live healthier lifestyles.

The UK Department of Health MORI Survey (2005a) identified that the majority of people with LTCs in the UK already feel that they play an active role in their own care and report that they would like to become more active 'self-carers'. The survey also showed that their confidence to do this is increased with professional guidance or support. However, in a public consultation of attitudes towards LTCs care, involving almost 1,000 participants at the National Citizen's Summit, half of those with LTCs felt that they did not have a clear plan which specified the things they could do for themselves to help them better manage their condition (Department of Health, 2006b). Nevertheless, the UK government agenda is focused on encouraging individuals to take steps towards maintaining their own health and wellbeing in the management of LTCs, through learning how to cope with difficulties, minimising or managing the way in which the condition affects their lives, and doing what they can to feel healthy, happy and fulfilled.

Self-care is referred to as:

> "The actions people take for themselves, their children and their families to stay fit and maintain good physical and mental health; meet social and psychological needs, prevent illness or accidents; care for minor ailments and long-term conditions; and maintain health and wellbeing after an acute illness or discharge from hospital." (Department of Health, 2005a).

Empowering individuals with LTCs to make healthy choices about physical activity for health benefit, psychological wellbeing, work ability and social inclusion is all part of the philosophy of self-care. In the UK, this philosophy is further recognised by the 'Expert Patient' approach to chronic disease management set out by our Department of Health, which outlines in its vision the plan for 'more patients with chronic diseases successfully using health-promoting strategies, for example, improving their diet, exercise and weight control' (Department of Health, 2007b).

The UK government has therefore demonstrated a clear commitment to promoting health and active lifestyles amongst people with LTCs. This is further evident in the UK Department of Health strategy for improving LTCs (Department of Health 2005b) which is set out in the 'National Health Service and Social Care Long-Term Conditions Model' to support people with LTCs (see figure 1). This model highlights 'promoting better health' and 'supporting patient self-care' as delivery systems leading to improved outcomes as patients become more informed and therefore empowered, with health and social care teams being prepared, proactive and responsive to need.

Promoting better health in this context means, 'To promote healthy lifestyles: by ensuring that the self-care support is in place for people to make healthier choices about diet, physical activity and lifestyle...'

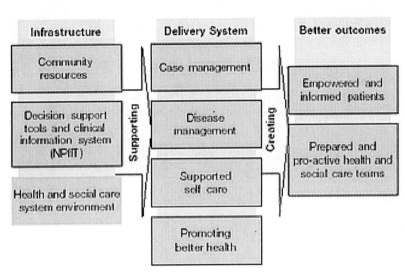

Figure 1. Supporting People with Long-Term Conditions: An NHS and Social Care Model to Support Local Innovation and Integration. Reproduced with permission. Crown Copyright, Department of Health.

PHYSICAL ACTIVITY IN LONG-TERM CONDITIONS

First, this chapter has shown that LTCs are prevalent and also, that non-communicable diseases are increasing at an alarming rate. Second, this chapter has demonstrated that certain risk factors account for a large proportion of disease burden in the western world and of these, physical inactivity and factors associated with inactivity (e.g. overweight) account for a significant proportion of disease alone. Third, this chapter has demonstrated that promoting healthy and more active lifestyles, and supporting people in managing their LTC and in making healthy lifestyle choices is clearly a key part of UK strategy for disease management.

The importance of physical activity for population health has already been outlined in chapter one. The following section reiterates the importance of physical activity for all, but clarifies the specific role of physical activity in the management of LTCs. The association between health behaviours, physical health and wellbeing outcomes in the general, healthy population is well established. We know that physical exercise makes an important contribution to a range of physical and psychological outcomes, including maintaining a healthy weight, building and maintaining a healthy bone density, muscle strength and joint mobility, improving cardiovascular health, promoting wellbeing and strengthening the immune system. This important role of physical activity in improving and maintaining good health is true for all individuals, including those with long-term conditions.

Levels of physical activity are positively associated with aerobic capacity (Berthouze et al., 1995). Aerobic capacity has been described as the capacity of the cardiorespiratory system to supply oxygen (i.e. cardiac output) and the capacity of the skeletal muscle to utilise oxygen (i.e. arterial-venous oxygen difference) (American College of Sports Medicine, 2000). It therefore follows that sustained physical inactivity or deconditioning for whatever reason, induces a reduction in aerobic capacity (Raven, Welch-O'Connor, & Shi, 1998). Poor aerobic fitness itself is a risk factor for the onset of various forms of chronic disease, such as cardiovascular disease and stroke (Guedes & Guedes, 2001; Kurl et al., 2003; Lakka et al., 2001; Rogers et al., 1987). However, sedentary lifestyles are common amongst those with diagnosed chronic health problems, such as high blood pressure, obesity, heart disease, Type 2 diabetes, osteoporosis and depression. The physical inactivity that often occurs in people with chronic conditions therefore means that these individuals are at risk of a decline in aerobic fitness and subsequent deconditioning, thus increasing their risk of developing secondary disease as a direct result of inactivity.

With this is mind is is established that physical activity directly contributes to chronic disease and the leading causes of death (Friedenreich & Orenstein, 2002; U.S. Department of Health and Human Services, 1996) and conversely, it is now widely accepted that physical activity is essential for population health and wellbeing, including those individuals living with a long-term condition. As outlined in chapter one, current recommendations for physical activity suggest that accumulating 30 minutes of moderate intensity physical activity on at least five days of the week is necessary for health benefit. Despite these recommendations, it was estimated that in the UK in 2003, only 37% of men and 24% of women achieved a level of physical activity required for health benefit (Department of Health, 2005d), a figure increasing to 40% of men and 28% of women by 2006 (Department of Health, 2006a). The overall proportion of people with long-term conditions who meet these guidelines for health benefit is unknown, although participation rates may be available for specific conditions, and also, specific determinants and barriers to physical activity participation have been investigated for people with a range of disabilities (e.g. Rimmer et al., 2004). However, we *do* know that inactivity is even more common in these groups for a variety of reasons, and therefore activity participation can be reasonably estimated to be much lower than the general population.

The reasons for this reduction in activity are diverse and often dependent on a range of factors including the nature of the condition and its associated impairments, individual needs, attitudes and preferences. People with chronic health conditions may be, or may perceive themselves to be, more limited than previously in the activities they are able to undertake. Or they may simply, and often unconsciously, reduce their physical activities for various reasons, such as fear of injury, worsening of symptoms or from the impact of their health condition on psychosocial factors including self-esteem or motivation. These issues are discussed in further detail in later chapters. With levels of physical activity estimated to be lower than that of the general 'healthy' population, individuals with LTCs are at particular risk of adverse outcomes from secondary complications of disease associated with inactivity. The may lead to increased disability, further loss of independence, poor quality of life and poor prognosis. It can also be costly, placing even more burden on an already strained healthcare system.

The extent of physical impairment is not always the only issue and poor outcomes in individuals with certain chronic health issues may be associated more with cognitive, behavioural or psychosocial factors than with physical or biomedical factors. Such factors are more amenable to lifestyle intervention, and supporting people to increase physical activity has already been associated with physical improvements in a wide range of health conditions including coronary artery disease, hypertension, stroke, chronic pain, insulin sensitivity, obesity, osteoporosis, cancer and depression (Alevizos, Lentzas, Kokkoris, Mariolis, Korantzopoulos, 2005; Brown, 1992; Bruce, Kriketos, Cooney, & Hawley, 2004; Dittrich et al., 2008; Hurley et al., 2007; Miller, Balady, & Fletcher, 1997; Schmitz et al., 2005; Speck & Looney, 2001; Toole, Thorne, Panton, Kingsley, & Haymes, 2007).

It is possible for most individuals living with a LTC to maintain an active lifestyle, although this depends on their specific needs being met. Aside from medical needs, people with LTCs also require psychological support, and often assistance is required with making lifestyle and health behaviour changes, working in collaboration with both professionals and peers. Since lifestyle behaviours frequently cluster, these may include changes to a whole range of health behaviours including physical activity, diet, alcohol consumption and smoking. Such lifestyle changes can be instrumental in supporting people, irrespective of disability or illness, to live independently, to recover from illness and stay as healthy as possible, to exercise maximum control over their lives, to have the best quality of life possible and to participate as active and equal citizens, as per the outcomes identified for UK adult care services in 'Putting People First' (HM Government, 2007).

Increasing physical activity levels is one important example of lifestyle change, and in order for individuals to implement such behavioural change, we need to know that there are the necessary facilities and services available, that the main barriers to physical activity are addressed, that there are support systems in place and that there is an evidence base which supports the promotion of physical activity as part of the rehabilitation or recovery process. However, exercise is increasingly being recognised as playing a key role in the rehabilitation of a range of LTCs and applications of exercise are presented for a range of specific conditions in the chapters which follow, which present a convincing argument. Furthermore, preventing secondary disabling conditions is now seen as a major component of health promotion activities for people with chronic disabilities and is becoming common practice in rehabilitation (Rimmer, 1999; Rimmer & Braddock, 2002).

So, it has long been known that exercise is associated with positive health outcomes in the general 'healthy' population. However, exercise has been discouraged in the past for some chronic conditions, particularly where there was a lack of knowledge about the contraindications of exercise for specific conditions, or where there was a known possibility of adverse health outcomes. Nevertheless, for many health problems, it is now thought that the *benefits* of physical exercise far outweigh the potential risks. When the condition is under control, there are strong arguments for promoting physical activity in people with LTCs, given the well-established links between physical activity participation, physical and mental health, and secondary disease risk.

The benefits of physical activity for those with chronic conditions are wide-ranging. Physical activity not only positively affects physical health and has even shown to slow disease progression in some cases, but has been shown to improve cognitive functioning or slow cognitive decline, improve psychological wellbeing, increase work ability and reduce social exclusion. For example, in neurological populations, exercise intervention has been associated with mild to moderate improvements in cognitive function, in brain injury (Szabo, Yong, Radak, and Gomez-Pinilla, 2009), stroke (Luo et al, 2007), and Alzheimer's disease (Lautenschlager et al, 2009). Medical practitioners frequently recommend increasing lifestyle physical activity, since even moderate increases in activity have been shown to improve psychological outcomes or quality of life in cancer

(Vallance, Courneya, Plotnikoff, Yasui, & Mackey, 2007), chronic pain (Sertpoyraz, Eyigor, Karapolat, Capaci, and Kirazli, 2009), injury (Hicks, Martin and Ditor et al, 2007), older adults (Blake, Mo, Malik and Thomas, 2009), neurological (Turner, Kivlahan and Haselkorn, 2009), cardiac (Crimi, Ignarro, Cacciatore and Napoli, 2009) or depressed (Haworth, Young, and Thornton, 2009; Blake, Mo, Malik and Thomas, 2009) populations. From a sociological perspective, it is known that people who have LTCs that affect their day-to-day activities are more than twice as likely to be unemployed when compared with those without LTCs (Department Of Health, 2007a). This can have devastating effects on mental health since it is known that people who are out of work long-term are twice as likely to suffer from depression, three times as likely to suffer from anxiety and have an increased risk of suicide (Department Of Health, 2007a), all of which further hamper the potential for gainful employment. The more long-term conditions a person has, the more limited they become in the amount or type of work that they are capable of. It follows that maintaining an active lifestyle has important implications not only for physical health, but for mental health, workability and social inclusion also.

EXERCISE IN REHABILITATION AND DISEASE PREVENTION

It is beyond the scope of this book to provide a detailed guide to the application of exercise in every chronic health condition. However, many chapters in this book concentrate on the application of exercise in a number of common health conditions, relating to either structured and supervised exercise rehabilitation programmes or encouragement of lifestyle physical activity.

This chapter presents a brief summary of the impact of exercise intervention in a range of common chronic conditions.

Hypertension

Hypertension is a chronic medical condition in which the blood pressure is elevated (high blood pressure), and is associated with increased risk of stroke and cardiovascular disease, heart failure and arterial aneurysm, and is a leading cause of chronic renal failure (Gordon et al., 2004). Regular physical activity has also been shown to be effective in reducing the relative risk of developing hypertension by 19 to 30 percent. Furthermore, resting blood pressure is known to be lower in individuals who exercise regularly than in those who exercise infrequently (US Department of Health & Human Services, 1996). For those with the diagnosed condition, whilst the tresearch evidence is limited, those studies published to date suggest that moderate-intensity activity (40 to 75 percent of the maximum oxygen uptake) may be most effective in lowering blood pressure. Research suggests that endurance exercise can lower blood pressure by an average of 3/2 mmHg more than controls (Cornelissen & Fagard, 2005). In those individuals with mildly or moderately elevated blood pressure, resistance training (particularly circuit training with low resistance and a high number of repetitions) may also exert similar positive effects although should be combined with endurance training rather than being the only form of exercise (Pescatello, 2004). In order to reduce resting blood pressure, it is suggested that training at an intensity of approximately 50% of VO2 max (moderate intensity) is sufficient (Fagard, 2001).

Coronary Heart Disease (CHD)

With regards primary prevention of coronary heart disease (CHD), there is an inverse relationship between CHD and physical activity or aerobic fitness and physical activity exerts a major influence on the primary risk factors for CHD such as obesity, hypertension, dyslipidaemias and insulin resistances. It has been proposed that regular endurance or aerobic exercise helps to improve overall stamina and the ability of the heart to pump oxygenated blood in patients with and without prior cardiovascular disease, with resistance training viewed as a complementary fitness programme rather than a substitute to endurance training (Meka, Katragadda, Cherian, & Arora, 2008).

In terms of secondary prevention, physical activity is now an integral part of rehabilitation for individuals with established CHD and this is an important point since rest and inactivity were previously recommended for patients with any form of cardiovascular disease. Systematic reviews and meta-analyses of 48 randomised clinical trials have shown that engaging in regular exercise can help to attenuate or reverse the disease process in patients with cardiovascular disease (Taylor et al., 2004). Research has shown that exercise-based cardiac rehabilitation reduces all-cause death by approximately 20%, and cardiac mortality by approximately a quarter compared with non-exercise based care of coronary heart disease, although rates of nonfatal myocardial reinfarction and the need for revascularisation surgery are not necessarily reduced (Taylor et al., 2004; Joliffe et al., 2001). Studies have shown that an energy expenditure of around 1600 kcal (6720 kj) per week can halt the progression of coronary artery disease and plaque reduction in patients with heart disease has been observed with an energy expenditure of around 2200kcal (9240 kj) (Hambrecht et al., 1993; Franklin et al., 2003). A more detailed discussion of the role of exercise in cardiac rehabilitation is presented in chapter seven, entitled: 'Exercise Based Cardiac Rehabilitation'.

Heart Failure

Heart failure is the final common stage of a range of heart diseases, such as myocardial infarction or cardiomyopathies. Chronic heart failure is increasing in prevalence (Bleumink et al., 2004) with clinical features including dyspnoea (breathlessness), fatigue and reduced exercise tolerance. Exercise has been established as an effective part of heart-failure management (Piepoli, Davos, Francis, Coats, & ExTraMatch Collaborative, 2004; Smart & Marwick, 2004; van Tol, Huijsmans, Kroon, Schothorst, & Kwakkel, 2006), with a recent Cochrane Review showing improvement to both exercise capacity and quality of life in patients with mild to moderate heart failure certainly in the short term with evidence lacking for assessment of long-term effects (Rees et al., 2009). Many studies examine the effects of exercise in a hospital setting (van Tol et al., 2006). Home-based exercise is often advocated in rehabilitation due to the lower cost and accessibility compared with exercise in the hospital environment. Home-based exercise has been shown to increase exercise capacity at both an impairment and activity level and has therefore been recommended as an alternative to hospital-based intervention (Chien et al., 2008), although adherence to home-based exercise in people with heart failure is lower than adherence to supervised exercise programmes and home based interventions may therefore not induce an equivalent training effect (de Mello Franco et al., 2006; McKelvie et al., 2002). Much of the evidence for home-based exercise interventions is based on studies incorporating low to moderate intensity exercise, predominantly with clinically stable individuals (Chien et al., 2008). Since individuals with heart failure are at higher risk of cardiovascular events (Corvera-Tindel, Doering, Woo, Khan, & Dracup, 2004), more information is needed about the safety of home-based exercise for higher risk individuals and those with severe co-morbidities since participants in study trials are often unrepresentative of the overall heart failure population (Rees et al., 2009). A more detailed account of the benefits and contraindications of exercise for people with heart failure is provided in chapter six, entitled: 'Aerobic and Resistance Exercise in Patients with Congestive Heart Failure'.

Stroke

A stroke is caused by a disruption in the flow of blood to the brain or spinal cord due to a blockage or haemorrhage, is a leading cause of disability worldwide, resulting in a range of physical, cognitive and/or emotional impairments. There is evidence to support lifestyle physical activity for the primary prevention of stroke and although optimal levels are at present unclear, general guidelines suggest that accumulating 30 minutes of moderate intensity exercise on most days of the week is necessary for health benefit. Stroke is associated with low levels of post-stroke physical activity and cardiovascular deconditioning (Michael, Allen, & Macko, 2005), therefore for stroke survivors, lifestyle modifications such as increasing physical activity levels are important in terms of reducing risk factors (Rothwell et al., 2005). Resistance training was once avoided in rehabilitation due to concern that such high exertion activity would increase spasticity. However, a recent review of the evidence has identified that resistance training produces increased strength, gait speed and functional outcomes, and improved quality of life without exacerbation of spasticity (Pak & Patten, 2008). Although more research is needed on exercise following stroke, the evidence seems to suggest that physical activity may be influential in brain health, in the prevention of secondary stroke, and is associated with increased physical function and improved general health and wellbeing. Specifically, it is thought that whilst therapeutic exercise can modify or reverse skeletal muscle abnormalities after stroke, aerobic exercise improves fitness, strength and ambulatory performance (Hafer-Macko, Ryan, Ivey, & Macko, 2008).

Exercise has been shown to build aerobic capacity in people with mild to moderate stroke and has been recommended as an important component of stroke rehabilitation (Pang, Eng, Dawson, & Glyfadóttir, 2006). It has also been demonstrated that task-specific rehabilitation intervention using treadmill training to improve gait speed not only serves to improve walking speed but may also be helpful in providing secondary benefits to stroke survivors by positively impacting on depression, mobility and social participation (Smith & Thompson, 2008). Indeed, it has been shown that the underlying cardiovascular and musculoskeletal impairments resulting from stroke are modifiable even years later with targeted exercise training (Lee et al., 2008). A more detailed account of the literature on physical activity, stroke and transient ischaemic attack (TIA) is provided in chapter three, entitled 'Exercise promotion and rehabilitation of neurological conditions'.

Treatment of Obesity and Weight Control

Physical exercise is key in the treatment of obesity and weight reduction or prevention of weight gain following weight reduction. Obesity is defined as a body mass index ≥30 and a sensible aim is often to permanently reduce body mass by 5-10%. In these treatments, exercise is always combined with a diet in which the intake of energy and saturated fats is restricted. For weight reduction, endurance exercise alone without dietary change may only reduce weight by a few kilograms (Shaw et al., 2006), but exercise reduces the intra-abdominal (i.e. visceral adipose tissue) more than diet alone even when weight loss is minor (Kay and Fiatarone Singh, 2006).

Making physical activity a part of everyday lifestyle is advocated as being preferable to fitness training on only a few occasions per week. Weight maintenance refers to the maintenance of body weight after a phase of weight reduction. This phase requires permanent lifestyle changes. Increased physical activity levels have been shown to decrease the amount of weight increase during the weight maintenance stage (Ross et al., 2000). Other studies have shown that physical activity compared with a low-energy diet can improve weight maintenance after weight loss when compared with diet al.one (Curioni & Lourenco, 2005). With obesity, poor compliance with physical activity programmes and weight loss regimes is a significant problem since these patients often demonstrate difficulty with adhering to permanent lifestyle changes.

However, even a minor increase in physical activity can reduce body mass index (Toole et al., 2007) and significantly improve cardiovascular risk factors for these patients (e.g. Shaw et al., 2006, Kelley, Kelley and Tran., 2005).

Type 2 Diabetes Mellitus (T2DM)

Exercise is significant in both primary and secondary prevention of T2DM. Whilst both aerobic and resistance exercise have been shown to be associated with decreased risk of type 2 diabetes (Helmrich, Ragland, Leung, & Paffenbarger, 1991), there is also strong evidence for the beneficial health effects of physical activity in the management of people with T2DM (Boulé. Kenny, Haddad, Wells, & Sigal, 2003; BjØrgaas et al., 2005). Fundamentally, there is an increased risk of death amongst inactive individuals with diabetes (Wei, Gibbons, Kampert, Nichaman, & Blair, 2000) and this relationship has also been observed in patients with metabolic syndrome (Katzmarzyk, Church, Janssen, Ross, & Blair, 2005). The impact of exercise on mortality is evident, since it has been shown that walking at least 2 hours per week has been associated with a reduction in the incidence of premature death of 39-54% from any cause and of 34-53% from cardiovascular disease amongst patients with diabetes (Gregg, Gerzoff, & Caspersen, 2003). In those with T2DM, physical activity can have positive effects on glycemic control, weight reduction and insulin resistance (Boulé, Haddad, Kenny, Wells, & Sigal, 2001; Bruce et al., 2004; Schneider, Amorosa, Khachadurian, & Ruderman, 1984; Yamanouchi et al., 1995). Whilst both aerobic and resistance training have shown to be of benefit in the control of diabetes, it has been suggested that resistance training may have greater effects on glycemic control than aerobic training (Dunstan et al., 2002). Further, a meta-analysis of controlled trials has shown that exercise interventions resulted in a significant reduction in glycosylated haemoglobin (0.66%) compared with no exercise intervention (Boulé et al., 2001).

As such, increasing physical activity levels is now presented as a cornerstone in treatment strategies. However, delivery of effective exercise intervention in this group can be challenging since people with T2DM often find it difficult to incorporate structured physical activity into their daily lives (Ford & Herman, 1995; Schneider, Khachadurian, Amorosa, Clemow, & Ruderman, 1992) and the majority of individuals with T2DM do not exercise regularly (Hays & Clark, 1999; Krug, Haire-Joshu, & Heady, 1991).

Although physical activity can reduce the risk of diabetic complications, such as coronary heart disease, it is important to take into account any possible complications when prescribing exercise for individuals with T2DM. Those who do engage in physical activity often find walking an acceptable form of physical activity (Krug et al., 1991). Although pedometer interventions can reflect aerobic fitness and be motivating in engaging individuals with physical activity, they have not consistently yielded positive findings in T2DM (BjØrgaas, Vik, Stolen, Lydersen, & Grill, 2008). One reason for this is that it is possible to accumulate high step counts using pedometers that do not take into account walking speed and duration, and it has been argued that pedometers alone may not yield the same improvements to cardiovascular fitness as structured forms of exercise intervention (Le Masurier, Sidman, & Corbin, 2003).

However, there is research suggesting that pedometer-based walking interventions can not only be helpful in T2DM, but those that are based on total accumulated daily steps ('lifestyle activity') are more acceptable to participants and can yield the same health benefits as 'structured' physical activity programmes which specify a minimum duration and moderate intensity of physical activity bouts (Richardson et al., 2007). This is important since attrition from exercise intervention in this group is high and unfortunately those that are less complaint with intervention are often the ones most in need of physical activity (BjØrgaas et al., 2008). A focus on interventions that are acceptable to participants and those which increase motivation is therefore required.

Osteoporosis and Bone Density

Osteoporosis is a bone disorder characterised by low bone mass and deterioration in the micro architecture of the bone. The result is bone fragility and an increased fracture risk, especially at the wrist, spine and hip. It has long been known that duration and force of muscle activity on bone are important in maintaining bone mass (Whedon, 1984). Primary prevention studies have provided evidence that routine physical activity, particularly weight bearing and impact exercise, prevent osteoporosis and loss of bone mineral density associated with ageing (Berard, Bravo, & Gauthier, 1997).

For those with established osteoporosis, there is some evidence to suggest that regular physical activity is an effective secondary prevention strategy which is important in the maintenance of bone health (Liu-Ambrose, Khan, Eng, Heinonen, & McKay, 2004; Kemmler et al., 2004). Regular exercise can help to reduce stiffness and pain associated with the condition.

Physical activity is important in order to maintain (or regain) mobility and prevent deterioration of the muscles. Low to moderate intensity exercise can improve posture and build muscle strength. Regular weight bearing exercise can improve bone density and improve fracture risk, with low impact exercises, such as swimming and Tai Chi, serving to prevent further bone loss, improve balance and coordination thus reducing the risk of falls and therefore fracturing (Todd & Robinson, 2003; Bassey, 1995). Hydrotherapy, or water-based exercises provide support and encourage relaxation of tight muscles and joints. Evidence for water-based exercise programmes is limited although non-significant trends in bone status of post-menopausal women have been demonstrated over seven months (Rotstein et al., 2008). Non-weight bearing exercises such as swimming and cycling do not directly influence bone mass although have general positive effects of health and wellbeing and help increase overall strength and flexibility. Research studies have shown significant gains in bone mass density in individuals with osteoporosis with aerobic exercise and muscle strengthening exercises (Iwamoto, Takeda, & Ichimura 2001; Chien, Wu, Hsu, Yang, & Lai, 2000; Hartard et al., 1996; Beverly, Rider, Evans, & Smith, 1989). Along with other life style measures (e.g. maintaining adequate body weight and calcium intake, modest alcohol consumption and cessation of smoking) exercise is encouraged in those with diagnosed osteoporosis as well as those at risk, for both the positive effects on bone density, prevention of osteoporotic fractures and the prevention of secondary complications (Todd & Robinson, 2003; Ernst, 1998).

Rheumatoid Arthritis

Rheumatoid arthritis (RA) is a chronic, systemic, inflammatory disease characterised by symmetric polyarticular pain and swelling, malaise and fatigue (Fleming, Benn, Corbett, & Wood, 1976). Physical inactivity is common with almost half of RA patients failing to meet recommendations for healthy levels of physical activity (Eurenius, Stenstrom, & The Para Study Group, 2005). Exercise is recognised as an important element in the management of patients with RA (deJong & Vlieland, 2005; van den Ende, Vliet Vlieland, Muneke, & Hazes, 2000). The majority of intervention studies have been conducted in clinical settings (Stenstrom & Minor, 2003), however, home-based interventions can also be effective although compliance with exercise regimes can be an issue (Jensen & Lorish, 1994). Much of the available evidence on exercise therapy and RA focuses on dynamic exercise, that is, exercise with sufficient intensity, duration and frequency to improve aerobic capacity and/or muscle strength.

Systematic reviews of dynamic exercise intervention studies conclude that exercise improves both aerobic capacity and muscle strength in RA, without detrimental effect on disease activity, pain or radiological joint damage (Van den Ende, Vliet Vlieland, Muneke, & Hazes, 1998; Stenstrom and Minor, 2003; Gaudin et al., 2008). Guidelines on the treatment of early RA recommend physical exercise and sports, muscle strengthening exercises and/or aerobic exercises (Gossec et al., 2006; Hennell & Luqmani, 2008) although intervention must be tailored to the needs and abilities of the individual. Recent research advocates the promotion of physical activity integrated into everyday life, and a one-year coaching programme for lifestyle physical activity in RA has shown improvements in perceived health status and muscle strength in intervention participants compared with controls (Brodin et al., 2008). For exercise maintenance outside of a healthcare environment it is important to identify the context and provide individualised support for the patient's needs and strengthen the patient's beliefs in their ability to exercise in different settings (Swärdh, Biguet, & Opava, 2008).

Long-Term or 'Chronic' Pain

The International Association for the Study of Pain (IASP Pain Terminology, 2001) have defined long-term or 'chronic' pain as 'an unpleasant sensory and emotional experience associated with actual or potential tissue damage, or described in terms of such damage…that which has lasted over 3 months, has poor outcome, arising out of complex aetiology and complex clinical presentation' (IASP Pain Terminology, 2001). Exercise has frequently been advocated in long-term pain to prevent or reverse the effects of deconditioning, to challenge fears regarding activity, to provide a safe and graded approach to activity, to improve functional capacity, and to help patients accept responsibility for improving their condition. Increasing general physical activity levels is thought to be more important than adopting specific exercise or any particular regime (Waddell & Watson, 2004). Studies have shown that aerobic exercise when combined with relaxation may help to reduce self-rated pain levels in migraine (Dittrich et al., 2008) and when combined with active coping strategies may help to improve self-reported function in chronic arthritic knee pain (Hurley et al., 2007). Overall, current thinking suggests that exercise is most effective when intervention is part of a 'toolkit' or package of treatment based on a biopsychosocial model of health, that includes paced activity, medication advice and relaxation training.

For a more detailed discussion of exercise in pain management, the reader is referred to chapter four, entitled: 'The role of exercise in the management of long term pain: a biopsychosocial approach'.

Chronic Obstructive Pulmonary Disease (COPD)

Chronic obstructive pulmonary disease (COPD) refers to chronic bronchitis and emphysema, which are two commonly co-existing diseases of the lungs in which the airways become narrowed. This leads to a limitation of the flow of air to and from the lungs causing shortness of breath, and these symptoms can worsen over time. Direct activity measures have shown that time spent in physical activities is reduced in patients with COPD compared with healthy controls of similar age (Pitta et al., 2006). The reason for this is that patients with COPD often experience fatigue and dyspnea (breathlessness) during physical exertion, the latter particularly is distressing and often leads to a reduction in physical activity levels in an attempt to reduce this symptom. This reduction in physical activity leads to deconditioning, which further increases breathlessness and has associated negative effects on health-related quality of life (Rearden, Lareau, & ZuWallack, 2006). Pulmonary rehabilitation programmes can be effective in reversing this process in the short-term (Lacasse et al., 1996) but patients can often return to the spiral of inactivity and deconditioning without an intensive maintenance strategy. Home-based rehabilitation, based on normal lifestyle physical activities, has shown to have long-lasting effects (Wijkstra et al., 1995; Wijkstra, ten Hacken, Wempe, & Koeter, 2003). More recently, it has been suggested that a physically active lifestyle of patients with COPD is essential for maintaining the benefits after rehabilitation, and that exercise counselling and stimulation of lifestyle physical activity such as stair-use, walking, gardening and so on, may be feasibly added to pulmonary rehabilitation (de Blok et al., 2006).

Cancer

With regards primary prevention, the evidence has established that routine physical activity is associated with reductions in the incidence of specific cancers, with epidemiologic studies showing that physically active men and women exhibit a 30-40% reduction in the relative risk of colon cancer, and physically active women a 20-30% reduction in the relative risk of breast cancer compared with inactive individuals (Lee, 2003). For those with a diagnosis of cancer, physical activity is increasingly being proposed as an appropriate intervention in cancer to enhance both physical and psychosocial outcomes. Cancer and its treatment can have a range of negative adverse effects that impact heavily on patient quality of life, and hormone therapies used in the treatment of breast and prostate cancer can drastically increase the risk of mortality and morbidity from other diseases such as obesity, type II diabetes, cardiovascular disease, osteoporosis and sarcopenia (Newton & Galvão, 2008).

Research has shown that increased levels of self-reported physical activity have been associated with a decreased recurrence of cancer and decreased death from breast and colon cancer (Hayden, Macinnis, English, & Giles, 2005; Holmes, Chen, Feskanich, Kroenke, & Colditz, 2005). The effect of physical activity on survival rates has been investigated further with regards the potential effects of exercise on chemotherapy treatment (Jones et al., 2005). The evidence supports the role of regular physical activity post-diagnosis in increasing survivorship by up to 50-60%, with positive effects on cardiovascular health, surgical outcomes, reducing symptom experience, managing side effects of radiation and chemotherapy, improving psychological health, maintaining physical function and reducing fat gain and muscle and bone loss (Newton & Galvão, 2008).

Regular physical activity confers a clear benefit to patients with established cancer since it is associated with an improved quality of life and overall health status (Adamsen et al., 2003; Galvão & Newton, 2005; Mackenzie & Kalda, 2003). For example, research has suggested that a combined health promotion approach using breast cancer-specific physical activity print materials and pedometers (n=377) may be an effective strategy for increasing both physical activity levels and quality of life in breast cancer survivors (Vallance et al., 2007). However, there is still scope for further research relating to secondary prevention of cancer.

Depression

Routine physical activity has been associated with improved psychological wellbeing through reduction of anxiety and depression (Dunn, Trivedi, & O'Neal, 2001). Common symptoms of depression typically include feelings of sadness, irritability, hopelessness, anxiety, reduced energy, loss of interest in enjoyable activities and diminished activity, and changes in eating and sleeping habits. It is thought that 121 million people worldwide are affected by depression (World Health Organisation, 2008) which can be chronic and recurrent.

The World Health Organisation (2008) states that depression is projected to become the second most common cause of disability adjusted life years in the world by 2020 and this is particularly significant since depression exerts an observable effect on health outcomes, and plays an important role in the prevention and management of a wide range of health conditions. Exercise has been proposed for both the prevention and treatment of depression and depressive symptoms. Traditional treatments for depression include antidepressant medications or 'talking therapies'. More recently, exercise therapy has received increasing attention as a potential alternative or supplementary treatment for diagnosed depression (Daley, 2002, Blake, Mo, Malik & Thomas, 2009) which is thought to be effective in reducing depressive symptoms in a range of age groups, and may even be as effective as antidepressant medication or psychotherapy. A more detailed discussion may be found in chapter eleven, entitled 'Exercise Interventions in the Treatment of Depression'.

CONCLUSION

There is now irrefutable evidence that regular physical activity is associated with a reduced risk of premature death and plays an important role in both primary and secondary prevention of many chronic diseases. There is a wealth of evidence in the literature to suggest that the risk of chronic disease begins early in childhood and increases with age, and this provides an evidence-based and common-sense argument for promoting healthy lifestyle choices from an early age. For those with an established chronic illness, the management of numerous health conditions is now rooted in the modification of multiple risk factors which combine appropriate medical and pharmacological treatments with comprehensive lifestyle interventions. Physical inactivity is viewed as the most prevalent of all the modifiable risk factors and is now targeted in the management of a range of chronic diseases.

Physical inactivity is not only damaging to the health of the individual, but impacts severely on hospital care and service use, thus presenting a considerable public health burden. As such there is an international drive to improve population health and increase levels of exercise in both healthy populations and in those with long-term conditions for both primary and secondary prevention. Increasing activity levels is particularly important for the latter group since those with long-term health problems can become deconditioned, and are at increased risk of secondary disease resulting from sedentary lifestyles.

There has been a shift in attitude over recent decades from discouraging certain populations to exercise, towards actively encouraging exercise in those for whom their condition is under control. In practice, this may include structured, supervised exercise intervention as part of a rehabilitation programme for example, cycle or treadmill training, flexibility training, aquatics, yoga or Tai Chi. Alternatively, this may include encouragement of 'lifestyle' physical activities which can be incorporated into the daily routine, such as walking, cycling, stair-climbing or gardening.

This chapter has provided a brief introduction to the evidence for promoting physical activity in selected chronic conditions, including hypertension, coronary heart disease and heart failure, stroke, obesity and type 2 diabetes, osteoporosis, rheumatoid arthritis, chronic pain, chronic obstructive pulmonary disease, cancer and depression. However, it must be recognised that people with LTCs are not a homogenous group and individuals have different physical and psychosocial needs that relate to their specific condition and the way in which they manage their lives. The benefits of exercise must outweigh any potential risks, and a process of screening and exercise programme design, monitoring and education of participants is strongly recommended. Exercise interventions are likely to be of most benefit when they are tailored to the needs and circumstances of the individual.

On a policy level, there is international diversity in the response of different countries to long-term conditions and non-communicable disease, with most in Europe for example, having accessible disease-based national protocols, guidelines and standards (e.g. heart disease, diabetes and cancer) but fewer having the corresponding policy instruments (e.g. weight control, physical activity)(World Health Organisation, 2006). At present the benefits of adopting an active lifestyle are recognised worldwide, although assimilating a wealth of evidence-based knowledge into clinical practice remains challenging, and there is not a universal international approach to the way in which exercise is managed in rehabilitation and recovery from illness. Nevertheless, it appears that physical activity is set to continue at the forefront of health promotion for people with chronic health problems.

KEY POINTS

- Over 15 million people in the UK live with a chronic condition, placing huge demands on health and social care services
- These people are at risk of physical deconditioning and secondary health complications due to inactivity.
- Promotion of healthy lifestyles is part of the overall strategy for the management of people with long-term conditions for both prevention and rehabilitation.
- Physical activity can help to reduce further disability, increase independence, improve prognosis, and psychosocial outcomes
- Rehabilitation and management of many long-term conditions should include structured exercise intervention or recommendation to increase lifestyle physical activity.
- Exercise programmes should be tailored to the needs of individuals. Physical activity has shown improvements in both health and quality of life in a diversity of conditions.

REFERENCES

Adamsen, L., Midtgaard, J., Rorth, M., Borregaard, N., Andersen, C., Quist, M., et al., (2003). Feasibility, physical capacity and health benefits of a multidimensional exercise program for cancer patients undergoing chemotherapy. *Supportive Care in Cancer, 11,* 707-716.

Alevizos, A., Lentzas, J., Kokkoris, S., Mariolis, A., & Korantzopoulos, P. (2005). Physical activity and stroke risk. *International Journal of Clinical Practice, 59,* 922-930.

American College of Sports Medicine (2000). *ACSM's Guidelines for exercise testing and prescription (6th edition).* Philadelphia: Lippincott, Williams and Wilkins.

Bassey, E. J. (1995). Exercise in primary prevention of osteoporosis in women. *Annals of the Rheumatic Disease, 54,* 861-862.

Berard, A., Bravo, G., & Gauthier, P. (1997). Meta-analysis of the effectiveness of physical activity for the prevention of bone loss in post-menopausal women. *Osteoporosis International, 7,* 331-337.

Beverly, M. C., Rider, T. A., Evans, M. J. & Smith, R. (1989). Local bone mineral response to brief exercise that stresses the skeleton. *BMJ, 299,* 233-235.

Berthouze, S. E., Minaire, P. M., Castells, J., Busso, T., Vico, L., & Lacour, J. R. (1995). Relationship between mean habitual daily energy expenditure and maximal oxygen uptake. *Medicine and Science in Sports and Exercise, 27,* 1170-1179.

Blake, H., Mo, P., Malik, S., Thomas, S. (2009) How effective are physical activity interventions for alleviating depressive symptoms in older people? A systematic review. *Clinical Rehabilitation,* 23, 10 873-887; DOI: 10.1177/0269215509337449.

Bleumink, G. S., Knetsch, A. M., Sturkenbaum, M. C., Strauss, S. M., Hofman, A., Deckers, J. W., et al., (2004). Quantifying the heart failure epidemic: prevalence, incidence rate, lifetime risk and prognosis of heart failure. The Rotterdam Study. *European Heart Journal, 25,* 1614-1619.

BjØrgaas, M., Vik, J. T., Saeterhaug, A., Langlo, L., Sakshaug, T., Mohus, R. M., et al., (2005). Relationship between pedometer registered activity, aerobic capacity and self-reported activity and fitness in patients with type 2 diabetes. *Diabetes, Obesity & Metabolism, 7,* 737-744.

BjØrgaas, M. R., Vik, J. T., Stolen, T., Lydersen, S., & Grill, V. (2008). Regular use of a pedometer does not enhance beneficial outcomes in a physical intervention study in type 2 diabetes mellitus. *Metabolism Clinical and Experimental, 57,* 605-611.

Boulé, N. G., Kenny, G. P., Haddad, E., Wells, G. A., & Sigal, R. J. (2003). Meta-analysis of the effect of structured exercise training on cardiorespiratory fitness in Type 2 Diabetes Mellitus. *Diabetologia, 46,* 1071-1081.

Boulé, N. G., Haddad, E., Kenny, G. P., Wells, G. A., & Sigal, R. J. (2001). Effects of exercise on glycaemic control and body mass in type 2 diabetes mellitus: a meta-analysis of controlled clinical trials. *JAMA, 286,* 1218-1227.

Brodin, N., Eurenius, E., Jensen, I., Nisell, R., Opava, C. H., & PARA Study Group. (2008) Coaching patients with early rheumatoid arthritis to healthy physical activity: a multicenter, randomised controlled study. *Arthritis and Rheumatism, 59,* 325-331.

Brown, D. R. (1992). Physical activity, ageing, and psychological wellbeing: an overview of the research. *Canadian Journal of Sport Sciences, 17,* 185-193.

Bruce, C. R., Kriketos, A. D., Cooney, G. J., & Hawley, H. A. (2004) Dissociation of muscle triglyceride content and insulin sensitivity after exercise training in patients with type 2 diabetes. *Diabetologia, 47,* 23-30.

Chien, M. Y., Wu, Y. T., Hsu, A. T., Yang, R. S., & Lai, J. S. (2000). Efficacy of a 24-week aerobic exercise programme for osteopenic post menopausal women. *Calcified Tissue International, 67,* 443-448.

Chien, C.L., Lee, C.M., Wu, Y.W., Chen, T.A., Wu, Y.T. (2008) Home-based exercise increases exercise capacity but not quality of life in people with chronic heart failure: a systematic review. *Aust J Physiother, 54,* 87-93.

Cornelissen, V.A., Fagard, R.H. (2005) Effect of resistance training on resting blood pressure: a meta-analysis of randomized controlled trials. *J Hypertens, 23,* 251-259.

Curioni, C.C., Lourenco, P.M. Long-term weight loss after diet and exercise: a systematic review. *Int J Obes (Lond), 29,* 1168-1174.

Corvera-Tindel, T., Doering, L. V., Woo, M. A., Khan, S., & Dracup, K. (2004) Effects of a home-walking exercise program on functional status and symptoms in heart failure. *American Heart Journal, 147,* 339-346.

Crimi, E., Ignarro, L.J., Cacciatore, F., Napoli, C. Mechanisms by which exercise training benefits patients with heart failure. *Nat Rev Cardiol, 6,* 292-300.

de Blok, B. M. J., de Greef, M. H. G., ten Hacken, N. H. T., Sprenger, S. R., Postema, K., & Wempe, J. B. (2006). The effects of a lifestyle physical activity counselling program with feedback of a pedometer during pulmonary rehabilitation in patients with COPD: a pilot study. *Patient Education and Counseling, 61,* 48-55.

de Jong, Z., & Vlieland, T. P. (2005). Safety of exercise in patients with rheumatoid arthritis. *Current Opinion in Rheumatology, 17,* 177-182.

de Mello Franco, F. G., Santos, A. C., Rondon, M. U., Trombetta, I. C., Stunz, C., Braga, A. M., et al., (2006). Effects of home-based exercise training on neurovascular control in patients with heart failure. *European Journal of Heart Failure, 8,* 851-855.

Daley, A. J. (2002). Exercise therapy and mental health in clinical populations: is exercise therapy a worthwhile intervention? *Advances in Psychiatric Treatment, 8,* 262-270.

Department of Health (2007a). *Raising the profile of long-term conditions care: A compendium of information.* London: Central Office of Information.

Department of Health (2007b). *The Expert Patients Programme.* UK: Department of Health.

Department of Health (2005a). *MORI Survey: Public attitudes to self-care baseline survey, February 2005.* UK: Department of Health.

Department of Health (2005b). *Supporting people with long-term conditions: an NHS and Social Care Model to support local innovation and integration.* London: Central Office of Information.

Department of Health (2005c). *The NHS Improvement Plan: Putting people at the heart of public services.* London: The Stationary Office.

Department of Health (2005d). *Health Survey for England.* London: The Stationary Office.

Department of Health (2006a). *Health Survey for England: Updating of Trend Tables to Include 2005 Data.* London: Information Centre.

Department of Health (2006b). Your Health, Your Care, Your Say: Research Report. UK: Opinion Leader Research.

Dittrich, S. M., Gunther, V., Franz, G., Burtscher, M., Holzner, B., & Kopp, M. (2008). Aerobic exercise with relaxation: influence on pain and psychological wellbeing in female migraine patients. *Clinical Journal of Sport Medicine, 18,* 363-365.

Dunn, A. L., Trivedi, M. H., & O'Neal, H. A. (2001). Physical activity dose-response effects on outcomes of depression and anxiety [discussion 609-610]. *Medicine and Science in Sports and Exercise, 33,* S587-S597.

Dunstan, D. W., Daly, R. M., Owen, N., Jolley, D., De Courten, M., Shaw, J., et al., (2002). High-intensity resistance training improves glycemic control in older patients with type 2 diabetes. *Diabetes Care, 25,* 1729-1736.

Ernst, E. (1998). Exercise for female osteoporosis: A systematic review of randomised clinical trials. *Sports Medicine, 25,* 359-368.

Eurenius, E., Stenstrom, C. H. & The Para Study Group (2005). Physical activity, physical fitness and general health perception amongst individuals with rheumatoid arthritis. *Arthritis & Rheumatism, 53,* 48-55.

Fagard, R.H. (2001). Exercise characteristics and the blood pressure response to dynamic physical training. *Med Sci Sports Exerc, 33:* S484-492; discussion S493-494.

Fleming, A., Benn, R. T., Corbett, M., & Wood, P. H. (1976). Early rheumatoid disease, II. Patterns of joint involvement. *Annals of the Rheumatic Disease, 35,* 361-364.

Ford, E. S., & Herman, W. H. (1995). Leisure-time physical activity patterns in the US diabetic population. Findings from the National Health Interview Survey – Health Promotion and Disease Prevention Supplement. *Diabetes Care, 18,* 27-33.

Franklin, B.A., Swain, D.P., Shephard, R.J. (2003). New insights in the prescription of exercise for coronary patients. *J Cardiovasc Nursing, 18,* 116-123.

Friedenreich, C., & Orenstein, M. (2002). Physical activity and cancer prevention: Etiologic evidence and biological mechanisms. *Journal of Nutrition, 132,* 3456S-3465S.

Galvão, D. A., & Netwon, R. U. (2005). Review of exercise intervention studies in cancer patients. *Journal of Clinical Oncology, 23,* 899-909.

Gaudin, P., Leguen-Guegan, S., Allenet, B., Baillet, A., Grange, L., & Juvin, R. (2008). Is dynamic exercise beneficial in patients with rheumatoid arthritis? *Joint, Bone, Spine, 75,* 11-17.

Office for National Statistics. General Household Survey, 2005. Social Surveys Division of the Office for National Statistics.

Gordon, N. F., Gulanick, M., Costa, F., Fletcher, G., Franklin, B. A., Roth, E. J., et al., (2004). Physical activity and exercise recommendations for stroke survivors. An American Heart Association Scientific Statement from the Council on Clinical Cardiology, Subcommittee on Exercise, Cardiac Rehabilitaion and Prevention; the Council on Cardiovascular Nursing; the Council on Nutrition, Physical Activity and Metabolism; and the Stroke Council. *Circulation, 109,* 2031-2041.

Gossec, L., Pavy, S., Pham, T., Constantin, A., Poiraudeau, S., Combe, B., et al., (2006). Nonpharmacological treatments in early rheumatoid arthritis: clinical practice guidelines based on published evidence and expert opinion. *Joint, Bone, Spine, 73,* 396-402.

Gregg, E. W., Gerzoff, R. B., & Caspersen, C. J. (2003). Relationship of walking to mortality among US adults with diabetes. *Archives of Internal Medicine, 163,* 1440-1447.

Guedes, D. P. & Guedes, J. E. (2001). Physical activity, cardiorespiratory fitness, dietary content, and risk factors that cause a predisposition towards cardiovascular disease. *Arquivos Brasileiros de Cardiologia, 77,* 243-257.

Hafer-Macko, C. E., Ryan, A. S., Ivey, F. M., Macko, R. F. (2008). Skeletal muscle changes after hemiparetic stroke and potential beneficial effects of exercise intervention strategies. *Journal of Rehabilitation Research and Devlopment, 45,* 261-272.

Hambrecht, R., Niebauer, J., Marburger, C., Grunze, M., Kälberer, B., Hauer, K., et al., (1993). Various intensities of leisure-time physical activity in patients with coronary artery disease: effects on cardiorespiratory fitness and progression of coronary atherosclerotic lesions. *Journal of American College of Cardiology, 22,* 468-477.

Hartard, M., Haber, P., Ilevia, D., Preisinger, E., Seifl, G., & Huber, J. (1996). Systematic strength training as a model of therapeutic intervention. A controlled trial in postmenopausal women with osteopenia. *American Journal of Physical Medicine & Rehabilitation, 75,* 21-28.

Haydon, A. M. M., Macinnis, R. J., English, D. R. & Giles, G. G. (2005). The effect of physical activity and body size on survival after diagnosis with colorectal cancer. *Gut, 1,* 62-67.

Hays, L. M., & Clark, D. O. (1999). Correlates of physical activity in a sample of older adults with type 2 diabetes. *Diabetes Care, 22,* 706-712.

Haworth, J., Young, C., Thornton, E (2009). The effects of an 'exercise and education' programme on exercise self-efficacy and levels of independent activity in adults with acquired neurological pathologies: an exploratory, randomized study. *Clinical Rehabilitation, 23,* 371-383.

Helmrich, S. P., Ragland, D. R., Leung, R. W. & Paffenbarger, R. S. (1991). Physical activity and reduced occurrence of non-insulin-dependent diabetes mellitus. *New England Journal of Medicine, 325,* 147-152.

Hennell, S., Luqmani, R. (2008). Developing multidisciplinary guidelines for the management of early rheumatoid arthritis. *Musculoskeletal Care, 6,* 97-107.

Hicks, A.L., Martin, K.A., Ditor, D.S., Latimer, A.E., Craven, C., Bugaresti, J., McCartney, N (2003). Long-term exercise training in persons with spinal cord injury: effects on strength, arm ergometry performance and psychological well-being. *Spinal Cord, 41,* 34-43.

Holmes, M. D., Chen, W. Y., Feskanich, D., Kroenke, C. H., & Colditz, G. A. (2005). Physical activity and survival after breast cancer diagnosis. *JAMA, 293,* 2479-2486.

Hurley, M. V., Walsh, N. E., Mitchell, H. L., Pimm, T. J., Patel, A., Williamson, E., et al., (2007). Clinical effectiveness of a rehabilitation program integrating exercise, self-management and active coping strategies for chronic knee pain: a cluster randomised trial. *Athritis and Rheumatism, 57,* 1211-1219.

IASP Pain Terminology (2001). International Association for the study of pain. Available on: http://www.iasp.pain.org/terms-p.html.2001 Last Accessed 17/05/09.

Iwamoto, J., Takeda, T., & Ichimura, S. (2001). Effect of exercise training and detraining on bone mineral density in post menopausal women with osteoporosis. *Journal of Orthopaedic Science, 6,* 128-132.

Jensen, G. M., & Lorish, C. D. (1994). Promoting patient cooperation with exercise programs: linking research, theory and practice. *Arthritis Care and Research, 7,* 181-189.

Jolliffe, J.A., Rees, K., Taylor, R.S., Thompson, D., Oldridge, N., Ebrahim, S. (2001) Exercise-based rehabilitation for coronary heart disease. *Cochrane Database Syst Rev.*CD 001800 Jones, L. W., Eves, N. D., Courneya, K. S., Chiu, B. K., Baracos, V. E., Hanson, J., et al., (2005). Effects of exercise training on antitumor efficacy of doxorubicin in MDA-MB-231 breast cancer xenografts. *Clinical Cancer Research, 11,* 6695-6698.

Katzmarzyk, P. T., Church, T. S., Janssen, I., Ross, R., & Blair, S. N. (2005). Metabolic syndrome, obesity and mortality: impact of cardiorespiratory fitness. *Diabetes Care, 28,* 391-397.

Kay, S.J., Fiatarone Singh, M.A. (2006) The influence of physical activity on abdominal fat: a systematic review of the literature. *Obes Rev, 7,* 183-200.

Kelley GA, Kelley KS, Tran ZV. Walking and Non-HDL-C in adults: a meta-analysis of randomized controlled trials. *Prev Cardiol, 8,* 102-107.

Kemmler, W., Lauber, D., Weineck, J. Hensen, J., Kalender, W., & Engelke, K. (2004). Benefits of 2 years of intense exercise on bone density, physical fitness, and blood lipids in early post-menopausal osteopenic women: results of the Erlangen Fitness Osteoporosis Prevention Study (EFOPS). *Archives of Internal Medicine, 164,* 1084-1091.

Krug, L. M., Haire-Joshu, D., Heady, S. A. (1991). Exercise habits and exercise relapse in persons with non-insulin dependent diabetes mellitus. *Diabetes Education, 17,* 185-188.

Kurl, S., Laukenen, J. A., Rauramaa, R., Lakka, T. A., Sivenius, J., Salonen, J. T. (2003). Cardiorespiratory fitness and the risk for stroke in men. *Archives of Intern Medicine, 163,* 1682-1688.

Lacasse, Y., Wong, E., Guyatt, G. H., King, D., Cook, D. J., & Goldstein, R. S, (1996). Meta-analysis of respiratory rehabilitation on chronic obstructive pulmonary disease. *Lancet, 348,* 1115-1119.

Lakka, T. A., Laukkenen, J., Rauramaa, R. Salonen, R., Lakka, H. M., Kaplan, G. A., et al., (2001). Cardiorespiratory fitness and the progression of carotid atherosclerosis in middle-aged men. *Annals of Internal Medicine, 134,* 12-20.

Lautenschlager, N.T., Cox, K.L., Flicker, L, Foster, J.K., van Bockxmeer, F.M., Xiao J, Greenop, K.R., Almeida, O.P.. Effect of physical activity on cognitive function in older adults at risk for Alzheimer disease: a randomized trial. *JAMA, 300,* 1027-1037.

Le Masurier, G. C., Sidman, C. L., Corbin, C. B. (2003). Accumulating 10,000 steps: does this meet the current physical activity guidelines? *Research Quarterly for Exercise and Sport, 74,* 389-394.

Lee, I. M. (2003). Physical activity and cancer prevention – data from epidemiologic studies. *Medicine and Science in Sports and Exercise, 35,* 1823-1827.

Lee, M. J., Kilbreath, S. L., Singh, M. F., Zeman, B., Lord, S. R., Raymond, J., et al., (2008). Comparison of effect of aerobic cycle training and progressive resistance training on walking ability after stroke: a randomised sham exercise-controlled study. *Journal of the American Geriatrics Society, 56,* 976-985.

Liu-Ambrose, T. Y., Khan, K. M., Eng, J. J., Heinonen, A., & McKay, H. A. (2004). Both resistance and agility training increase cortical bone density in 75-85 year old women with low bone mass: a 6 month randomised controlled trial. *Journal of Clinical Densitometry, 7,* 390-398.

Luo, C.X., Jiang, J, Zhou Q.G, Zhu, X.J., Wang, W, Zhang, Z.J, Han X, Zhu, D.Y. (2007) Voluntary exercise-induced neurogenesis in the postischemic dentate gyrus is associated with spatial memory recovery from stroke. *J Neurosci Res, 85, 8,* 1637-1646.

McKelvie, R. S., Teo, K. K., Roberts, R., McCartney, N., Humen, D., Montague, T., et al., (2002). Effects of exercise training in patients with heart failure: the Exercise Rehabilitation Trial (EXERT). *American Heart Journal, 144,* 23-30.

McKenzie, D. C., & Kalda, A. L. (2003). Effect of upper extremity exercise on secondary lymphedema in breast cancer patients: a pilot study. *Journal of Clinical Oncology, 21,* 1653-1659.

Meka, N., Katragadda, S., Cherian, B., & Arora, R. R. (2008). Endurance exercise and resistance training in cardiovascular disease. *Therapeutic Advances in Cardiovascular Disease, 2,* 115-121.

Michael, K. M., Allen, J. K., & Macko, R. F. (2005). Reduced ambulatory activity after stroke: The role of balance, gait, and cardiovascular fitness. *Archives of Physical Medicine and Rehabilitation, 86,* 1552-1556.

Miller, T. D., Balady, G. J., & Fletcher, G. F. (1997). Exercise and its role in the prevention and rehabilitation of cardiovascular disease. *Annals of Behavorial Medicine, 19,* 220-229.

Newton, R. U., & Galvão, D. A. (2008). Exercise in prevention and management of cancer. *Current Treatment Options in Oncology, 9,* 135-146.

Pak, S., & Patten, C. (2008). Strengthening to promote functional recovery post-stroke: an evidence-based review. *Topics in Stroke Rehabilitation, 15,* 177-199.

Pang, M. Y. C., Eng, J. J., Dawson, A. S., & Glyfadóttir, S. (2006). The use of aerobic exercise training in improving aerobic capacity in individuals with stroke: a meta-analysis. *Clinical Rehabilitation, 20,* 97-111.

Pescatello, L.S., Franklin, B.A., Fagard, R., Farquhar, W.B., Kelley, G.A., Ray, C.A.; American College of Sports Medicine (2004). American College of Sports Medicine position stand. Exercise and hypertension. *Med Sci Sport Exerc, 36,* 533-553.

Piepoli, M. F., Davos, C., Francis, D. P., Coats, A. J. S., & ExTraMatch Collaborative. (2004). Exercise training meta-analysis of trials in patients with chronic heart failure (ExTraMatch). *British Medical Journal, 328,* 189-192.

Pierdomenico SD, Di Nicola M, Esposito AL, *et al.* (2009). Prognostic Value of Different Indices of Blood Pressure Variability in Hypertensive Patients. *American Journal of Hypertension.* doi:10.1038/ajh.2009.103.

Pitta, F., Troosters, T., Probst, V. S., Spruitt, M. A., Decramer, M., & Gosselink, R. (2006). Physical activity and hospitalisation for exacerbation of COPD. *Chest, 129,* 536-544.

HM Government (2007). *Putting people first: a shared vision and commitment to the transformation of adult social care.* UK: HM Government.

Quality and Outcomes Framework (QOF) 2006/07. More information on QOF prevalence counts can be found at www.ic.nhs.uk . Last accessed 17/05/09.

Raven, P. B., Welch-O'Connor, R. M., & Shi, X. (1998). Cardiovascular function following reduced aerobic activity. *Medicine and Science in Sports and Exercise, 30,* 1041-1052.

Rearden, J. Z., Lareau, S. C., & ZuWallack, R. (2006). Functional status and quality of life in chronic obstructive pulmonary disease. *The American Journal of Medicine, 119,* S32-S37.

Rees, K., Taylor, R. R. S., Singh, S., Coats, A. J. S. & Ebrahim, S. (2009). Exercise based rehabilitation for heart failure. *Cochrane Database of Systematic Reviews, 2.*

Richardson, C. R., Mehari, K. S., McIntyre, L. G., Janney, A. W., Fortlage, L. A., Sen, A., et al., (2007). A randomised trial comparing structured and lifestyle goals in an internet-mediated walking program for people with type 2 diabetes. International *Journal of Behavioural Nutrition and Physical Activity, 4,* 59.

Rimmer, J. H. (1999). Health promotion for people with disabilities: the emerging paradigm shift from disability prevention to prevention of secondary conditions. *Physical Therapy, 79,* 496-502.

Rimmer, J. H., Braddock, D. (2002). Health promotion for people with physical, cognitive and sensory disabilities: an emerging national priority. *American Journal of Health Promotion, 16,* 220-224.

Rimmer, J. H., Riley, B., Wang, E., Rauworth, A., & Jurkowski, J. (2004). Physical activity participation among persons with disabilities: barriers and facilitators. American Journal of Preventive Medcine, 26, 419-425.

Rogers, M. A., Yamamoto, C., Hagberg, J. M., Holloszy, J. O., Ehsani, A. A. (1987). The effects of 7 years of intense exercise training in patients with coronary artery disease. *Journal of the American College of Cardiology, 10,* 321-326.

Ross, R., Dagnone, D., Jones, P.J., Smith, H., Paddags, A., Hudson, R., Janssen, I. (2000).Reduction in obesity and related comorbid conditions after diet-induced weight loss or exercise-induced weight loss in men. A randomized, controlled trial. *Ann Intern Med, 133,* 92-103.

Rothwell, P. M., Coull, A. J., Silver, L. E., Fairhead, J. F., Giles, M. F., Lovelock, C. E., et al., (2005). Population-based study of event-rate, incidence, case fatality, and mortality for all acute vascular events in all arterial territories (Oxford Vascular Study). *Lancet, 366,* 1773-1783.

Rotstein, A., Harush, M., & Vaisman, N. (2008). The effect of a water exercise program on bone density of post-menopausal women. *Journal of Sports Medicine and Physical Fitness, 48,* 352-359.

Schmitz, K. H., Holtzman, J., Courneya, K. S., Mâsse, L. C., Duval, S., & Kane, R. (2005). Controlled physical activity trials in cancer survivors: a systematic review and meta-analysis. *Cancer Epidemiology Biomarkers & Prevention, 14,* 1588-1595.

Schneider, S. H., Amorosa, L. F., Khachadurian, A. K. & Ruderman, N. B. (1984). Studies on the mechanism of improved glucose control during regular exercise in type 2 diabetes. *Diabetologia, 26,* 355-360.

Schneider, S. H., Khachadurian, A. K., Amorosa, L. F., Clemow, L., & Ruderman, N. B. (1992). Ten year experience with an exercise-based outpatient lifestyle modification program in the treatment of diabetes mellitus. *Diabetes Care, 15,* 1800-1810.

Shaw K, Gennat H, O'Rourke P, Del Mar C. (2006). Exercise for overweight or obesity. *Cochrane Database Syst Rev., 18,* CD003817.

Smart, N., Marwick, T.H. (2004). Exercise training for patients with heart failure: a systematic review of factors that improve mortality and morbidity. *Am J Med, 116,* 693-706.

Sertpoyraz, F., Eyigor, S., Karapolat, H., Capaci, K., Kirazli, Y (2009). Comparison of isokinetic exercise versus standard exercise training in patients with chronic low back pain: a randomized controlled study. *Clinical Rehabilitation, 23,* 238-247.

Smith, P. S., & Thompson, M. (2009). Treadmill training post-stroke: are there any secondary benefits? A pilot study. *Clinical Rehabilitation, 22,* 997-1002.

Speck, B. J., & Looney, S. W. (2001). Effects of a minimal intervention to increase physical activity in women: daily activity records. *Nursing Research, 50,* 374-378.

Stenstrom, C. H., & Minor, M. A. (2003). Evidence for the benefit of aerobic and strengthening exercise in rheumatoid arthritis. *Athritis & Rheumatism, 49,* 428-434.

Swärdh, E, Biguet, G., & Opava, C. H. (2008). Views on exercise maintenance: variations among patients with rheumatoid arthritis. *Physical Therapy, 88,* 1049.

Szabo, Z, Yong Z, Radak Z, Gomez-Pinilla F (2009). Voluntary exercise may engage proteasome function to benefit the brain after trauma. *Brain Res,* Jan 30 (EPub ahead of print).

Taylor, R.S., Brown, A., Ebrahim, S., Jolliffe, J., Noorani, H., Rees, K., Skidmore B., Stone, J.A., Thompson, D.R., Oldridge, N. (2004) Exercise-based rehabilitation for patients with coronary heart disease: systematic review and meta-analysis of randomized controlled trials. *Am J Med. 116,* 682-692.

Todd, J. A., & Robinson, R. J. (2003). Osteoporosis and exercise: review. *Postgraduate Medical Journal, 79,* 320-323.

Toole, T., Thorne, J. E., Panton, L. B., Kingsley, D., & Haymes, E. M. (2007). Effects of a 12-month pedometer walking program on gait, body mass index and lower extremity function in obese women. *Perceptual and Motor Skills, 104,* 212-220.

Turner, A.P., Kivlahan, D.R., Haselkorn, J.K. (2009). Exercise and quality of life among people with multiple sclerosis: looking beyond physical functioning to mental health and participation in life. *Arch Phys Med Rehabil, 90,* 420-428.

U.S. Department of Health and Human Services. (1996). *Physical activity and health: A report of the Surgeon General.* Atlanta, GA: Author.

van Tol, B. A., Huijsmans, R. J., Kroon, D. W., Schothorst, M., & Kwakkel, G. (2006). Effects of exercise training on cardiac performance, exercise capacity and quality of life in patients with heart-failure: a meta-analysis. *European Journal of Heart Failure, 8,* 841-850.

Vallance, J. K. H., Courneya, K. S., Plotnikoff, R. C., Yasui, Y., & Mackey, J. R. (2007). Randomised controlled trial of the effects of print materials and step pedometers on physical activity and quality of life in breast cancer survivors. *Journal of Clinical Oncology, 25,* 2352-2359.

Van den Ende, C. H., Vliet Vlieland, T. P., Muneke, M., & Hazes, J. M. (1998). Dynamic exercise therapy for rheumatoid arthritis: a systematic review. *British Journal of Rheumatology, 37,* 677-687.

Van den Ende, C. H., Vliet Vlieland, T. P., Muneke, M., & Hazes, J. M. (2000). Dynamic exercise therapy for rheumatoid arthritis. Cochrane Database Systematic Review, CD000322.

Waddell, G. & Watson, P. (2004). Rehabilitation. In G. Waddell (Ed.) *The Back Pain Revolution (2nd edition)* (pp. 371-400). Edinburgh, UK: Churchill Livingstone.

Wei, M., Gibbons, L. W., Kampert, J. B. Nichaman, M. Z., & Blair, S. N. (2000). Low cardiorespiratory fitness and physical inactivity as predictors of mortality in men with type 2 diabetes. *Annals of Internal Medicine, 132,* 605-611.

Whedon, G. D. (1984). Disuse osteoporosis: physiological aspects. *Calcified Tissue International, 36,* S151-154.

Wijkstra, P. J., ten Vergert, E. M., van Altena, R., Otten, V., Kraan, J., Postema, D. S., et al., (1995). Long term benefits of rehabilitation at home on quality of life and exercise tolerance in patients with chronic obstructive pulmonary disease. *Thorax, 50,* 824-828.

Wijkstra, P. J., ten Hacken, N., Wempe, J. B., Koeter, G. H. (2003). What is the role of rehabilitation in COPD? In: M. Pearson & W. Wedzicha (eds). *Chronic Obstructive Pulmonary Disease: Critical Debates* (pp.147-167). Massachusetts: Blackwell Science.

World Health Organisation. (2008). *Depression.* Retrieved 5 May, 2008, from http://www.who.int/mental_health/management/depression/definition/en/

World Health Organisation (2006). *Gaining health. The European strategy for the prevention and control of non-communicable diseases.* Geneva: World Health Organisation

Yamanouchi, K., Shinozaki, T., Chikada, K., Nishikawa, T., Ito, K., Shimizu, S., et al., (1995) Daily walking combined with diet therapy is a useful means for obese NIDDM patients not only to reduce body weight but also to improve insulin sensitivity. *Diabetes Care, 18,* 775-778.

In: Physical Activity in Rehabilitation and Recovery   ISBN: 978-1-60876-400-6
Editor: Holly Blake   © 2010 Nova Science Publishers, Inc.

Chapter 3

EXERCISE PROMOTION AND REHABILITATION OF NEUROLOGICAL CONDITIONS

Helen Dawes[*]

School of Life Sciences, Oxford Brookes University & Dept. of Clinical
Neurology, University of Oxford, UK.

ABSTRACT

This chapter explores the effect of an active lifestyle on the general
health, well being and role in prevention of the primary disease and
occurrence of secondary diseases for selected conditions affecting the central
nervous system. It will give an initial overview of neurological conditions,
consider the barriers and facilitators for engagement and long term
maintenance of physical activity, and finally explore physical activity levels
and interventions in people with stroke, Parkinson's disease (PD) and
Multiple Sclerosis (MS). The aim is not to cover detailed discussion of
exercise prescription for attainment of specific functional recovery within
rehabilitation, but rather to scrutinise exercise prescription for health and
wellbeing in primary and secondary prevention.

[*] Tel:+44(0)1865 483293; Fax:+44(0)1865 483242; Email: hdawes@brookes.ac.uk

NEUROLOGICAL POPULATIONS

Over two million people in the UK and an estimated 1 billion people worldwide according to the World Health Organization (WHO) are affected by neurological disorders (World Health Organisation, 2009). Common neurological disorders include dementia, epilepsy, headache disorders, multiple sclerosis, neuroinfections, Parkinson's disease, stroke and traumatic brain injuries(WHO 2009). Neurological disorders kill an estimated 6.8 million people each year, equating to 12 percent of global deaths (World Health Organisation, 2009). These conditions have a growing human, societal and economic cost as the elderly population increases worldwide. Indeed there is evidence that pinpoints neurological disorders as one of the greatest threats to public health (World Health Organisation, 2009). This section will give an overview of physical activity in neurological conditions, but will cover in detail multiple sclerosis (MS), stroke and Parkinson's disease (PD).

A detailed awareness of the basic structure and function of the neuromuscular system and the pathological processes will enable better exercise prescription in these conditions. Detailing underlying pathological process is outside the remit of this text, however for a quick summary of these conditions readers may wish to consider *Mosby's Crash Course in Neurology* (Turner, 2006), *Neurology an Illustrated Colour Text* (Fuller, 2005) or some of the excellent publications on the society websites of the *Stroke Association, Parkinson's Disease Associations and Multiple Sclerosis Society or Trust.* The underlying pathology affecting neurological and neuromuscular function should be taken into account when considering safe participation in physical activities. Conditions affecting the nervous system can be categorised into the following (Fuller, 2005):

1   Systemic pathology (metabolic, toxic, nutritional, immunological or endocrine disorders)
2   Intrinsic pathology (metabolic, infectious, neoplastic, degenerative, paroxysmal, immunological and genetic disorders)
3   Vascular pathology
4   Extrinsic pathology

Many systems including those affecting movement, continence, cognition and mood may be affected by neurological pathology, which result in a range of possible symptomatic presentations and progressions. Some conditions are progressive (such as Parkinson's disease and Motor Neuron Disease), some have a sudden onset and variable levels of recovery (such as a stroke or transient ischaemic attack), whilst others may relapse and remit at any time point over a number of years (Multiple Sclerosis). The type and level of impairment of body function will impact on the choice of activity and its delivery and needs to be considered to enable safe, effective and sympathetic exercise prescription. However, whilst the observed impairments will affect exercise prescription independent of underlying condition, for successful exercise participation, health and fitness professionals may also need to consider the underlying pathology and adapt exercises appropriately whatever the chosen exercise modality or setting. Day to day performance in people with neurological conditions may be more variable than that observed in healthy individuals. Condition specific pathology affecting physical, cognitive, social and emotional factors, medication and its timing in relation to exercise sessions may all affect participation on a given day.

A consideration for health and fitness professionals when supporting exercise in people with neurological conditions is the wide range of possible body systems affected as shown in figure 1. The practicalities of dealing with symptoms such as fatigue, continence, attention and behaviour within exercise prescription programmes are discussed elsewhere (Dawes, 2008a) and not the focus of this chapter. The impact of exercise on body function, activity and participation will be considered later.

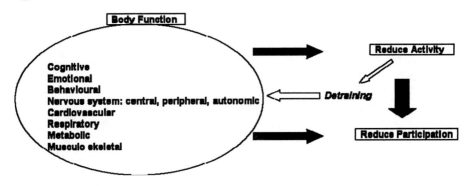

Figure 1.

As shown in figure 1 neuromuscular systems may be disrupted by neurological diseases affecting coordination, balance, muscle strength, power, speed, flexibility and endurance. The reduction in neuromuscular function may limit mobility and participation in physical activities and lead to detraining of cardiovascular and neuromuscular systems, further reducing performance and activity. The impact on mobility and physical activity can thus result in a downward spiral of inactivity and detraining as shown in figure 1.

As outlined above these effects may be observed to directly affect neuromuscular (muscular atrophy) and cardiovascular systems (cardiovascular fitness) but reduced mobility may also greatly affect the functioning of skeletal, urinary and gastro-intestinal systems.

The complex relationship between primary pathology and the secondary effects of inactivity may present a confusing picture to practitioners working with people with neurological disorders. Practitioners may have difficulty distinguishing between symptoms that result directly from pathological impairment and those that are secondary to disuse and inactivity and may more readily respond to exercise interventions. When monitoring exercise prescription, clinicians need to consider that observed improvements in function may be due to recovery/remission of underlying pathology, or a response to training. Thus for optimal prescription in this clinical group, a fusion of skills of both health and exercise professionals may be required.

In Summary

- Conditions affecting the neurological system can present with symptoms affecting many systems.
- Changes in function in components of fitness such as strength, power, speed and endurance may be due to the primary disease process or occur as a secondary consequence of enforced physical inactivity and detraining.
- Knowledge of the underlying pathology is needed for safe effective exercise prescription.
- Impairments of body function will also impact on the choice of activity and its delivery independent of underlying pathology.
- Change in performance in response to physical activity programmes may be due to changes in fitness and/or in underlying pathology.

INTRODUCTION TO PHYSICAL ACTIVITY IN NEUROLOGICAL POPULATIONS

Two thousand years have passed since Plato commented "Lack of activity destroys the good condition of every human being, while movement and methodical physical exercise save it and preserve it"(Dawes, 2008b).

Now the scientific evidence for regular participation for all in physical activity is compelling (Dawes, 2008b). Physical activity contributes to well-being and good health, whilst the risks associated with participating in physical activity at levels that promote health are low for all (Department of Health, 2004a). People who are physically active reduce their risk of developing a list of major chronic diseases including coronary heart disease, stroke and type 2 diabetes – by up to 50 percent, and the risk of premature death by about 20-30 percent (Department of Health, 2004a). Further evidence confirms the importance of strong muscles and more vigorous activities for health(O'Donovan & Shave, 2007; Ruiz et al., 2008). However, even within normal populations there is an ongoing debate as to the optimal exercise dose, frequency, intensity and duration for health and wellbeing benefits(O'Donovan & Shave, 2007).

In neurological populations, exercise prescription has swung into fashion over recent years and is now a more common component of rehabilitation programmes. People with a range of long-term neurological conditions would appear to be no different from the general population, with participation in a range of physical activities having demonstrated benefits at international classification of function (ICF) levels of body function, activity and participation (Dawes, 2008b). It may be that many people with neurological conditions, many of whom are extremely detrained, could potentially gain from increasing their physical activity and mobility. For many neurological conditions, participation in physical activity and exercise prescription has been evaluated within the rehabilitation setting, with outcome measures tending to focus mainly on physical functions directly affected by their condition. In many ways research in these populations has lagged behind other long-term conditions where there has been a paradigm shift towards a focus of exercise as an intervention for prevention of secondary conditions(Rimmer, 1999). There is limited evidence as to the effect of participation in regular exercise on long-term general health and wellbeing within individuals with disabilities' daily lives, in particular those with neurological conditions (Rimmer, Rowland, & Yamaki, 2007). It is unclear whether benefits accrue as a result of changes in the pathological process, effects on health and wellbeing, or both. Certainly there is now accumulating evidence of the importance that exercise and activity may play in modifying inflammatory responses and so benefit health(Cotman, Berchtold, & Christie, 2007; DeLegge & Smoke, 2008; Smith, Carr, Dorozynski, & Gomashe,2009; White & Castellano, 2008a). In neurological conditions, characterised by varied patterns of inflammation, these benefits may be even more important as disease mediators as well as providing secondary health benefits (DeLegge & Smoke, 2008). Many important questions remain regarding implementing safe effective exercise for neurological conditions within rehabilitation and community settings.

SPECIFICALLY

1. What exercise content is optimal?
    How long, hard and frequently should people exercise?
    What activities and muscles should be targeted?
    Which physiological components should be trained (cardiovascular fitness, flexibility, balance, coordination and skill, muscle strength, speed and power or muscle endurance)?

2. For best uptake of exercise and successful implementation into peoples' lives where and how should exercise be undertaken?
    What types of exercise (swimming, cycling, circuits)?
    What setting (home, gym or hospital)?
    Who should lead/instruct the sessions?
    Which mode of delivery/social setting is better (individual or special group sessions)?

3. How can exercise be safely and accurately prescribed?
    How can exercise intensity, duration and frequency be accurately measured in neurological populations?

Simple fitness and activity targets (such as achieving a particular heart rate or counting steps) that can be utilised by everyone in any setting are a central tenet for effective exercise prescription in normal populations (Department of Health, 2004a). However many of these models of measuring and promoting activity and fitness may not be appropriate for people with neurological conditions (Dawes, 2008b; Elsworth et al, 2009a).

MEASURING PHYSICAL ACTIVITY LEVELS

Physical activity occurs within social, work, transport and home domains. Although in healthy populations most physical activity is undertaken socially or as a means of transport, for the elderly and in neurological populations most physical activity would appear to occur in the home (Elsworth et al., 2009). This presents a challenge if attempting to accurately determine activity levels. A further consideration is that models of exercise prescription and monitoring developed for healthy individuals (Bravata et al., 2007), such as heart rate estimates, metabolic equivalents (METS) or pedometer step counts, may not be appropriate (Dawes et al., 2003) or accurate (valid or reliable) (Elsworth et al, 2009a) for all individuals with neurological conditions. For example; pedometers have been shown to be accurate in adolescents with Down Syndrome (Stanish, 2004), but to undercount in people with neurological conditions (Elsworth et al, 2009a). A simple marker of walking speed does not appear to be related to pedometer accuracy if used in neurological populations (Elsworth, In Press). Thus, individuals will require assessing to determine if a pedometer can be accurately used on them (Elsworth et al, 2009a). This is a challenge for both researchers and clinicians when attempting to validly and reliably quantify how active people are. For capturing activity levels (frequency, intensity and duration), activity questionnaires (van der Ploeg et al., 2008) or diaries can be utilised with the known limitations of other self report measures (Dawes et al., 2006) (Elsworth, Patel et al., in press).

Technological measurement tools, such as accelerometer devices (Busse et al., 2006a; Mudge, & Stott, 2008; Hale, Pal, & Becker, 2008) which have been shown to be accurate in neurological populations may be utilised. However, as yet, expense may prohibit use of the latter within many clinical settings. Heart rate and rating of perceived exertion (RPE) should be used with caution if monitoring intensity levels in this group. Heart rate may give an indication of activity intensity, but reduced capacity and possible effect of medications should be considered (ACSM, 2003). RPE may offer a less sensitive and more variable measure of intensity than when used in healthy populations (Dawes et al, 2006) and thus may not be accurate or reliable (Dawes et al, 2006) particularly if used not just to monitor but to direct the intensity of performing exercises. Evidence to date is limited in people with neurological conditions, but there is a general picture of low activity levels performed at low exercise intensities (Dawes et al, 2008a) with most physical activity occurring within home domains(Dawes et al, 2008a; Motl et al., 2008a). Specific evidence in neurological conditions will be discussed in the later sections on: Parkinsons disease, multiple sclerosis and stroke or transient ischemic attack (TIA).

Summary

- Measures utilised for exercise prescription and monitoring in healthy populations may not be valid and accurate in people with neurological conditions.
- Activity diaries/questionnaires will indicate general levels of overall activity (duration) and the domain in which they are carried out.
- Pedometers may be used to determine number of steps, but may undercount in people with neurological populations and accuracy will need to be determined individually prior to use.
- Heart rate can indicate intensity of activities, though care should be taken if using perceptual ratings of intensity.

BARRIERS AND FACILITATORS TO PHYSICAL ACTIVITY

The observation of overall activity levels in the general population being lower than the currently recommended weekly five 30 minute sessions indicates there are barriers to being active for all of us. The barriers for healthy people are outside the remit of this chapter, however there are additional contextual, physical, social and personal factors that affect participation in exercise for people with neurological conditions. On a daily basis people with neurological conditions have to tackle environmental factors (suitable transport, access and facilities) (Rimmer et al., 2004), negative attitudes of people in fitness and community centres (their beliefs about risk and benefit) and may rely on a high level of family support in order to be able to participate (Wiles, In Press).

Whilst, as discussed in earlier chapters, there are often national policies pursuing increases in activity in the population as a whole (Department of Health, 2004a) with local targets to increase exercise participation, there are often no specific targets for people with disabilities or neurological conditions in many countries. When considering sporting opportunities for people with disabilities, the Paralympic movement is extensive with a massive worldwide impact, whereas exercise opportunities for people with disabilities receive less attention. Environmental and social barriers (transport, access, equipment, staff attitudes and awareness) may require strategic policies such as those addressed by the Inclusive Fitness Initiative http://www.inclusivefitness.org/, a charitable programme initiated in the UK now gaining global coverage (inclusive fitness coalition), that was set up to support the fitness industry to become more inclusive and cater for the needs of disabled alongside non-disabled people. The initiative provides a charter mark to facilities so that that users know that a centre is equipped and staffed with people with skills to cater for their needs. However there is still a general paucity of optimal facilities in the community for people with disabilities and low levels of participation for people with neurological conditions are observed generally within community facilities.

People with a range of disabilities have been researched in order to determine factors affecting their participation in physical activities (Rimmer et al., 2004). For people with disabilities, barriers include:

- Environmental barriers
- Economic issues
- Emotional and psychological barriers
- Equipment barriers
- Barriers related to the use and interpretation of guidelines, codes, regulations, and laws
- Information-related barriers
- Professional knowledge, education, and training issues
- Perceptions and attitudes of persons who are not disabled, including professionals
- Policies and procedures both at the facility and community level
- Availability of resources (Rimmer et al., 2004).

In people with neurological conditions including those with multiple sclerosis, motor neurone disease, neuromuscular conditions and Parkinson's disease, specific issues to being physically active have been categorised under individuals' general opinions of physical activity, barriers to physical activity, and factors that would facilitate increased physical activity involvement'(Elsworth, Patel et al., in press). Reported secondary conditions of physical de-conditioning and feelings of isolation have been shown to be inversely related to the ability of moderately impaired women with physical disabilities to participate in leisure time physical activities, independent of their functional ability (Santiago & Coyle, 2004). Enabling participation would appear to be extremely important for health promoting behaviour (Santiago & Coyle, 2004). In general, people with neurological conditions report enjoying exercise "quite a lot" with only 15% of individuals, albeit in a small sample, reporting to enjoy exercise "not at all" (Elsworth, Patel et al., in press). Preferred activities reported in this heterogenous sample of people included swimming, stretching and walking.

Some of these activities may not always be readily available to people with neurological conditions, particularly those with greater levels of impairment. The most common barriers to participating in physical activity in neurological conditions are similar to those observed in a range of other long term conditions (Rimmer et al., 2004; Rimmer, 2005.) but more specifically include those of:

- Concern regarding appropriate facilities
- Embarrassment issues when using community venues
- Perceived lack of knowledge of fitness or health professionals about their neurological disease and the impact of the condition on exercise prescription (Elsworth, Patel et al., in press).

Additional issues specifically measured in a group of women with MS observed in the literature on normal populations, are self-efficacy to perform activities and functional limitations (Morris et al., 2008a). Indeed in this large study of 173 women with MS, environmental factors seemed to have less of an impact on activity levels than in a healthy elderly female sample (Morris et al., 2008a). Engaging people following a stroke in physical activity also continues to be a major challenge (Rimmer, Wang, & Smith, 2008). People following stroke ranked similar barriers to other groups; the five most common being (Rimmer et al., 2008):

- Cost of exercise programs (61%)
- Lack of awareness of a fitness centre in the area (57%)
- No means of transportation to a fitness centre (57%)
- No knowledge of how to exercise (46%)
- No knowledge of where to exercise (44%).

The least common barriers were:

- Lack of interest (16%)
- Lack of time (11%)
- Concern that exercise would worsen their condition (1%).

It is notable when considering the delivery of exercise that in contrast to opinions reported by people with other disabilities, the majority of individuals in a sample of people with neurological conditions including MS and PD indicated that they would prefer to exercise in a group of people with disabilities (not necessarily their own condition), with relatively few people indicating they would like to exercise alone (Elsworth, Patel et al., in press). The presence of specifically trained staff is perceived as particularly important, with the majority of individuals indicating they would prefer to exercise with the support of health or fitness professionals with expertise relevant to their condition (Dawes et al., 2006). Certainly there is now a need to develop specific courses for health and fitness professionals in order to develop the necessary skills. Another major challenge is the issue of providing transport in all people with disabilities. People with greater disability, some of whom may have cognitive, speech and physical impairments, report finding public and private transport systems difficult to use and expensive. Furthermore people with conditions affecting the nervous system may be unable to use typical gym equipment such as a treadmill or cycle ergometer in a standard way (Wiles et al., in press). A flexible approach for individuals is thus required, adapting postures or using additional equipment when necessary such as reclining ergometers, theraband, upper limb systems and adapted weight machines. Facilities need to be adequately equipped and those that are need to be well marketed so they can easily be found.

To date there is limited evidence of the cost/ benefit in people with neurological conditions (Salvetti, Oliveira, Servantes, & Vincenzo de Paola, 2008). Individuals and families have different desires and needs, but certainly for some people, possibly those with greater levels of impairment, the cost of being physically active within the community in financial, physical and emotional terms may be prohibitive when weighed up against the benefits. Other options for home activity are available and whilst possibly not providing the same social enrichment as that provided by participating in activities outside the home they can be extremely effective and desirable for some people.

Summary

People with neurological conditions express a desire to be able to participate in a range of activities including those that are not just gym-based and in a range of environments. People with neurological conditions highlight many barriers and facilitators in common with other people with disabilities and some individual concerns. Factors affecting participation in physical activity are different for each individual, however major themes affecting regular ongoing participation are:

- Friendly welcoming facilities with good access and appropriate equipment.
- The exercise provider should be knowledgeable of the individual's neurological condition and appropriate exercise prescription.
- People have expressed a desire to have the opportunity to exercise with other people and to be able to participate in group exercise sessions or sessions where there are other people with disabilities.
- Good reliable transport and parking.
- Support initially attending sessions and becoming familiar with the exercise environment.
- The cost of the activity, though in general community gym costs do not appear to be prohibitive.
- A lack of awareness of appropriate local resources

Facilities need to be well marketed and advertised so that individuals know what is available and where. An approach that utilises charitable support groups, general practitioners and medical centres would appear to be essential for providing such information in order to reach as many people as possible.

ATTAINING AND MAINTAINING PHYSICAL ACTIVITY

When setting out to attain and maintain physical activity levels we know from our own experiences and backed by the literature in healthy adults and children that simply informing people what is good for them and leaving it at that is not effective. Attaining adequate physical activity for health benefit even in the normal population is complex. Research into the application of exercise attainment and maintenance models is a relatively new field in neurological conditions. Indeed previous research into physical activity in elderly populations has suggested mixed models may more appropriately explain adherence in populations with a range of abilities and situations (Cohen-Mansfield, Marx, & Guralnik, 2006). Although it is possible to increase activity in people with disabilities (Froehlich-Grobe & White, 2004), exercise adherence often varies considerably, which is not unsurprising when considering the factors affecting participation (Romberg et al., 2004). With limited research in this area, it is not surprising that health professionals have expressed difficulty finding ways to keep people with disabilities engaged in community-based physical activity/rehabilitation programs (Rimmer, 2006).

Low community activity levels are reported in long-term neurological conditions (Busse, Pearson, van Deursen, & Wiles, 2004; Busse et al., 2006a; Elsworth et al, 2009b) and after stroke (Shaughnessy, Resnick, & Macko, 2006). Sixty nine percent of people after a stroke report being unable to exercise at a level suggested by the ACSM to give health benefits, ie four times or more a week, even when this included therapeutic support systems (Shaughnessy et al., 2006). After stroke, factors that have been shown to relate to low activity levels are a lack of clarity of expected therapeutic exercise levels, as in MS a poor self-efficacy for exercise, and a pre-illness history of low activity levels (Shaughnessy et al., 2006).

There are many factors that promote and inhibit the successful integration of physical activities into people's everyday lives (Elsworth et al, 2009b). These include individual likes and dislikes, perceived benefits and difficulties (family, work and home commitments) that affect regular physical activity involvement. Individuals may find greater difficulty re-engaging with exercise when prevented from participating for a period of time than healthy individuals. Individuals have reported previous difficulties (such as difficulties safely negotiating the exercise environment after a lay off), sometimes embarrassing, as an emotional barrier when attempting to reengage (Elsworth et al, 2009b). When maintaining physical participation, understanding an individual's motivation is critical and the extensive theoretical literature from normal healthy populations should inform the area of not only engaging people with exercise but in successfully maintaining their level of activity. Clinicians working with people with neurological conditions will know that individuals are not just motivated by improving their disability or function (Dawes, Roach, Wade, & Scott, 1999). An early study looking at people with brain injury found a range of motivating factors for people with stroke and brain injury (Dawes et al., 1999). A range of motivating factors has also been confirmed in people with PD (Steffen, Boeve, Mollinger-Riemann, & Petersen, 2007) and in people with MS (McAuley et al., 2007) . These factors include as well as physical, social and environmental influences those psychological factors such as enjoyment and self efficacy. People in rehabilitation are not just motivated to improve their condition and function, but would appear to be motivated by most of the factors the general population are motivated including a desire to:

- Lose or control weight
- Improve appearances
- Build up muscles
- Handle stress and anxiety

- Make individuals feel good about themselves
- Improve health
- Increase endurance
- Enjoy themselves and have fun
- Social engagement reasons

Although clinicians may instigate exercise and activity in order to improve function, there may be other factors motivating people to attain/maintain physical activity participation. This should be considered when attempting to integrate physical activity into people's everyday lives. Evidence from the general population has shown that whilst self efficacy to be active is important (McAuley & Blissmer, 2000), enjoyment of an activity is also significant for long-term adherence (Dishman, 1988). Enjoyment of the activity would also appear to be key for engagement with exercise and rehabilitation activities (Colombo et al., 2007).

Certainly engaging people in physical activities in the longer term is also complex and has been modeled with self determination, stress, coping, and motivational theories (Ntoumanis, Edmunds, & Duda, 2008). The reasons for participation are individual and affected by many factors at body function, activity and participation levels (Rimmer, 2006) . However other factors affecting engagement in long-term conditions include previous exercise experiences (Borkoles, Nicholls Bell, Butterly, & Polman, 2008) and issues of age and gender (Ntoumanis et al., 2008; Tappe, Duda, & Ehrnwald, 1989; 1990).

Attaining long-term engagement in people with neurological conditions may require an approach that encompasses both a medical and social model when considering the barriers and facilitators for participation in this group. Research utilising a community physical activity support system (PASS) for neurological conditions, modeled loosely on cardiac rehabilitation programmes, but structured as an expert patient self managing system, in pilot testing has achieved an increase in activity levels of 25% in the short term, but requires further examination in a controlled trial and in the longer term(Elsworth, Patel et al., in press). Such a support system, whilst encouraging an expert patient self determined approach to exercise, does provide medical support for optimal safe prescription. Its effectiveness has yet to be shown but the model is supported by qualitative data (Zalewski, 2007) which emphasizes the importance of medical support to reintegrate individuals to community exercise. Certainly novel approaches may be required in order to engage people in the long term and 'top ups' of support would appear to help maintain ongoing participation. Further evidence would suggest that, following rehabilitation, individuals with neurological conditions who are supported by counseling will have an increase in physical activity behaviour compared to those without this support at both nine weeks(van der Ploeg et al., 2006) and one year (van der Ploeg et al., 2007a)after rehabilitation. In a follow on study, determinants of the intervention-induced improvement in physical activity behaviour at both nine weeks and one year were observed to include the participants attitude; their perceived benefits "improved health and reduced risk of disease", "better feeling about oneself," and "improved fitness,". Again, mirroring the evidence of barriers to participation, a major barrier to ongoing participation was the effect of "limited local environmental possibilities(van der Ploeg et al., 2008).

In Summary

- Factors affecting ongoing physical activity participation integration into peoples' lives are multiple and complex and this is true in people with neurological conditions.
- Long-term engagement in physical activity may require both a medical and social model, utilising community facilities but using medical support as required, possibly from a self management system.
- Clinicians should be aware that people with neurological conditions may be motivated to be active by a number of motivators that reflect those observed in the healthy population.

EXERCISE PRESCRIPTION IN NEUROLOGICAL POPULATIONS

Physical activity targets to promote health and wellbeing for healthy adults of five or more sessions of 30 minutes aerobic activity a week are well established (Department of Health, 2004a). However for many neurological conditions there is no clear evidence base for the optimal amount or content of exercise, either within rehabilitation or as part of a healthy lifestyle. Guidance for modes of delivery, general approaches and the actual amount of exercise for exercise prescription has often been developed from consensus of expert opinion and best evidence for many neurological conditions (ACSM, 2003). When considering the evidence for exercise prescription aimed at maintaining an active lifestyle for general health, well being and prevention of secondary disease this is particularly limited. Clinicians working with clients with neurological conditions are faced with prescribing exercise programmes from relatively limited evidence, however there is an increasing amount of ongoing research and a fast developing evidence base.

CHOOSING PHYSICAL ACTIVITIES

When considering engaging with physical activity for health benefits it is important to consider what, how often, how frequently and how hard. Certain questions remain:

1 Which fitness components should be trained (cardiovascular, muscle endurance, power, strength, speed, balance, skill, coordination or flexibility)?
2 Which activity is optimal? An activity with a functional goal (walking), one with a skill attainment goal (dancing) or one with a social goal (swimming) or combination of these.
3 When and what dose (frequency, intensity and duration) of exercise should be performed?

Research into exercise prescription in healthy populations is extensive and ongoing but safe, minimal doses and expected dose responses are not yet well described in many clinical groups. Exercise dose response and effect at an activity/participation level may be dependent on the threshold level of ability in body functions, such as strength, flexibility and endurance. There still remain many questions about participating in physical activity for people with neurological conditions (Dawes, 2008a).

This chapter will focus on stroke and transient ischaemic attack, Parkinson's disease and multiple sclerosis, considering briefly the role of exercise in primary prevention and then the role of exercise for heath and wellbeing and prevention of secondary disorders.

STROKE AND TRANSIENT ISCHAEMIC ATTACK

Stroke is the second leading cause of death and leading cause of disability worldwide (Rothwell, 2004). People are often left dependent in activities of daily living with moderate to severe disability and vulnerable to an increased risk of falling (Department of Health, 2007). A stroke or transient ischemic attack is caused by a disruption in the flow of blood to the brain or spinal cord (Fuller, 2005). The terms "transient ischaemic attack (TIA)" and "minor stroke" are often used synonymously, but with TIA there should be no residual impairments 24 hours after an episode. A stroke will most commonly affect the cerebral hemispheres and subcortical structures. Stroke is grouped into two major categories that reflect the mechanism of the insult: primary ischaemia (a blood clot occludes an artery interrupting the brain's blood supply) and primary haemorrhage (a blood vessel ruptures causing bleeding, the resulting pressure directly damaging cells or preventing blood flow). Primary ischaemic stroke accounts for approximately 80% and haemorrhagic stroke for 20% of cases (Fuller, 2005). The effect of a cerebral vascular event on body function health and wellbeing depends on the size and location of the area of the brain affected (Schiemanck et al., 2005; Stinear et al., 2007). Commonly one side of the body will be affected, with function generally more affected in the arm than the leg (Schiemanck et al., 2005) . Longitudinal studies show that generally stroke patients experience most functional recovery in the first three months(Wade, Wood, & Hewer, 1985) although functional changes may occur later. Following the acute recovery period, likelihood of response to rehabilitation and exercise interventions appears to be independent of an individual's age or level of impairment (Dawes et al., 2007).

STROKE AND TRANSIENT ISCHEMIC ATTACK: PREVENTION

In primary prevention of cerebrovascular incidents strong evidence supports the benefits of participation in physical activity for all (Kozakova et al., 2007; Lee et al, 2003; Wendel-Vos Get al., 2004) and specifically for both men and women (Wisloff et al., 2006), people with hypertension (Hu et al., 2007a), diabetis (Blonde, Dempster, Gallivan, & Warren-Boulton, 2006) and for people of different ages (Kozakova et al., 2007). Evidence from two meta-analysis studies suggest that activity performed within work or leisure time is preventative, and that activity should be of a high or moderate level to attain a significant decrease in risk of stroke (Lee et al., 2003; Wendel-Vos et al., 2004). To date, no further evidence is available of the optimal dose or form of the activity, current advice suggesting thirty minutes of moderate daily exercise for at least five times a week should be recommended to lower both cardiovascular and cerebrovascular risk factors in healthy adults (Department of Health, 2004a). However a single weekly bout of exercise of high intensity has been shown to reduce the risk of cardiovascular death in men and women compared with those who reported no activity, with no additional benefit from increasing the duration or the number of exercise sessions per week (Wisloff et al., 2006). It has been suggested that UK physical activity guidelines should be amended to state that vigorous activity offers greater health benefits than moderate levels (O'Donovan & Shave, 2007). However for some individuals this may not be recommended, as participation in vigorous activities may be associated with a trend for increased risk of an adverse event of a stroke in people with asymptomatic coronary heart disease (Yu, Patterson, & Yarnell, 2008).

Summary

- Evidence supports physical activity for prevention of cerebrovascular accidents.
- The optimal content of activity is unclear, but as little as one intense session a week may be of benefit. General recommendations would be for five 30 minute sessions a week of moderate intensity exercise.

STROKE AND TRANSIENT ISCHAEMIC ATTACK: SECONDARY PREVENTION, HEALTH AND WELLBEING

About a third of people following a stroke or TIA go on to suffer a further, often more severe, cerebrovascular event. People surviving a stroke often live with moderate to severe disability (Rothwell et al, 2004) and are dependent in activities of daily living (Mayo et al, 1999). Thus stroke survivors may be predisposed to lead a sedentary lifestyle with an increased likelihood of detraining of musculoskeletal and cardiovascular systems (Wolfe, 2000), risk of falling and fracturing (AGSPF, 2001) and a high risk of recurrent stroke and cardiovascular disease2. The Royal College of Physicians recommend minimal levels of therapy for stroke rehabilitation (stroke), and the National Stroke Strategy 6 promotes the development of appropriately tailored long-term services, but most rehabilitation currently ends six months after a stroke11 although people following a TIA may receive no physical activity advice or support.

There are no guidelines for physical activity targets for health and wellbeing and secondary prevention of cerebrovascular events within UK clinical guidelines (stroke), although the American Stroke Association and American Heart Association guidelines for the secondary prevention of stroke in 2006 provide helpful guidelines and recommendations for physical activity after stroke, with the aim of preventing a secondary event (Gordon et al., 2004; Rincon & Sacco, 2008).

When considering how physically active people are six months following a stroke, profound cardiovascular deconditioning and extremely low ambulatory activity profiles have been observed; 2837 steps a day (Michael, Allen, & Macko, 2005) versus 5000-6000 steps a day in sedentary older adults (Bohannon, 2007) . Over two thirds of individuals perform less than four exercise sessions a week (Shaughnessy et al., 2006). There is no data regarding activity levels following a TIA. Restoration of mobility and an independent, secure, fast, and safe gait is a major challenge and aim for clinicians following a stroke (Jorgensen et al., 1995) as well as a major focus of patients (Jette et al., 2005). Although important, when considering factors affecting activity levels after a stroke, they do not appear to just be related to physical impairments such as weakness, spasticity affecting mobility (Welmer, von Arbin, Widen Holmqvist, & Sommerfeld, 2006) but also due to a combination of other factors including cognition (Luk, Chiu, & Chu, 2008) and difficulty in performing simultaneous physical and cognitive tasks (Hyndman, Ashburn, & Stack, 2002; Shumway-Cook, Woollacott, 2007). Psychological factors such as self-identity, social support and self-efficacy have been shown to affect physical activity levels, and these constructs have been shown to be affected by people's exercise experiences (Plow, Mathiowetz, & Resnik, 2008) .

When considering ongoing health and wellbeing for people following a cerebrovascular incident, current strategies to reduce further events in these individuals include controlling for risk factors, introducing appropriate pharmacological therapy and lifestyle modification (Rothwell et al., 2005). The UK National Service Framework for Coronary Heart Disease recommends that cardiac patients should have access to a multi-disciplinary programme of secondary prevention and rehabilitation. Indeed, reductions in cardiac mortality of 26%, and all cause mortality of 20% have been claimed in response to cardiac rehabilitation. There is increasing evidence that participation in regular physical activity could reduce the risk of a second stroke (Lennon, Carey, Gaffney, Stephenson, & Blake, 2008; Tanne et al., 2008). In general, reductions in functional ability have been linked with reductions in health related quality of life (Langhammer, Stanghelle, & Lindmark, 2008; Muren et al., 2008) and health (Rincon & Sacco, 2008) following a stroke.

We know that physical activity and exercises can improve fitness (Tanne et al., 2008), mobility and function in the short-term following stroke (Saunders, Greig, Young, & Mead, 2004; Dawes, in press) and that participation in physical activity would appear to benefit brain health in general (Tang, Chu, Hui, Helmeste, & Law, 2008). Whilst evidence from systematic reviews observes there is no strong evidence yet that participation in physical activity benefits health (Karmisholt & Gotzcshe, 2005), a recent study observed that participation in half hour cycle sessions twice per week for 10 weeks reduced secondary event risk factors, including blood pressure, for people with existing cerebrovascular disease (Lennon, Carey, Gaffney, Stephenson, & Blake, 2008). Reduced mobility after stroke may cause a reduction in muscle mass and strength, further affecting mobility and function. It would appear that attaining appropriate physical activity levels after a stroke or TIA may help prevent this detraining spiral, secondary health problems including falls and fractures (Carin-Levy et al., 2006) and improve wellbeing.

Researchers have explored different approaches to enhance physical activity but exercise programmes for secondary prevention of cerebrovascular events or disease modification are not well-established within clinical practice (Lennon et al., 2008). Attaining physical activity levels that are high enough to benefit health and wellbeing is a constant challenge, particularly in neurological populations where minimal levels for health have not been established. Good physical activity participation has been observed in community circuits in younger stroke victims (Stibrant Sunnerhagen, 2007) and in a group of older adults, including stroke victims when a community based physical activity programme was combined with a self efficacy enhancing support system (Resnick, Luisi, & Vogel, 2008). However the increased physical activity levels did not transfer to improved physical functioning, health and wellbeing (Resnick, Luisi, & Vogel, 2008). This work highlights the importance of establishing minimal activity and exercise dose responses for health and wellbeing benefits in these clinical groups in order to offer clear guidance for people following a stroke or TIA.

The benefit of short term rehabilitation and a range of different exercise interventions (aerobic training, motor relearning, strengthening, balance, jumping) have been extensively explored, particularly when evaluating functional effects (Dawes 2008b; Eser, Yavuzer, Karakus, & Karaoglan, 2008; Macko et al., 2005; van de Port, Wood-Dauphinee, Lindeman, & Kwakkel, 2007). Generally training specific tasks has been shown to most benefit the task trained (van de Port et al., 2007). There is evidence for a range of endurance and strengthening activities benefiting functional performance (Ada, Dorsch, & Canning, 2006; Pang, Eng, Dawson, & Gylfadottir, 2006) with programmes that combine both elements suggested to better prepare people for everyday activities and so offer greater functional benefit (M. J. Lee et al., 2008). Different delivery approaches have also been explored ranging from medical, community to home environments. Intensive rehabilitation delivered to patients with chronic stroke have been shown to improve physical and social function as well as reduce disability (Aprile et al., 2008). Outpatient supervised exercise training program after a minor ischemic stroke has been shown to be feasible, well tolerated and to improve exercise capacity (Tanne et al., 2008). Simple community delivered exercise interventions, such as circuits, have also been shown to improve mobility following stroke (Sherrington et al., 2008).

Maintaining physical activity over the longer term when intensive support is not viable is harder. In a trial of therapeutic exercise, effects were observed in both health and wellbeing, but these had reduced six months after completing the supported intervention (Studenski et al., 2005). Repeated cycles of treatment have been shown to be a means of helping to maintain activity levels and improvements reached within rehabilitation over the longer term (Aprile et al., 2008; Studenski et al., 2005). An approach that combines group and home programmes may incorporate the best of both systems and offer both social and practical benefits and thus provide the potential for longer term integration of physical activity into peoples' lives. This form of approach has been shown to improve gait, balance, basic activities of daily living, mood and quality of life in the short term (Macko et al., 2008). Another approach to promote continued exercise may be to provide additional counseling (van der Ploeg et al., 2007a) or other psychological interventions to boost self efficacy for being active (Shaughnessy et al., 2006). Gender differences may in turn affect the approach, since within a small study, women following stroke were observed to adhere better to supervised and men to unsupervised programmes (Olney et al., 2006). Psychological support can be provided within a clinical or a community setting (Tanne et al., 2008; van der Ploeg et al., 2007a).

Interventions specifically aimed at improving community mobility, that could potentially attain ongoing physical activity, have attained some success in increasing activity in the shorter term although carry over to changes in quality of life was not investigated in this study (Lord, McPherson, McNaughton, Rochester, & Weatherall, 2008). Home-based walking, whilst not suitable for all, has been proposed as a cheap, effective and feasible method to improve physical fitness and quality of life (QoL) among community living people (Okamoto, Nakatani, Morita, Saeki, & Kurumatani, 2007; Pohl et al., 2007; Rosie & Taylor, 2007). An interesting study comparing structured exercise with self initiated exercise observed much greater improvements in health related quality of life in the longer term in people who were in the self initiated exercise group (Langhammer et al., 2008). These findings support the importance of an individualized self directed approach for attaining longer term physical activity.

It is apparent that there is much work to be done in this area but the initial indicators are positive. Physical ability and participation levels do relate to a higher quality of life (Hudson et al., 2008; Naess, Beiske, & Myhr, 2008). As such, participation in regular physical activity appears to provide functional, health and wellbeing benefits following a stroke. Following a stroke, we know that a wide range of physical activities can benefit function (Eser et al., 2008) even in the elderly (Rosie & Taylor, 2007) . We know that a minimal dose of at least 16-hours therapy treatment time have to be attained for greater functional recovery to be observed than that expected from the passing of time alone (Kwakkel et al., 2004). Whilst lower intensity exercise appears to be of benefit (Cramp, Greenwood, Gill, Rothwell, & Scott, 2006), there is also a suggestion that interventions set at a higher intensity may be more effective at improving lower limb (Sullivan, Knowlton, & Dobkin, 2002; Wing, Lynskey, & Bosch, 2008) and upper limb function (Patten, Dozono, Schmidt, Jue, & Lum, 2006). However, the research evidence is limited and as yet there is no evidence as to the minimal or optimal setting, delivery, approach and content for health and wellbeing following a stroke or TIA. We do not know what dose of physical activity should be encouraged or what is the minimal dose and dose response (frequency, intensity, duration). Contrary to current thinking that aerobic exercise, five times a week is optimal, it may be that a single session of exercise is enough, or that short hard anaerobic (strengthening) sessions or a combination of both aerobic and anaerobic programmes are better when aiming for health and wellbeing.

Overwhelming evidence would suggest that training specific functional tasks will impact most on performance of the task trained, but for longer term participation and health and wellbeing benefits the selection of the mode of activity delivery is more complex. There is much we do not know when considering how best to attain long term successful integration of physical activity into the lives of people with cerebrovascular disease who present with a wide range of abilities. But the possible human, societal and economic benefits to be attained from regular participation, considered alongside the substantial barriers to continued participation in regular activity for people following stroke, endorse the need for the development of an evidence base for physical activity guidelines for stroke and TIA. Such guidelines for success would then need to be supported by structured governmental policy (Stuart, Chard, & Roettger, 2008).

Summary

- Physical activity appears to improve function, health and wellbeing and reduce the likelihood of secondary disease and cerebrovascular events.
- The minimal and optimal dose (frequency, duration and intensity) of physical activity for health and wellbeing are not known.
- Endurance, strengthening and balance training appear to benefit individuals following a stroke, but the optimal content of sessions is not known.
- The optimal mode (individual, group, disease specific, community or home) of delivery for health and wellbeing is not known.
- The optimal approach for different disability/ability levels is not known.
- Attainment of appropriate physical activity may require support for long-term successful integration within everyday lives.
- Ongoing injections of support may offer additional benefit but self directed exercise would appear to attain better long-term participation and health related quality of life.

PARKINSON'S DISEASE

Parkinson's disease (PD), named after Dr James Parkinson (1755–1824), is a progressive condition affecting the nervous system (Fuller, 2005; Turner, 2006). Parkinson's disease is a neurodegenerative disorder seriously affecting the physical, psychological, social, and functional status of individuals (Goodwin, Richards, Taylor, Taylor, & Campbell, 2008). Usually symptoms affecting walking, talking and writing first appear after the age of 50, although UK figures show that one in 20 of people diagnosed will be aged under 40(http://www.parkinsons.org.uk). Prevalence increases with age, affecting 0.3 percent of the 55–64 age group, 10 percent of the 65–74 age group, 3.1 percent of the 75–84 age group, and 4.3 percent of the 85–94 age and is greater in males (http://www.parkinsons.org.uk). Parkinson's disease occurs when neurons in the substantia nigra of the basal ganglia die or become impaired (Fuller, 2005). Normally, these cells produce dopamine, a neurotransmitter that signals to the striatum within the basal ganglia (Fuller, 2005) . When 60–80 percent of these dopamine-producing cells are lost, symptoms develop (Grillner, Helligren, Menard, Saitoh, & Wikstrom, 2005).

The reason why the loss of dopamine occurs in the brains of people with Parkinson's is currently unknown, although possible causes include both genetic and environmental factors. At present there is no cure for Parkinson's, but there are a range of treatments available to help control the symptoms and maintain quality of life for people with the condition. Approaches include: drug treatments such as Levodopa, often in combination with other medications, surgery such as deep brain stimulation of the thalamus, globus pallidus or subthalamic nucleus, and rarely lesioning of cells in the thalamus or globus pallidus.

PD is often classified by Hoehn and Yahr Staging (Goetz et al., 2004) to give an indication of functional ability.

- Stage One
  - Signs and symptoms on one side only
  - Symptoms mild
  - Symptoms inconvenient but not disabling
  - Usually presents with tremor of one limb
  - Friends have noticed changes in posture, locomotion and facial expression
- Stage Two
  - Symptoms are bilateral
  - Minimal disability
  - Posture and gait affected
- Stage Three
  - Significant slowing of body movements
  - Early impairment of equilibrium on walking or standing
  - Generalized dysfunction that is moderately severe
- Stage Four
  - Severe symptoms
  - Can still walk to a limited extent
  - Rigidity and bradykinesia
  - No longer able to live alone
  - Tremor may be less than earlier stages
- Stage Five
  - Cachectic stage
  - Invalidism complete
  - Cannot stand or walk
  - Requires constant nursing care

The more complicated Unified Parkinson's Disease Rating Scale, a more sensitive measure, may also be used (Martinez-Martin et al., 1994) by clinicians to grade disease progression.

PARKINSON'S DISEASE PREVENTION

Although environmental factors are suggested with PD, no strong link has been formed in the primary prevention or cause of physical activity in relation to PD (Logroscino, Sesso, Paffenbarger, & Lee, 2006). It has been suggested that higher levels of physical activity (jogging/running, lap swimming, tennis/racquetball, bicycling/stationary bike, aerobics/calisthenics) could be instrumental in lowering the risk of PD (Radak, Chung, & Goto, 2008; Thacker et al., 2008) and in PD men specifically (Chen, Zhang, Schwarzschild, Hernan, & Ascherio, 2005). Certainly people associated with low activity levels such as those with type 2 diabetes have a higher risk of developing PD (Hu et al., 2007b). It has been posited that men predisposed to PD are those who perform less strenuous physical activity in their early adult years (Chen et al., 2005). High total cholesterol has also been associated with PD (Hu, Antikainen, Jousilahti, Kivipelto, Tuomilehto, 2008) although the possibility that cholesterol levels may simply reflect low physical activity levels has not been investigated.

Summary

- A weak relationship has been proposed between low physical activity and the occurrence of PD with a suggestion that vigorous exercise may be more protective than moderate exercise. (Radak et al., 2008; Thacker et al., 2008)

PARKINSON'S DISEASE : SECONDARY PREVENTION, HEALTH AND WELLBEING

People with PD present with a range of physical, psychological, social, and functional symptoms (Goodwin et al., 2008). Severity of PD, self-reported mood symptoms and postural and gait impairments have been associated with poorer quality of life (QoL) in people with PD (Hirayama, Gobbi, Gobbi, & Stella, 2008;

Muslimovic, Post, Speelman, Schmand, & de Haan, 2008) as have gender with females reporting lower QoL (Zhao et al., 2008). The effect of symptoms on quality of life would appear to be stronger in transitional phases from mild to moderate and moderate to advanced stages of the disease (Hirayama et al., 2008). Physical activity interventions that aim to improve function and mobility would logically appear to be an appropriate part of therapeutic approaches to improve quality of life. Certainly physical therapy has long been considered alongside medication (Paciaroni & Raspa, 1970) as part of the therapeutic approach for people with PD (Bilowit, 1956). Although early therapeutic exercise was suggested over 20 years ago (Schenkman et al., 1989), individuals when receiving a diagnosis of PD may not all be routinely referred for therapy within clinical practice.

People with PD appear to be less active than their healthy counterparts (Hale et al., 2008). Indeed metabolic muscle changes indicative of reduced activity levels, muscle endurance and aerobic capacity have been described (Landin Hagenfeldt, Saltin, & Wahren, 1974; Saltin & Landin, 1975). When physical activity levels were observed longitudinally in 32 people with PD compared with age matched healthy controls at first diagnosis, people with PD did not differ from controls. As the disease progressed, physical activity levels declined in the PD group (Fertl, Doppelbauer, & Auff, 1993). When considering the most popular activities, swimming, hiking and gym based exercises were favoured (Fertl et al., 1993). Interestingly, when interviewed, participants expressed concern in the difficulty they found in learning new physical activities (Fertl et al., 1993). PD patients with more severe fatigue may be more sedentary and have poorer functional capacity and physical function compared with patients with less fatigue (Garber & Friedman, 2003) although results are conflicting (Hoff, Van Hilten, Middelkoop, & Roos, 1997). When considering activity and exercise, care should be taken to ensure participants can safely participate. In a study examining stress testing in people with PD, one third were observed to need cardiac evaluation prior to safe participation (Skidmore, Patterson, Shulman, Sorkin, & Macko, 2008). Further considerations are the timing of exercise in relation to medication (Muller & Muhlack, 2008). Certainly fear of ensuring that medication levels will be adequate throughout, has been highlighted as a factor that people with PD consider carefully prior to participation in physical activities (Elsworth et al., 2009).

General exercise and therapeutic exercise interventions have been shown to be well tolerated (Bloomer et al., 2008), benefit functional performance for people with PD (Crizzle & Newhouse 2006; Palmer, Mortimer, Webster, Bistevins, & Dickinson, 1986) and possibly reduce falls risk (Ashburn et al., 2007).

Certainly it appears exercise therapy may benefit the health (Kamide, Fukuda, & Miura, 2008) and function (Ellis et al., 2005; Smidt, de Vet, Bouter, & Dekker, 2005) of people with mild-to-moderate Parkinson's disease. Early exercise interventions have been shown to benefit function (Fisher et al., 2008), whilst interventions delivered in later stages of the condition within the home by nursing staff have been shown to benefit health (Hurwitz, 1989). Physical activity participation has also been shown to benefit quality of life, in people with Parkinson's disease at light to moderate stages resulting in improvements in their perception of QoL, mainly in social interaction and physical activity domains. In a recent systematic review, which included fourteen randomised controlled trials, evidence supported exercise as benefiting physical functioning, health-related quality of life, strength, balance and gait speed for people with PD (Goodwin et al., 2008). The health and wellbeing benefits of physical activity in people with PD are generally less researched, but provisional studies look promising.

The choice of venue for exercise delivery for people with PD can vary from home (Hurwitz, 1989), to medical (Morris, Iansek, & Kirkwood, 2008) and community environments, but exercise can effectively be delivered in the community (Lun, Pullan, Labelle, Adams, & Suchowersky, 2005) early or late in relation to diagnosis (Van Oteghen, 1987), individually, or within groups (Minnigh, 1971). Strategies to encourage long term physical activity participation need to be explored for people with PD, but evidence from other neurological conditions of a sustainable affordable approach would support community settings. From focus group work we observed that more impaired individuals stated a preference for home delivery but that other populations were content with various community venues (Elsworth et al., 2009b).

Consideration of the content of therapy is important, as not all interventions have been shown to be effective (Pedersen, Oberg, Insulander, & Vretman, 1990). We know that in order to best benefit a functional task, training at that task should give the greatest effect and that combined approaches (utilising a range of techniques) may be effective (Hirsch, Toole, Maitland, & Rider, 2003). In PD it would appear that cued task-specific training may attain a greater effect than task training alone (Mak & Hui-Chan, 2008). People with PD may have difficulty in learning new physical activities (Fertl et al., 1993) and so encouraging activities already or previously engaged in may be preferable. People with PD have been observed to co-activate muscles particularly when weakness is present in the lower limb (Busse et al 2006b). Thus it would appear that strength training would appear to be both enjoyable (O'Brien, Dodd, & Bilney, 2008) and to benefit function in people with PD (Falvo, Schilling, & Earhart, 2008).

Aerobic training has been shown to improve mobility but the effect on self-sufficiency or quality of life has been shown to vary (Burini et al., 2006; Morris et al., 2008).

When considering dose, the evidence of direct comparison of different exercise doses is limited, but higher intensity exercise in the early stages of PD (within three years of diagnosis) may be better (Fisher et al., 2008). The findings suggest the dose-dependent benefits of exercise and that high-intensity exercise can normalize corticomotor excitability in early PD (Fisher et al., 2008). However, minimal and dose response (intensity, frequency, duration) to exercise interventions at different stages of the disease has not been investigated. As with other neurological conditions, to date, research has not been able to sensitively describe the exercise dose (amount) and often studies ascertaining the effect of vigorous compared to moderate exercise is based on self report measures rather than being carefully controlled. As such, there is a need at this time to cautiously interpret findings.

Summary

- The results of the present research synthesis support the hypothesis that patients with PD improve their physical performance and activities of daily living through participation in exercise (Crizzle & Newhouse 2006; Reuter, Engelhardt, Stecker, & Baas, 1999).
- Although less clearly described, physical activity would appear to benefit health and wellbeing.
- The optimal delivery, content, mode and dose of physical activity interventions has not been well described.
- There is also a need for longer term studies (over 1 year) to assess if improvements achieved during interventions are retained in the long term (Crizzle & Newhouse 2006).

MULTIPLE SCLEROSIS

Multiple sclerosis (MS) is a complex disease of the central nervous system (Coyle, 2000; Fuller, 2005). It can be characterised by its course (Coyle, 2000; Ebers, 2001; Fuller, 2005). Benign MS is characterized by mild intermittent relapses with nearly complete resolution(Ebers, 2001). Secondary progressive MS starts with a relapsing–remitting course, with symptoms becoming more severe with less complete recovery of function after each exacerbation (Ebers, 2001) . Patients may then enter a chronic progressive phase, characterized by a step-like downhill course. MS that begins with a slow progression of signs and symptoms is classified as "primary progressive MS" (Ebers, 2001). MS is thought to be an "immune-mediated" inflammatory disease (Coyle, 2000; DeLegge & Smoke, 2008). MS is a chronic demyelinating disorder in which axon insulation, myelin, is lost from nerves in the central nervous system (CNS). The disease may affect various parts of the CNS, including the spinal cord, brainstem, cerebellum, cerebrum and optical nerves, but not peripheral nerves (Thompson, 2001; Fuller, 2005; Turner, 2006). Although the aetiology is unknown, an abnormal immune response against oligodendrocytes and myelin is believed to contribute to the disease. Lesions are scattered throughout the CNS white matter, with a loss of the myelin sheath, perivascular inflammation and relative sparing of the axons (Thompson, 2001; Fuller, 2005; Turner, 2006). The following symptoms have been suggested to affect more than 50% of patients: problems using legs, problems using arms, fatigue/lack of energy, spasms, pain, and feeling sleepy (Higginson, Hart, Silber, Burman, & Edmonds, 2006). Recovery from symptoms during remissions has been suggested to mainly be due to the restoration of axonal function, either by remyelination, resolution of inflammation, or paradoxical restoration of conduction to axons that persist in the demyelinated state (Thompson, 2001).

MS is progressive, characterized by exacerbations and remissions. Nerve conduction alters with variations in sclerosis and inflammation. Symptoms and the rate of progression of the disease differ between people. At times there may be a plateau or slight improvement in symptoms due to reduction of inflammation, whereas at other times a sudden deterioration may occur due to rapid demyelination.

MULTIPLE SCLEROSIS: PREVENTION

The role of environmental factors such as physical activity has not been strongly implicated as a possible cause or preventative measure for multiple sclerosis. However exercise exposure has been suggested as a model to enhance stress resistance and support neuronal survival under heightened stress conditions by upregulating anti-oxidant defences and neurotrophic support that could attenuate CNS vulnerability to neuronal degeneration and reduce long-term disability for people with MS (White & Castellano, 2008a; 2008b).

Summary

- To date, there is no evidence for physical activity to be implicated as causative or preventative of MS

MULTIPLE SCLEROSIS: SECONDARY PREVENTION HEALTH AND WELLBEING

Many people with MS do not receive regular exercise or physical therapy and may have been advised in the past to be careful or avoid exercising in an effort to help minimise the risk of exacerbations and symptoms of fatigue (Solari et al., 1999). These factors, alongside other physical and environmental barriers, may be related to the low physical activity levels observed in people with MS (Ansved, 2003; Creange et al., 2007; Eagle, 2002; Philips & Mastaglia, 2000). Activity levels appear to be lower in people with more severe symptoms and in those with lower levels of exercise self efficacy (Motl et al., 2008c). The relationship between neurological symptoms and physical activity levels (Motl et al., 2008f) can also in part be explained by walking difficulty affecting ability to engage in exercise (Motl et al., 2008d).

A conceptual model has been proposed that connects exercise and brain health and suggests the benefit of physical activity participation for all (White & Castellano, 2008a). With axonal loss and cerebral atrophy occur early in MS, considering the possible link of exercise to both local and systemic alterations in cytokine production and immune function, exercise prescription is proposed to be particularly effective in the acute stages of the disease as a promoter of neuroprotection, neuroregeneration and neuroplasticity (White & Castellano, 2008a; 2008b). Physical activity may benefit health and wellbeing as it has also been shown to up-regulate hippocampal brain derived neurotrophin factor (BDNF), which may play a role in mood states, learning and memory and lessen the general decline in cognitive function associated with MS (White & Castellano, 2008a; 2008b).

Exercise (Khan, Pallant, Brand, & Kilpatrick, 2008) and therapy interventions (Rietberg, Brooks, Uitdehaag, & Kwakkel, 2005; Taylor, Dodd, Shields, & Bruder, 2007) improve disability levels. A Cochrane review of exercise therapy in general by Reitberg et al., (2005) found exercise therapy compared to no exercise therapy improved muscle strength, exercise tolerance and mobility-related activities, thus benefiting functional performance with no evidence of deleterious effects. Improvements have been attained in people with moderate (Kileff & Ashburn, 2005) and more severely affected individuals (van den Berg, Newman, Dawes, & Wade, 2005). The importance of physical activity for both functional benefit and social health has more recently been emphasized in this group (McDonald, 2002) with physical ability and participation having been observed to relate to perceived quality of life in people with MS (Hudson et al., 2008; Naess et al., 2008). Higher activity levels have been related to both physical and psychological related quality of life (Motl & Snook, 2008d), with activity levels possibly improving quality of life by influencing self efficacy (Motl & Snook, 2008d). Exercise training is associated with a small improvement in QoL among individuals with MS (Motl & Gosney, 2008b) that last beyond the intervention period (McCullagh, Fitzgerald, Murphy, & Cooke, 2008) with worsening of MS symptoms related to reductions in physical activity independently of condition deteriation (Motl et al., 2008d).

Short and long term therapy interventions may improve health for people with MS not experiencing an exacerbation (Romberg et al., 2004; van den Berg et al., 2006). Unfortunately fatigue and physical limitations may in themselves hinder exercise participation (Becker & Stuifbergen, 2004) as may psychological barriers (Morris, McAuley, & Motl., 2008). Physical activity programmes have been successfully delivered within the community, which offer a model for long-term integration into peoples' lives. Programmes that are enjoyable and promote confidence to exercise may be more effective (McAuley et al., 2007). Water based exercise is one such approach as it is known to be a preferred modality for people with MS (Elsworth et al, 2009b) and has been shown to benefit people with MS (Pariser, Madras, & Weiss, 2006).

When considering optimising functional performance the optimal content of fitness components has not been established. Balance training (Cattaneo, Jonsdottir, Zocchi, & Regola, 2007) strengthening (Gutierrez et al., 2005; Taylor, Dodd, Prasad, & Denisenko, 2006) stretching (Bovend'Eerdt et al., 2008) and aerobic/endurance training (Newman et al., 2007; Rampello et al., 2007) have all been shown to benefit function, but have not been directly compared. Whether endurance, strengthening, or functional training or a combination of these is optimal has not been established for functional, health and wellbeing benefits (Dalgas, Stenager, & Ingemann-Hansen, 2008; Rasova et al., 2006). However specific training benefits, such as aerobic training affecting fatigue and task training affecting function have been observed (Rasova et al., 2006), supporting the importance of investigating exercise content.

When considering dose, optimal or dose response has not yet been established for function, health and wellbeing in people with MS. Moderate intensity exercise has been shown to be of functional benefit (Bjarnadottir, Konradsdottir, Reynisdottir, & Olafsson, 2007) and with people with MS detrimentally affected by heat, sessions that lead to less heating are less stressful and enable participation in people with MS (Grahn, Murray, & Helle, 2008). However in other neurological conditions higher intensity sessions have been shown to be more effective (Dawes, in press).

Summary

- The results of the present research synthesis support the hypothesis that patients with MS improve their physical performance and activities of daily living through exercise.
- Less clearly described exercise would appear to benefit health and wellbeing.
- The optimal delivery, content, mode and dose of physical activity interventions has not been well described.
- There is also a need for longer term studies (over 1 year) to assess if improvements achieved during interventions are retained in the long term.

OVERALL CONCLUSION

For people with neurological conditions:

- Physical activity benefits brain and body health.
- Physical activity is likely to benefit function, wellbeing and health through underlying physiological, psychological and sociological effects.
- Participation in moderate intensity physical activities is associated with low risk and unlikely to do harm.
- The optimal or most effective setting, mode and format for delivery for health and wellbeing has not been established.
- The optimal or most effective content and dose of physical activity for health and wellbeing has not been established.
- The optimal or most effective timing and physical activity content for health and wellbeing for people at different stages of neurological conditions is not established.

Whilst there has as yet been limited research investigating participation in physical activity for health and wellbeing benefits in neurological conditions, it would appear that the being active offers benefits for many. There is much work to be done in this area and initial findings would indicate that governments may need to enforce policies that positively support activity in people with disabilities alongside those introduced for healthy populations. This chapter has covered specifically MS, PD, stroke and TIA but there is emerging evidence supporting exercise in a range of long-term neurological conditions. In summary the possible benefits of being active appear substantial, and to date there is no indication that attaining a level of moderate activity is harmful for people with neurological disease.

REFERENCES

ACSM (2003) .ACSM's Exercise Management for Persons with Chronic Diseases and Disabilities. Champaign, IL: Human Kinetics.

AGSPF. (2001) Guideline for the prevention of falls in older persons. *J Am Geriatr Soc, 49,* 664-72.

Ada, L., Dorsch, S., & Canning, C. G. (2006). Strengthening interventions increase strength and improve activity after stroke: a systematic review. *Australian Journal of Physiotherapy, 52,* 241-248.

Ansved, T. (2003). Muscular dystrophies: influence of physical conditioning on the disease evolution. *Current Opinion in Clinical Nutrition and Metabolic Care, 6,* 435-439.

Aprile, I., Di Stasio, E., Romitelli, F., Lancellotti, S., Caliandro, P., & Tonali, P., (2008). Effects of rehabilitation on quality of life in patients with chronic stroke. *Brain Injury, 22,* 451-456.

Ashburn, A., Fazakarley, L., Ballinger, C., Pickering, R., McLellan, L. D., & Fitton, C. (2007). A randomised controlled trial of a home based exercise programme to reduce the risk of falling among people with Parkinson's disease. *Journal of Neurology, Neurosurgery, and Psychiatry, 78,* 678-684.

Becker, H., & Stuifbergen, A. (2004). What makes it so hard? Barriers to health promotion experienced by people with multiple sclerosis and polio. *Family & Community Health, 27,* 75-85.

Bilowit, D. S. (1956). Establishing physical objectives in the rehabilitation of patients with Parkinson's disease; gymnasium activities. *Physical Therapy Review 36,* 176-178.

Bjarnadottir, O. H., Konradsdottir, A. D., Reynisdottir, K., & Olafsson, E. (2007) Multiple sclerosis and brief moderate exercise. A randomised study. *Multiple Sclerosis, 13,* 776-782.

Blonde, L., Dempster, J., Gallivan, J. M., & Warren-Boulton, E. (2006). Reducing cardiovascular disease risk in patients with diabetes: a message from the National Diabetes Education Program. *Journal of the American Academy of Nurse Practitioners, 18,* 524-533.

Bloomer, R. J., Schilling, B. K., Karlage, R. E., Ledoux, M. S., Pfeiffer, R. F., & Callegari, J. (2008). Effect of resistance training on blood oxidative stress in Parkinson disease. *Medicine and Science in Sports and Exercise, 40,* 1385-1389.

Bohannon, R. (2007). Number of pedometer-assessed steps taken per day by adults: a descriptive meta-analysis. *Physical Therapy, 87,* 1642-1650.

Borkoles E, Nicholls A., Bell, K., Butterly, R., Polman, R. (2008) The lived experiences of people diagnosed with multiple sclerosis in relation to exercise. *Psychology and Health, 23,* 427-441.

Bovend'Eerdt, T. J., Newman, M., Barker, K., Dawes, H., Minelli, C., & Wade, D. T. (2008). The effects of stretching in spasticity: A systematic review. *Archives of Physical Medicine and Rehabilitation, 89,* 1395-1406.

Bravata, D. M., Smith-Spangler, C., Sundaram, V., Gienger, A. L., Lin, N., Lewis, R., et al. (2007). Using pedometers to increase physical activity and improve health: a systematic review. *JAMA, 298,* 2296-2304.

Burini, D., Farabollini, B., Iacucci, S., Rimatori, C., Riccardi, G., & Capecci, M., et al. (2006). A randomised controlled cross-over trial of aerobic training versus Qigong in advanced Parkinson's disease. *Europa Medicophysica, 42,* 231-238.

Busse, M. E., Pearson, O. R., Van Deursen, R., & Wiles, C. M. (2004). Quantified measurement of activity provides insight into motor function and recovery in neurological disease. *Journal of Neurology Neurosurgery and Psychiatry, 75,* 884-888.

Busse, M. E, Wiles, C. M., & van Deursen, R. W. (2006a). Community walking activity in neurological disorders with leg weakness. *Journal of Neurology and Neurosurgery Psychiatry, 77,* 359-362.

Busse, M. E., Wiles, C. M., & van Deursen, R. W. (2006b). Co-activation: its association with weakness and specific neurological pathology. *Journal of Neuroengineering and Rehabilitation, 3,* 26.

Carin-Levy, G., Greig, C., Young, A., Lewis, S, Hannan, J., & Mead, G. (2006). Longitudinal changes in muscle strength and mass after acute stroke. *Cerebrovascular Diseases, 21,* 201-207.

Cattaneo, D., Jonsdottir, J., Zocchi, M., & Regola, A. (2007). Effects of balance exercises on people with multiple sclerosis: a pilot study. *Clinical Rehabilitation, 21,* 771-781.

Chen, H., Zhang, S. M., Schwarzschild, M. A., Hernan, M. A., & Ascherio, A. (2005). Physical activity and the risk of Parkinson disease. *Neurology, 64,* 664-9.

Cohen-Mansfield, J., Marx, M. S., Guralnik, J. M. (2006). Comparison of exercise models in an elderly population. *Aging Clinical and Experimental Research,18,* 312-319.

Colombo, R., Pisano, F., Mazzone, A., Delconte, C., Micera, S., Carrozza, M. C., et al. (2007). Design strategies to improve patient motivation during robot-aided rehabilitation. *Journal of Neuroengineering and Rehabilitation, 4,* 3.

Cotman, C. W., Berchtold, N. C., & Christie, L. A. (2007). Exercise builds brain health: key roles of growth factor cascades and inflammation. *Trends in Neuroscience, 30,* 464-472.

Coyle, P. (2000). Diagnosis and classification of inflammatory demyelinating disorders. In J. Burks, & K. Johnson (eds.) *Multiple Sclerosis Diagnosis, Medical Management, and Rehabilitation* (pp. 81-98). New York: Demos.

Cramp, M. C., Greenwood, R. J., Gill, M., Rothwell, J. C., & Scott, O. M. (2006). Low intensity strength training for ambulatory stroke patients. *Disability and Rehabilitation, 28,* 883-889.

Creange, A., Serre, I., Levasseur, M., Audry, D., Nineb, A., Boerio, D., et al. (2007). Walking capacities in multiple sclerosis measured by global positioning system odometer. *Multiple Sclerosis, 13,* 220-223.

Crizzle, A. M., & Newhouse, I. J. (2006). Is physical exercise beneficial for persons with Parkinson's disease? *Clinical Journal of Sport Medicine, 16,* 422-425.

Dalgas, U., Stenager, E., & Ingemann-Hansen, T. (2008). Multiple sclerosis and physical exercise: recommendations for the application of resistance-, endurance- and combined training. *Multiple Sclerosis, 14,* 35-53.

Dawes, H. (2008a). Exercise in Neurological Populations. In J. P. Buckley (ed.), *Exercise Physiology in Special Populations: Advances in Sport and Exercise Science.* Oxford: Elsevier 269-308.

Dawes, H. (2008b). The role of exercise in rehabilitation. *Clinical Rehabilitation, 22,* 67-70.

Dawes, H. Bateman, A., Culpan, J., Scott, O. M., Roach, N. K. & Wade, D. (2003). Heart rate as a measure of exercise testing early after acquired brain injury. *Physiotherapy, 89,* 10-15.

Dawes, H., Enzinger, C., Johansen-Berg, H., Bogdanovic, M., Guy, C., Collett, J., et al. (2007) Walking performance and its recovery in chronic stroke in relation to extent of lesion overlap with the descending motor tract. *Experimental Brain Research, 186,* 325-333.

Dawes, H., Korpershoek, N., Freebody, J., Elsworth, C., van Tintelen, N., & Wade, D. T., et al. (2006). A pilot randomised controlled trial of a home-based exercise programme aimed at improving endurance and function in adults with neuromuscular disorders. *Journal of Neurology, Neurosurgery, and Psychiatry 77,* 959-962.

Dawes, H., et al. (2006) Exertional symptoms and exercise capacity in individuals with brain injury. Disabil Rehabil 28, 1243-1250

Dawes, H., Roach, N., Wade, D., & Scott, O. M. (1999) Measurement of exercise motives after brain injury. *Journal of Sports Science, 17,* 27-28.

DeLegge, M. H., & Smoke, A. (2008). Neurodegeneration and inflammation. *Nutrition in Clinical Practice, 23,* 35-41.

Department of Health (2004a). At least five a week. Evidence on the impact of physical activity and its relationship to health. UK: Department of Health, Health Improvement and Prevention.

Department of Health (2004b). Physical Activity, Health Improvement and Prevention At least five a week: evidence on the impact of physical activity and its relationship to health. UK: Department of Health

Department of Health (2007). *National Stroke Strategy.* London: Central Office of Information

Dishman, R. K. (1988). *Exercise adherence: its impact on public· health.* Leeds: Human Kinetics Publishers.

Eagle, M. (2002). Report on the muscular dystrophy campaign workshop: Exercise in neuromuscular diseases Newcastle, January 2002. *Neuromuscular Disorders, 12,* 975-983.

Ebers, G. C. (2001). Natural history of multiple sclerosis. *Journal of Neurology Neurosurgery and Psychiatry, 71,* II16-II19.

Ellis, T., de Goede, C. J., Feldman, R. G., Wolters, E. C., Kwakkel, G., & Wagenaar, R. C. (2005). Efficacy of a physical therapy program in patients with Parkinson's disease: A randomized controlled trial. *Archives of Physical Medicine and Rehabilitation, 86,* 626-632.

Elsworth, C., Dawes, H., Winward, C., Howells, K., Collett, J., Dennis, A., et al. (2009a). Pedometer step counts in individuals with neurological conditions. *Clinical Rehabilitation*

Elsworth, C., Dawes, H., Sackley, C., Soundy, A., Howells, K., Wade, D., et al. (2009b) A study of perceived facilitators to physical activity in neurological conditions. *International Journal of Therapy and Rehabilitation, 16,* 17-24.

Elsworth, C., Dawes, H., Sackley, C., Soundy, A., Howells, K., Wade, D. et al. (in press) Perceived facilitators to physical activity in individuals with progressive neurological conditions; a focus group and questionnaire study. *Journal of Sport Sciences.*

Elsworth, C., Patel, S., Meek, C., Sackley, C., & Dawes, H. (in Press). Long Term individual fitness enablement intervention for people with Multiple sclerosis. *Clinical Rehabilitation conference proceedings.*

Eser, F., Yavuzer, G., Karakus, D., & Karaoglan, B. (2008). The effect of balance training on motor recovery and ambulation after stroke: a randomized controlled trial. *European Journal of Physical Rehabilitation Medicine, 44,* 19-25.

Falvo, M. J., Schilling, B. K., & Earhart, G. M. (2008). Parkinson's disease and resistive exercise: rationale, review, and recommendations. *Movement Disorders, 23,* 1-11.

Fertl, E., Doppelbauer, A., & Auff, E. (1993). Physical activity and sports in patients suffering from Parkinson's disease in comparison with healthy seniors. *Journal of Neural Transmission: Parkinson's Disease and Dementia Section, 5,* 157-61.

Fisher, B. E., Wu, A. D., Salem, G. J., Song, J., Lin, C. H., Yip, J., et al. (2008) The Effect of Exercise Training in Improving Motor Performance and Corticomotor Excitability in People With Early Parkinson's Disease. *Archives of Physical Medicine and Rehabilitation, 7,* 1221-1229.

Froehlich-Grobe, K., & White, G. W (2004). Promoting physical activity among women with mobility impairments: A Randomized controlled trial to assess a home- and community-based intervention. *Archives of Physical Medicine and Rehabilitation 85,* 640-648.

Fuller, G. (2005). *Neurology: An Illustrated Colour Text.* Oxford: Elsevier Health Sciences.

Garber, C. E., & Friedman, J. H. (2003). Effects of fatigue on physical activity and function in patients with Parkinson's disease. *Neurology, 60,* 1119-1124.

Goetz, C. G., Poewe, W., Rascol, O., Sampaio, C., Stebbins, G. T., Counsell, C., et al. (2004). Movement Disorder Society Task Force report on the Hoehn and Yahr staging scale: status and recommendations. *Movement Disorders, 19,* 1020-1028.

Goodwin, V. A., Richards, S. H., Taylor, R. S., Taylor, A. H., & Campbell, J. L. (2008). The effectiveness of exercise interventions for people with

Parkinson's disease: a systematic review and meta-analysis. *Movement Disorders, 23,* 631-640.

Gordon, N. F., Gulanick, M., Costa, F., Fletcher, G., Franklin, B. A., Roth, E. J., et al. (2004). Physical activity and exercise recommendations for stroke survivors - An American Heart Association scientific statement from the Council on Clinical Cardiology, Subcommittee on Exercise, Cardiac Rehabilitation, and Prevention; the Council on Cardiovascular Nursing; the Council on Nutrition, Physical Activity, and Metabolism; and the Stroke Council. *Stroke, 35,* 1230-1240.

Grahn, D. A., Murray, J. V., & Heller, H. C. (2008). Cooling via one hand improves physical performance in heat-sensitive individuals with multiple sclerosis: a preliminary study. *BMC Neurology, 8,* 14.

Grillner, S., Helligren, J., Menard, A., Saitoh, K., & Wikstrom, M. A. (2005). Mechanisms for selection of basic motor programs - roles for the striatum and pallidum. *Trends in Neurosciences, 28,* 364-370.

Gutierrez, G. M., Chow, J. W., Tillman, M. D., McCoy, S. C., Castellano, V., & White, L. J. (2005). Resistance training improves gait kinematics in persons with multiple sclerosis. *Archives of Physical Medicine and Rehabilitation, 86,* 1824-1829.

Hale, L. A., Pal, J., & Becker, I. (2008). Measuring free-living physical activity in adults with and without neurologic dysfunction with a triaxial accelerometer. *Archives of Physical Medicine and Rehabilitation, 89,* 1765-1771.

Higginson, I. J., Hart, S., Silber, E., Burman, R., & Edmonds, P. (2006). Symptom prevalence and severity in people severely affected by multiple sclerosis. *Journal of Palliative Care, 22,* 158-165.

Hirayama, M. S., Gobbi, S., Gobbi, L. T., & Stella, F. (2008). Quality of life (QoL) in relation to disease severity in Brazilian Parkinson's patients as measured using the WHOQOL-BREF. *Archives of Gerontology and Geriatrics, 46,* 147-160.

Hirsch, M. A., Toole, T., Maitland, C. G., & Rider, R. A. (2003). The effects of balance training and high-intensity resistance training on persons with idiopathic Parkinson's disease. *Archives of Physical Medicine and Rehabilitation, 84,* 1109-1117.

Hoff, J. I., Van Hilten, J. J., Middelkoop, H. A., & Roos, R. A. (1997). Fatigue in Parkinson's disease is not associated with reduced physical activity. *Parkinsonism & Related Disorder, 3,* 51-54.

Hu, G., Antikainen, R., Jousilahti, P., Kivipelto, M., & Tuomilehto, J. (2008). Total cholesterol and the risk of Parkinson disease. *Neurology, 70,* 1972-1979.

Hu, G., Jousilahti, P., Antikainen, R., & Tuomilehto, J. (2007a). Occupational, commuting, and leisure-time physical activity in relation to cardiovascular mortality among finnish subjects with hypertension. *American Journal of Hypertension, 20,* 1242-1250.

Hu, G., Jousilahti, P., Bidel, S., Antikainen, R., & Tuomilehto, J. (2007b). Type 2 diabetes and the risk of Parkinson's disease. *Diabetes Care, 30,* 842-847.

Hudson, M., Thombs, B. D., Steele, R., Watterson, R., Taillefer, S., & Baron, M. (2008). Clinical correlates of quality of life in systemic sclerosis measured with the World Health Organization Disability Assessment Schedule II. *Arthritis & Rheumatism, 59,* 279-84.

Hurwitz, A. (1989). The benefit of a home exercise regimen for ambulatory Parkinson's disease patients. *Journal of Neuroscience Nursing, 21,* 180-184.

Hyndman, D., Ashburn, A., & Stack, E. (2002). Fall events among people with stroke living in the community: Circumstances of falls and characteristics of fallers. *Archives of Physical Medicine and Rehabilitation, 83,* 165-170.

Jette, D. U. Latham, N. K., Smout, R .J., Gassaway, J., Slavin, M. D., & Horn, S. D. (2005). Physical therapy interventions for patients with stroke in inpatient rehabilitation facilities. *Physical Therapy, 85,* 238-248.

Jorgensen, H. S., Nakayama, H., Raaschou, H. O., & Olsen, T. S. (1995). Recovery of walking function in stroke patients: the Copenhagen Stroke Study. *Archives of Physical Medicine & Rehabilitation, 76,* 27-32.

Kamide, N., Fukuda, M., Miura, H. (2008). The relationship between bone density and the physical performance of ambulatory patients with Parkinson's disease. *Journal of Physiological Anthropology, 27,* 7-10.

Karmisholt, K., & Gotzcshe, P. C. (2005). Physical activity for secondary prevention of disease - Systematic reviews of randomised clinical trials. *Danish Medical Bulletin, 52,* 90-94.

Khan, F., Pallant, J. F., Brand, C., & Kilpatrick, T. J. (2008). Effectiveness of rehabilitation intervention in persons with multiple sclerosis: a randomised controlled trial. *Journal of Neurology, Neurosurgery, and Psychiatry, 79,* 1230-1235.

Kileff, J., & Ashburn, A. (2005). A pilot study of the effect of aerobic exercise on people with moderate disability multiple sclerosis. *Clinical Rehabilitation, 19,* 165-169.

Kozakova, M., Palombo, C., Mhamdi, L., Konrad, T., Nilsson, P., Staehr, P. B., et al. (2007). Habitual physical activity and vascular aging in a young to middle-age population at low cardiovascular risk. *Stroke ,38,* 2549-2555.

Kwakkel, G., van Peppen, R., Wagenaar, R. C., Dauphinee, S. W., Richards, C., Ashburn, A., et al. (2004). Effects of augmented exercise therapy time after stroke - A meta-analysis. *Stroke, 35,* 2529-2536.

Landin, S., Hagenfeldt, L., Saltin, B., & Wahren, J. (1974). Muscle metabolism during exercise in patients with Parkinson's disease. *Clinical Science and Molecular Medicine, 47,* 493-506.

Langhammer, B., Stanghelle, J. K., & Lindmark, B. (2008). Exercise and health-related quality of life during the first year following acute stroke. A randomized controlled trial. *Brain Injury, 22,* 135-145.

Lee, C. D., Folsom, A. R., & Blair, S. N. (2003). Physical activity and stroke risk - A meta-analysis. *Stroke, 34,* 2475-2481.

Lee, M. J., Kilbreath, S. L., Singh, M. F., Zeman, B., Lord, S. R., Raymond, J., et al. (2008). Comparison of effect of aerobic cycle training and progressive resistance training on walking ability after stroke: a randomized sham exercise-controlled study. *Journal of American Geriatrics Society, 56,* 976-985.

Lennon, O., Carey, A., Gaffney, N., Stephenson, J., & Blake, C. (2008). A pilot randomized controlled trial to evaluate the benefit of the cardiac rehabilitation paradigm for the non-acute ischaemic stroke population. *Clinical Rehabilitation, 22,* 125-133.

Logroscino, G., Sesso, H. D., Paffenbarger, R. S. Jr., & Lee, I. M. (2006). Physical activity and risk of Parkinson's disease: a prospective cohort study. *Journal of Neurology, Neurosurgery, and Psychiatry, 77,* 1318-1322.

Lord, S., McPherson, K. M., McNaughton, H. K., Rochester, L., & Weatherall, M. (2008). How feasible is the attainment of community ambulation after stroke? A pilot randomized controlled trial to evaluate community-based physiotherapy in subacute stroke. *Clinical Rehabilitation, 22,* 215-225.

Luk, J. K., Chiu, P. K., & Chu, L. W. (2008). Rehabilitation of older Chinese patients with different cognitive functions: How do they differ in outcome? *Archives of Physical Medicine and Rehabilitation, 89,* 1714-1719.

Lun, V., Pullan, N., Labelle, N., Adams, C., & Suchowersky, O. (2005). Comparison of the effects of a self-supervised home exercise program with a physiotherapist-supervised exercise program on the motor symptoms of Parkinson's disease. *Movement Disorders, 20,* 971-975.

Macko, R. F., Benvenuti, F., Stanhope, S., Macellari, V., Taviani, A., & Nesi, B., (2008). Adaptive physical activity improves mobility function and quality of life in chronic hemiparesis. *Journal of Rehabilitation Research and Development, 45,* 323-328.

Macko, R. F., Ivey, F. M., Forrester, L. W., Hanley, D., Sorkin, J. D., & Katzel, L. I., (2005). Treadmill exercise rehabilitation improves ambulatory function and cardiovascular fitness in patients with chronic stroke: a randomized, controlled trial. *Stroke, 36,* 2206-2211.

Mak, M. K., & Hui-Chan, C. W. (2008). Cued task-specific training is better than exercise in improving sit-to-stand in patients with Parkinson's disease: A randomized controlled trial. *Movement Disorders, 23,* 501-509.

Martinez-Martin, P., Gil-Nagel, A., Gracia, L. M., Gomez, J. B., Martinez-Sarries, J., & Bermejo, F. (1994). Unified Parkinson's Disease Rating Scale characteristics and structure. The Cooperative Multicentric Group. *Movement Disorders, 9,* 76-83.

Mayo NE, Wood-Dauphinee S, Ahmed S, Gordon C, Higgins J, McEwen S, et al (1999). Disablement following stroke. Disability and Rehabilitation, 21,:258-68 99

McAuley E, Blissmer B (2000). Self-efficacy determinants and consequences of physical activity. *Exercises and Sport Sciences Reviews, 28,* 85-88.

McAuley, E., Motl, R. W., Morris, K. S., Hu, L., Doerksen, S. E., Elavsky, S. et al. (2007). Enhancing physical activity adherence and well-being in multiple sclerosis: a randomised controlled trial. *Multiple Sclerosis, 13,* 652-659.

McCullagh, R., Fitzgerald, A. P., Murphy, R. P., & Cooke, G. (2008). Long-term benefits of exercising on quality of life and fatigue in multiple sclerosis patients with mild disability: a pilot study. *Clinical Rehabilitation, 22,* 206-214.

McDonald, C. M. (2002). Physical activity, health impairments, and disability in neuromuscular disease. *American Journal Physical Medicine & Rehabilitation, 81,* S108-S120.

Michael, K. M., Allen, J. K., & Macko, R. F. (2005). Reduced ambulatory activity after stroke: The role of balance, gait, and cardiovascular fitness. *Archives of Physical Medicine and Rehabilitation, 86,* 1552-1556.

Minnigh, E. C. (1971). The changing picture of parkinsonism. II. The Northwestern University concept of rehabilitation through group physical therapy. *Rehabilitation Literature, 32,* 38-39 passim.

Morris, K. S., McAuley, E., & Motl, R. W. (2008). Self-efficacy and environmental correlates of physical activity among older women and women with multiple sclerosis. *Health Education Research, 23,* 744-752.

Morris, M. E., Iansek, R., & Kirkwood, B. (2008b). A randomized controlled trial of movement strategies compared with exercise for people with Parkinson's disease. *Movement Disorders, 24,* 64-71.

Motl, R.W. (2008a) Physical activity and its measurement and determinants in multiple sclerosis. Minerva Med 99, 157-165

Motl, R. W., & Gosney, J. L. (2008b). Effect of exercise training on quality of life in multiple sclerosis: a meta-analysis. *Multiple Sclerosis, 14,* 129-135.

Motl, R. W., & Snook, E. M. (2008c). Physical activity, self-efficacy, and quality of life in multiple sclerosis. *Annals of Behavorial Medicine, 35,* 111-115.

Motl, R. W., Arnett, P. A., Smith, M. M., Barwick, F. H., Ahlstrom, B., & Stover E. (2008d). Worsening of symptoms is associated with lower physical activity levels in individuals with Multiple Sclerosis. *Multiple Sclerosis, 14,* 140-142.

Motl, R. W., Snook, E. M., & Schapiro, R. T. (2008e). Symptoms and physical activity behavior in individuals with multiple sclerosis. *Research in Nursing & Health, 31,* 466-475.

Motl, R. W., Snook, E. M., Wynn, D. R., & Vollmer, T. (2008f). Physical activity correlates with neurological impairment and disability in multiple sclerosis. *Journal of Nervous and Mental Disease, 196,* 492-495.

Mudge, S., & Stott, N. S. (2008) Test-retest Reliability of the StepWatch Activity Monitor Outputs in Individuals with Chronic Stroke measure. *Clinical Rehabilitation, 22,* 871-877

Muller, T., & Muhlack, S. (2008). Impact of endurance exercise on levodopa-associated cortisol release and force increase in patients with Parkinson's disease. *Journal of Neural Transmission, 115,* 851-855.

Muren, M. A., Hutler, M., & Hooper, J. (2008). Functional capacity and health-related quality of life in individuals post stroke. *Topics in Stroke Rehabilitation, 15,* 51-58.

Muslimovic, D., Post, B., Speelman, J. D., Schmand, B., & de Haan, R. J. (2008). Determinants of disability and quality of life in mild to moderate Parkinson disease. *Neurology, 70,* 2241-2247.

Naess, H., Beiske, A. G., & Myhr, K. M. (2008). Quality of life among young patients with ischaemic stroke compared with patients with multiple sclerosis. *Acta Neurologica Scandinavica, 117,* 181-185.

Newman, M. A., Dawes, H., van den Berg, M., Wade, D. T., Burridge, J., & Izadi, H. (2007). Can aerobic treadmill training reduce the effort of walking and fatigue in people with multiple sclerosis: a pilot study. *Multiple Sclerosis, 13,* 113-119.

Ntoumanis, N., Edmunds, J., & Duda, J. L. (2008). Understanding the coping process from a self-determination theory perspective. *British Journal of Health Psychology, 14,* 249-260.

O'Brien, M., Dodd, K. J., & Bilney, B. (2008). A qualitative analysis of a progressive resistance exercise programme for people with Parkinson's disease. *Disability & Rehabilitation, 30,* 1350-1357.

O'Donovan, G., & Shave, R. (2007). British adults' views on the health benefits of moderate and vigorous activity. *Preventive Medicine, 45,* 432-435.

Okamoto, N., Nakatani, T., Morita, N., Saeki, K., & Kurumatani, N. (2007). Home-based walking improves cardiopulmonary function and health-related QOL in community-dwelling adults. *International Journal of Sports Medicine, 28,* 1040-1045.

Olney, S. J., Nymark, J., Brouwer, B., Culham, E., Day, A., Heard, J., et al. (2006). A randomized controlled trial of supervised versus unsupervised exercise programs for ambulatory stroke survivors. *Stroke, 37,* 476-481.

Paciaroni, E., & Raspa, E. G. (1970). Results of treatment with levodopa and rehabilitative therapy in 10 cases of Parkinson's disease. *Sistema Nervoso, 22,* 153-161.

Palmer, S. S., Mortimer, J. A., Webster, D. D., Bistevins, R., & Dickinson, G. L. (1986) Exercise therapy for Parkinson's disease. *Archives of Physical Medicine & Rehabilitation, 67,* 741-745.

Pang, M. Y. C., Eng, J. J., Dawson, A. S., & Gylfadottir, S. (2006), The use of aerobic exercise training in improving aerobic capacity in individuals with stroke: a meta-analysis. *Clinical Rehabilitation, 20,* 97-111.

Pariser, G., Madras, D., &Weiss, E. (2006). Outcomes of an aquatic exercise program including aerobic capacity, lactate threshold, and fatigue in two individuals with multiple sclerosis. *Journal of Neurologic Physical Therapy, 30,* 82-90.

Patten, C., Dozono, J., Schmidt, S., Jue, M., & Lum, P. (2006). Combined functional task practice and dynamic high intensity resistance training promotes recovery of upper-extremity motor function in post-stroke hemiparesis: a case study. *Journal of Neurologic Physical Therapy, 30,* 99-115.

Pedersen, S. W., Oberg, B., Insulander, A., & Vretman, M. (1990). Group training in parkinsonism: quantitative measurements of treatment. *Scandinavian Journal of Rehabilitation Medicine, 22,* 207-211.

Philips, B. A., & Mastaglia, F. L. (2000). Exercise therapy in patients with myopathy. *Current Opinions in Neurology, 13,* 547-552.

Plow, M. A., Mathiowetz, V., & Resnik, L. (2008). Multiple sclerosis: impact of physical activity on psychosocial constructs. *American Journal of Health Behavior, 32,* 614-626.

Pohl, M., Werner, C., Holzgraefe, M., Kroczek, G., Mehrholz, J., Wingendorf , I., et al. (2007). Repetitive locomotor training and physiotherapy improve walking and basic activities of daily living after stroke: a single-blind, randomized multicentre trial (DEutsche GAngtrainerStudie, DEGAS). *Clinical Rehabilitation, 21,* 17-27.

Radak, Z., Chung, H. Y., & Goto, S. (2008). Systemic adaptation to oxidative challenge induced by regular exercise. *Free Radical Biology & Medicine, 44,* 153-159.

Rampello, A. Marco, F., Piepoli, M., Antenucci, R., Lenti, G., & Olivieri, D. (2007). Effect of aerobic training on walking capacity and maximal exercise tolerance in patients with multiple sclerosis: a randomized crossover controlled study. *Physical Therapy, 87,* 545-559.

Rasova, K., Havrdova, E., Brandejsky, P., Zalisova, M., Foubikova, B., & Martinkova, P. (2006). Comparison of the influence of different rehabilitation programmes on clinical, spirometric and spiroergometric parameters in patients with multiple sclerosis. *Multiple Sclerosis, 12,* 227-234.

Resnick, B., Luisi, D., & Vogel, A. (2008). Testing the Senior Exercise Self-efficacy Project (SESEP) for use with urban dwelling minority older adults. *Public Health Nursing, 25,* 221-234.

Reuter, I., Engelhardt, M., Stecker, K., & Baas, H. (1999). Therapeutic value of exercise training in Parkinson's disease. *Medicine and Science in Sports and Exercise, 31,* 1544-1549.

Rietberg, M. B., Brooks, D., Uitdehaag, B. M. J., & Kwakkel, G. (2005). Exercise therapy for multiple sclerosis. *Cochrane Database of Systematic Reviews, 1.*

Rimmer, J. H. (1999). Health promotion for people with disabilities: the emerging paradigm shift from disability prevention to prevention of secondary conditions. *Physical Therapy, 79,* 495-502.

Rimmer, J. H. (2005). Exercise and physical activity in persons aging with a physical disability. *Physical Medicine and Rehabilitation Clinics of North America, 16,* 41-56.

Rimmer, J. H. (2006). Use of the ICF in identifying factors that impact participation in physical activity/rehabilitation among people with disabilities. *Disability and Rehabilitation, 28,* 1087-1095.

Rimmer, J. H., Riley, B., Wang, E., Rauworth, A., & Jurkowski, J. (2004). Physical activity participation among persons with disabilities: barriers and facilitators. *American Journal of Preventive Medicine, 26,* 419-425.

Rimmer, J. H., Rowland, J. L., & Yamaki, K. (2007). Obesity and secondary conditions in adolescents with disabilities: addressing the needs of an underserved population. Journal of Adolescent Health, 41, 224-229.

Rimmer, J. H., Wang, E., Smith, D. (2008). Barriers associated with exercise and community access for individuals with stroke. *Journal of Rehabilitation Research & Development, 45,* 315-322.

Rincon, F., Sacco, R. L. (2008). Secondary stroke prevention. *Journal of Cardiovascular Nursing, 23,* 34-41; quiz 42-3.

Romberg, A., Virtanen, A., Ruutiainen, J., Aunola, S., Karppi, S. L., Vaara, M., et al. (2004). Effects of a 6-month exercise program on patients with multiple sclerosis: a randomized study. *Neurology, 63,* 2034-2038.

Rosie, J., & Taylor, D. (2007), Sit-to-stand as home exercise for mobility-limited adults over 80 years of ageGrandStand System(TM) may keep you standing? *Age and Ageing, 36,* 555-562.

Rothwell PM, Coull AJ, Giles MF. Change in stroke incidence,. mortality, case-fatality, severity and risk factors in Oxfordshire, UK from 1981 to 2004 (Oxford Vascular Study). Lancet 2004;363:1925-33.

Rothwell, P. M., Coull, A. J., Silver, L. E., Fairhead, J. F., Giles, M. F., Lovelock, C. E., et al. (2005). Population-based study of event-rate, incidence, case fatality, and mortality for all acute vascular events in all arterial territories (Oxford Vascular Study). *Lancet, 366,* 1773-1783.

Ruiz, J. R., Sui, X., Lobelo, F., Morrow, J. R. Jr., Jackson, A. W., Sjostrom, M., et al. (2008). Association between muscular strength and mortality in men: prospective cohort study. *BMJ, 337,* a439.

Saltin, B., & Landin, S. (1975). Work capacity, muscle strength and SDH activity in both legs of hemiparetic patients and patients with Parkinson's disease. *Scandinavian Journal of Clinical and Laboratory Investigation, 35,* 531-538.

Salvetti, X. M., Oliveira, J. A., Servantes, D. M., & Vincenzo de Paola, A. A., (2008) How much do the benefits cost? Effects of a home-based training programme on cardiovascular fitness, quality of life, programme cost and adherence for patients with coronary disease. *Clinical Rehabilitation, 22,* 987-996.

Santiago, M. C., Coyle, C. P. (2004). Leisure-time physical activity and secondary conditions in women with physical disabilities. *Disability and Rehabilitation, 26,* 485-494.

Saunders, D. H., Greig, C. A., Young, A., & Mead, G. E. (2004). Physical fitness training for stroke patients. *Cochrane Database Systematic Review, 1.*

Schenkman, M., Donovan, J., Tsubota, J., Kluss, M., Stebbins, P., & Butler, R. B. (1989). Management of individuals with Parkinson's disease: rationale and case studies. *Physical Therapy, 69,* 944-955.

Schiemanck, S. K., Post, M. W. M., Kwakkel, G., Witkamp, T. D., Kappelle, L. J., & Prevo, A. J. H. (2005). Ischemic lesion volume correlates with long-term functional outcome and quality of life of middle cerebral artery stroke survivors. *Restorative Neurology and Neuroscience, 23,* 257-263.

Shaughnessy, M., Resnick, B. M., & Macko, R. F. (2006). Testing a model of post-stroke exercise behavior. *Rehabilitation Nursing, 31,* 15-21.

Sherrington, C., Pamphlett, P. I., Jacka, J. A., Olivetti, L. M., Nugent, J. A., Hall, J. M., et al. (2008). Group exercise can improve participants' mobility in an outpatient rehabilitation setting: a randomized controlled trial. *Clinical Rehabilitation, 22,* 493-502.

Shumway-Cook, A., & Woollacott, M. H. (2007). *Motor Control: Translating Research into Clinical Practice.* Baltimore, MD: Lippincott, Williams & Wilkens,.

Skidmore, F. M., Patterson, S. L., Shulman, L. M., Sorkin, J. D., Macko, R. F. (2008). Pilot safety and feasibility study of treadmill aerobic exercise in Parkinson disease with gait impairment. *Journal of Rehabilitation Research and Development, 45,* 117-124.

Smidt, N., de Vet, H. C. W., Bouter, L. M., & Dekker, J. (2005). Effectiveness of exercise therapy: A best-evidence summary of systematic reviews. *Australian Journal of Physiotherapy, 51,* 71-85.

Smith, D. T., Carr, L. J., Dorozynski, C., & Gomashe, C. (2009) Internet-delivered lifestyle physical activity intervention: limited inflammation and antioxidant capacity efficacy in overweight adults. *Journal of Applied Physiology, 106,* 49-56.

Snook, E. M., & Motl, R. W. (2008). Physical activity behaviors in individuals with multiple sclerosis: roles of overall and specific symptoms, and self-efficacy. *Journal of Pain and Symptom Management, 36,* 46-53.

Solari, A. Filippini, G., Gasco, P., Colla, L., Salmaggi, A., & La Mantia, L. et al. (1999). Physical rehabilitation has a positive effect on disability in multiple sclerosis. *Neurology, 52,* 57-62.

Stanish, H. I. (2004). Accuracy of pedometers and walking activity in adults with mental retardation. *Adapted Physical Activity Quarterly, 21,* 167-179.

Steffen, T. M., Boeve, B. F., Mollinger-Riemann, L. A., & Petersen, C. M. (2007). Long-term locomotor training for gait and balance in a patient with mixed progressive supranuclear palsy and corticobasal degeneration. *Physical Therapy, 87,* 1078-1087.

Stibrant Sunnerhagen, K. (2007). Circuit training in community-living "younger" men after stroke. *Journal of Stroke and Cerebrovascular Diseases, 16,* 122-129.

Stinear, C. M., Barber, P. A., Smale, P. R., Coxon, J. P., Fleming, M. K., & Byblow, W. D. (2007). Functional potential in chronic stroke patients depends on corticospinal tract integrity. *Brain, 130,* 170-180.

Stuart, M., Chard, S., & Roettger, S. (2008). Exercise for chronic stroke survivors: A policy perspective. *Journal of Rehabilitation Research and Development, 45,* 329-336.

Studenski, S., Duncan, P. W., Perera, S., Reker, D., Lai, S. M., & Richards, L. (2005). Daily functioning and quality of life in a randomized controlled trial of therapeutic exercise for subacute stroke survivors. *Stroke, 36,* 1764-1770.

Sullivan, K. J., Knowlton, B. J., Dobkin, B. H. (2002). Step training with body weight support: Effect of treadmill speed and practice paradigms on poststroke locomotor recovery. *Archives of Physical Medicine and Rehabilitation, 83,* 683-691.

Tang, S. W., Chu, E., Hui, T., Helmeste, D., & Law, C. (2008) Influence of exercise on serum brain-derived neurotrophic factor concentrations in healthy human subjects. *Neuroscience Letters, 431,* 62-65.

Tanne, D., Tsabari, R., Chechik, O., Toledano, A., Orion, D., Schwammenthal, Y., et al. (2008). Improved exercise capacity in patients after minor ischemic stroke undergoing a supervised exercise training program. *Israel Medical Association Journal, 10,* 113-116.

Tappe , M. K., Duda, J. L., & Ehrnwald, P. M (1990). Personal investment predictors of adolescent motivational orientation toward exercise. *Canadian Journal of Sport Science, 15,* 185-192.

Tappe, M. K., Duda, J. L., & Ehrnwald, P. M. (1989). Perceived barriers to exercise among adolescents. *Journal of School Health, 59,* 153-155.

Taylor, N. F. Dodd, K. J., Prasad, D., & Denisenko, S. (2006). Progressive resistance exercise for people with multiple sclerosis. *Disability & Rehabilitation, 28,* 1119-1126.

Taylor, N. F., Dodd, K. J., Shields, N., & Bruder, A. (2007). Therapeutic exercise in physiotherapy practice is beneficial: a summary of systematic reviews 2002-2005. *Australian Journal of Physiotherapy, 53,* 7-16.

Thacker, E. L., Chen, H., Patel, A. V., McCullough, M. L., Calle, E. E., Thun, M. J., et al. (2008). Recreational physical activity and risk of Parkinson's disease. *Movement Disorders, 23,* 69-74.

Thompson, A. J. (2001). Symptomatic management and rehabilitation in multiple sclerosis. *Journal of Neurology Neurosurgery and Psychiatry 71,* II22-II27.

Turner, P. R. (2006). *Mosby's Crash Course: Neurology.* London: Mosby.

van de Port, I. G., Wood-Dauphinee, S., Lindeman, E., & Kwakkel, G. (2007). Effects of exercise training programs on walking competency after stroke: a systematic review. *American Journal of Physical Medicine and Rehabilitation, 86*, 935-951.

van den Berg, M., Dawes, H., Wade, D. T., Newman, M., Burridge, J., Izadi, H., et al. (2006). Treadmill training for individuals with multiple sclerosis: a pilot randomised trial. *Journal of Neurology, Neurosurgery, and Psychiatry, 77*, 531-533.

van den Berg, M., Newman, M., Dawes, H., & Wade, D. (2005) A randomised crossover trial: the effects of aerobic treadmill training on gait characteristics, walking speed and enndurance and fatigue in individuals with multiple sclerosis. *Gait & Posture, 21*, S135.

van der Ploeg, H. P. Streppel, K. R., van der Beek, A. J., van der Woude, L. H., van Harten, W. H., & van Mechelen, W. (2008). Underlying mechanisms of improving physical activity behavior after rehabilitation. *International Journal of Behavorial Medicine, 15*, 101-108.

van der Ploeg, H. P. Streppel, K. R., van der Beek, A. J., van der Woude, L. H., Vollenbroek-Hutten, M. M., van Harten, W. H., et al. (2006). Counselling increases physical activity behaviour nine weeks after rehabilitation. *British Journal of Sports Medicine, 40*, 223-229.

van der Ploeg, H. P. Streppel, K. R., van der Beek, A. J., van der Woude, L. H., Vollenbroek-Hutten, M. M., van Harten, W. H., et al. (2007a) Successfully improving physical activity behavior after rehabilitation. *American Journal of Health Promotion, 21*, 153-159.

van der Ploeg, H. P. Streppel, K. R., van der Beek, A. J., van der Woude, L. H., Vollenbroek-Hutten, M. M., & van Mechelen, W. (2007b) The Physical Activity Scale for Individuals with Physical Disabilities: test-retest reliability and comparison with an accelerometer. *Journal of Physical Activity & Health, 4*, 96-100.

Van Oteghen, S. L. (1987). An exercise program for those with Parkinson's disease. *Geriatric Nursing, 8*, 183-184.

Wade, D. T., Wood, V. A., & Hewer, R. L. (1985). Recovery after stroke--the first 3 months. *Journal of Neurology, Neurosurgery, and Psychiatry, 48*, 7-13.

Welmer, A. K., von Arbin, M., Widen Holmqvist, L., & Sommerfeld, D. K. (2006). Spasticity and its association with functioning and health-related quality of life 18 months after stroke. *Cerebrovascular Diseases, 21*, 247-253.

Wendel-Vos, G. C., Schuit, A. J. Feskens, E. J., Boshuizen, H. C., Verschuren, W. M., Saris, W. H. et al. (2004). Physical activity and stroke. A meta-analysis of observational data. *International Journal of Epidemiology, 33*, 787-798.

White, L. J., Castellano, V. (2008a) Exercise and brain health--implications for multiple sclerosis: Part 1--neuronal growth factors. *Sports Medicine, 38,* 91-100.

White, L. J., Castellano, V. (2008b) Exercise and brain health--implications for multiple sclerosis: Part II--immune factors and stress hormones. *Sports Medicine, 38,* 179-186.

Wiles, R., Demain, S., & Robison, J. (in press). Exercise on prescription for stroke patients post-discharge from physiotherapy. *Disability & Rehabilitation.*

Wing, K., Lynskey, J. V., & Bosch, P. R. (2008). Whole-body intensive rehabilitation is feasible and effective in chronic stroke survivors: a retrospective data analysis. *Topics in Stroke Rehabilitation, 15,* 247-255.

Wisloff, U., Nilsen, T. I., Droyvold, W. B., Morkved, S., Slordahl, S. A., & Vatten, L. J. (2006). A single weekly bout of exercise may reduce cardiovascular mortality: how little pain for cardiac gain? 'The HUNT study, Norway'. *European Journal of Cardiovascular Prevention & Rehabilitation, 13,* 798-804.

Wolfe CDA. (2000). The impact of Stroke. *British Medical Bull,* 56:275-86.

World Health Organisation (2009). *Neurological Disorders: Public Health Challenges.* Geneva: World Health Organisation.

Yu, S., Patterson, C. C., & Yarnell, J. W. (2008). Is vigorous physical activity contraindicated in subjects with coronary heart disease? Evidence from the Caerphilly study. *European Heart Journal, 29,* 602-608.

Zalewski, K. (2007). Exploring barriers to remaining physically active: a case report of a person with multiple sclerosis. *Journal of Neurologic Physical Therapy, 31,* 40-45.

Zhao, Y. J., Tan, L. C., Lau, P. N., Au, W. L., Li, S. C., & Luo, N. (2008). Factors affecting health-related quality of life amongst Asian patients with Parkinson's disease. *European Journal of Neurology, 15,* 737-742.

In: Physical Activity in Rehabilitation and Recovery   ISBN: 978-1-60876-400-6
Editor: Holly Blake   © 2010 Nova Science Publishers, Inc.

Chapter 4

THE ROLE OF EXERCISE IN THE MANAGEMENT OF LONG TERM PAIN: A BIOPSYCHOSOCIAL APPROACH

Paula Banbury, Caroline Neal* and Elizabeth Johnson*
Nottingham Back & Pain Team,
Nottingham University Hospitals NHS Trust, UK.

ABSTRACT

The benefits of exercise and activity in the management of long term pain are well documented. A wealth of information exists about the most effective treatments for this complaint. It is generally accepted that the evolution of a new model for understanding the complex phenomenon of persistent pain has been more useful to patients and professionals working in this clinical area. The limitations of a purely medical approach have been acknowledged and a biopsychosocial model is proposed, applying principles of cognitive behavioural therapy to achieve more effective results for patients. Exercise has always been considered a pivotal feature of pain management programmes but evidence for which type or style has varied, and researchers continue to debate this issue. However a body of evidence has been building to explore the involvement of beliefs, thoughts and feelings in influencing prognosis for patients with long term pain. This is reflected in this chapter and it is acknowledged that a biopsychosocial

* Tel:+44 115 9936626; Fax:+44 115 9936627; Paula.Banbury@nuh.nhs.uk
* Tel:+44 115 9936626; Fax:+44 115 9936627; Email:Caroline.Neal@nuh.nhs.uk

approach should be employed when treating people with long term pain who present with barriers to increasing their activity levels.

INTRODUCTION

This chapter will explore the role of exercise in the management of long term pain, with particular focus upon the importance of adopting a biopsychosocial approach. Having defined long term pain and exercise, there will be a review of the history and policy surrounding the emergence of graded activity and the demise of bed rest in the management of persistent pain. The chapter will then focus upon the specific use of exercise in Pain Management Programmes and evaluate the literature, concluding that the medical model is now outdated for this multi-faceted phenomenon and that a biopsychosocial approach should be utilised. The central focus of the chapter is the application of this model in recommending exercise to people with long term pain. The biological, psychological and social aspects of the model will be explored as well as the obstacles faced by individuals trying to increase activity with long term pain. Case studies will be used to provide the reader with practical examples of how the model can be applied. Finally, the chapter will explore any implications that this approach may have in practice and the benefits of working within an interdisciplinary team to employ this model as effectively as possible.

DEFINITIONS

For the purpose of both this chapter and for clarity, it is necessary to define the terms 'exercise' and 'pain'. There are many and varied definitions that could be used, but the authors consider these to be the most widely recognised and acknowledged. Marcus and Forsyth (2003) describe exercise as *'any activity, which involves training, to improve physical capacity through stamina, strength or flexibility'*. It should be noted that when the authors refer to the term exercise, this includes generalised activity, which can improve physical function.

The International Association for the Study of Pain's (IASP, 2001) definition of long-term or 'chronic' pain is *'an unpleasant sensory and emotional experience associated with actual or potential tissue damage, or described in terms of such damage...that which has lasted over 3 months, has poor outcome, arising out of complex aetiology and complex clinical presentation'* (IASP, 2001). The IASP recognises that long-term pain is a multifaceted phenomenon and a challenging topic to research rigorously due to the subjectivity of the experience itself. For example, there will be a varied physical and emotional response amongst the general population to 'stubbing a toe' regarded as a relatively minor and acute pain experience. Pain, which persists, is further clouded by the growing influence of cognitive, emotional, and behavioural responses; and by environmental and social influences. This chapter will be focussing upon the unique role that the biopsychosocial model plays in utilising and applying exercise in pain rehabilitation.

HISTORY AND POLICY

Recognition of the value of exercise in the treatment of pain has manifested itself in the United Kingdom (UK) since the Second World War. In order to appreciate the pivotal role exercise plays in an individual's rehabilitation, it is necessary to examine and critique interventions which have previously been utilised and now condemned.

The Promotion of Bed Rest as a Treatment for Pain

Historically, episodes of pain, in particular spinal pain have been treated with bed rest, based largely on the belief that movement caused more harm (Fordyce, 1976). Health professionals who have promoted 'rest' and subsequent avoidance of any activities, which produce pain, have reinforced these beliefs over time. Bed rest was first proposed as a treatment for management of various ailments by a surgeon John Hunter in 1794. His recommendations were based upon the theory that inflammation in a wound would reduce if rested. This theory remained largely unchallenged throughout the 19th and indeed most of the 20th century by researchers and clinicians who ardently advocated rest for a variety of conditions, but predominantly pain. It was not until the 1990's that the value of bed rest began to be questioned by researchers. In 1995, two large Scandinavian randomised control trials (RCT) concluded that returning to normal activity as soon as possible led to a more rapid recovery from injury (Indahl, et al., 1995; Malmivara, et al., 1995). The Royal College of General Practitioners (RCGP, 1996) subsequently issued guidelines about the treatment of acute low back pain as a result of the impact of these studies. The overriding recommendation being that bed rest should be kept to a minimum and that an individual should return to normal activity as soon as possible.

Waddell reinforced these findings in 1998 and thus contradicted the existing evidence by arguing that bed rest was indeed *'harmful'* and a *'potent cause of iatrogenic disability'* (Waddell, 1998). This emphatic conclusion marked the beginning of the end of rest, and began to question the role of the medical model in the treatment of long-term pain.

The Harmful Effects of Rest

In order to endorse the value of an early return to activity in the management of long term pain, it is useful to highlight some of the harmful effects of prolonged rest. Whilst the primary focus for researchers appears to be on the 'bed rest versus activity' debate, few authors make any direct comment about the physical and emotional effects of inactivity. Mayer and Gatchel (1988) define the process by which people with pain become less 'fit' as the 'deconditioning syndrome'. This relates to the stiffening of joints, weakening of muscles and a notable reduction in cardiovascular ability, which occurs in people with low back pain in particular. Smorawinski et al (2001) published a detailed study that analysed the effect of bed rest on athletes. They concluded that after just 3 days there were noticeable changes in exercise performance as a result of impaired oxygen transportation and adverse alterations in musculoskeletal function. These findings were reinforced by Main and Williams (2002) who strongly endorsed the abandonment of prolonged bed rest and the early restoration of activity in order to maximise the rehabilitation of low back pain. The benefits of regular physical activity for our general health are well documented. Thirty minutes of sustained exercise or activity [at] 60-70% of an individual's maximum heart rate, making the heart beat faster and breathing heavier is advised by the British Heart Foundation (2003) and reinforced internationally. Frequent exercise can help reduce the risk or cardiovascular disease, improve mild to moderate depression and have positive effects on persistent pain (Taylor, 2002). Despite this, there is evidence to suggest that 60% of the population in the UK find reasons not to participate in regular, sustained aerobic activity (Main & Williams 2002). The effects of long term inactivity can be demonstrated in the following case study:

Case study: Mrs G

Mrs G is a 42-year-old lady who attended an assessment, reporting a 3-month history of low back pain. She had consulted her G.P who had advised her to rest and signed her off work for a 3-month period. In her opinion, this had led to worsening lumbar stiffness, reduced muscle strength and an inability to walk long distances anymore. She was no longer able to put her socks on and found she was out of breath when climbing the stairs.

The subjective findings were endorsed by objective examination and Mrs G was given analgesic advice, a Home Exercise Programme and guidance on gradually increasing activity levels. She returned to work within 4 weeks and her pain was much improved.

This section has briefly outlined the post war policy changes that have developed regarding bed rest and activity for back pain, highlighting the potential adverse effects of prolonged rest and advocate a shift from rest to activity. This chapter will now focus in more detail upon the history, role and value of exercise in Pain Management Programmes.

THE ROLE OF EXERCISE IN PAIN MANAGEMENT PROGRAMMES

In their trials of patients with persistent low back pain, Frost (1995, 2000) and Klaber Moffett (1999) found some benefit of patients undertaking exercise in functional restoration programmes. Main and Spanswick (2000) describe the origin of Pain Management Programmes used to treat long term pain. These multidisciplinary programmes were developed after the Second World War to treat complicated pain problems and were developed over subsequent years. The traditional medical model was replaced by the biopsychosocial model, which took into account, not only tissue-based pathology, but also the resulting suffering and pain. In the 1970s and 80s, modification of behaviour was considered an important component and more recently the cognitive aspect was added as it became more widely recognised that thought processes can drive behavioural change. Modern pain management programmes contain elements of pain control, education, activation, functional restoration, and some element of psychological therapy (British Pain Society, 2007).

Treatment is conducted in groups, it focuses on 'disease management' rather than a 'cure', and the emphasis is on self-management of the condition. With regards to exercise on these pain programmes, aims were to overcome the effects of physical deconditioning resulting from long term pain, challenge fears regarding activity, provide a safe and graded approach to activity, improve functional capacity, and help patients accept responsibility for improving their condition (Watson, 2000). This refers to exercises consisting of aerobic conditioning, paced up to 60-70% intensity for maximum advantage, stretching to counteract limited range of movement, and strengthening. Additionally, Watson (2000) recommends functional strength training with the purpose of counteracting deconditioning, rather than any particular regime.

One of the earliest pain management programmes in the UK was at St.Thomas's Hospital in London. Williams, et al. (1996) found that their 4 week inpatient pain management programme demonstrated better outcome than the 8 half days a week outpatient programme, although both recorded improvements over the waiting list control group. As anticipated, pain intensity was not affected, but there were significant improvements in physical performance and psychological function, which was maintained at the one-year follow-up. These findings appear to be confirmed by the international review of multi-disciplinary biopsychosocial rehabilitation on chronic low back pain patients, carried out by Guzman, et al. (2001), in which it was shown that intensive rehabilitation of more than 100 hours reduces pain and improves function, whereas less than 30 hours of therapy was not effective, when compared with non-multidisciplinary outpatient rehabilitation or usual care. Paradoxically, Johnson, et al. (2007) found that a brief programme of exercise and education, delivered over 16 hours in total, produced minimal benefit on pain overall, but patients who had a expressed a preference for it had clinically significant reductions in pain and disability.

Lack of agreement among researchers is often attributed to persistent pain being treated as if it has a common origin. The proposed argument is that it is necessary to classify cases, as they will not all respond to the same treatment. For example McCarthy (2005) argues that patients treated by physiotherapists are a large, diverse group and the clinical presentations are extremely heterogeneous, and therefore sub-classification is necessary before treatment. The European Guidelines (2004) for long term non-specific low back pain recommend Cognitive Behavioural Therapy (CBT), brief educational interventions, and multidisciplinary (bio-psychosocial) treatment. They advise that back schools, and short courses of manipulation can also be considered.

The most promising approaches seem to be cognitive-behavioural interventions encouraging activity / exercise, and they recommend supervised exercise therapy as a first-line treatment. The next section will identify three different types of exercise that are commonly used to treat people with persistent pain.

MCKENZIE EXERCISES

Robin McKenzie, a New Zealand Physiotherapist was popularised by devising a theoretical framework for exercises for the treatment of back pain throughout the 1980's. His approach followed a medical model establishing cause and effect. This regime of treatment proposed that there are three syndromes in low back pain: postural, dysfunctional and derangement (McKenzie, 2006). Treatment involved a remedial home exercise programme prescribed, and reviewed by a specialist physiotherapist and progressed as required. McKenzie exercises have been the subject of many research trials. Long (2004) established "directional preference" exercise for 230 subjects (i.e. an immediate, lasting improvement in pain from performing repeated lumbar flexion, extension, or side-glide/rotation tests) and found that subjects performing exercises related to their directional preference made significant improvements over either, subjects doing exercises opposite to their directional preference, or "non-directional" exercises. However Peterson (2007) found that there was no significant difference between groups of patients with persistent low back pain, who were given either McKenzie therapy or strength training. Although some controversy exists around the benefit of the McKenzie style of exercises, what it clearly established was a move towards active treatment, the hands off approach, providing the opportunity for patients to begin taking responsibility for their own pain management.

CORE STABILITY

Over the last twenty years, the concept of lumbar instability and the necessity to remedy this has received a lot of attention. O'Sullivan (2000) reports that spinal inter-segmental injury and intervertebral disc degeneration increases laxity around the 'neutral zone' of the spine. It is considered necessary to have adequate control in both the large trunk muscles and the smaller local muscles. There is evidence that the deep abdominals and lumbar multifidus muscles are preferentially adversely affected in low back pain and lumbar instability.

Persistent low back pain often results in general loss of function and deconditioning, in addition to changes in the neural control system to the muscles. Retraining of the musculature consists of three stages:

1   Simultaneous contraction of transversus abdominis with lumbar multifidus at low levels of maximal voluntary contraction
2   The contraction system described above is activated repeatedly during specific exercises.
3   Subjects then apply this combination of movements to stabilise their spines automatically during functional activities of daily living.

Some of the research using stability training has been positive (Hides, Jull, & Richardson, 2001; Rasmussen-Barr, Nilsson-Wikmar, & Arvidsson, 2003; O'Sullivan, Twomey, & Allison, 1997), but some doubts remain about the effectiveness of this treatment (Standaert & Herring, 2007). These findings are reinforced by May and Johnson (2008) who found that there was no evidence that stabilisation exercises for back pain were any more effective than other active interventions, although they conceded there may be a role for them with some patients.

GENERAL ACTIVITY

Waddell and Watson (2004) argue that specific exercises are not as important as general physical activity, and improving performance may be as much a matter of changing beliefs and behaviour as any physiologic change. There is increasing evidence that encourages individuals not to avoid any activity as long as it is approached in a paced manner. The best exercises for back pain are *"the one(s) which you actually do!"* and exercise programmes that also address psychosocial issues are more likely to be more effective.

Having reviewed the evidence for types of activity that can be utilised to treat persistent pain, this chapter will now focus upon the biopsychosocial approach, detailing its biological, psychological and social elements, highlighting common barriers to exercise.

THE BIOPSYCHOSOCIAL APPROACH

This chapter has already alluded to the fact that the medical model is too narrow to meet the complex needs of a population with long term non-malignant pain (Main & Spanswick, 2000). It does not encompass the multidimensional nature of this condition and the limitations of it are widely accepted. The table below outlines key stages of the medical model, and highlights it's inefficiencies in assessing and treating long term pain.

Table 1. The Medical Model applied to long term Pain

Medical Model	Long term pain
Specific symptoms reported	Symptoms might be widespread, changeable and intractable
History	History of the current condition may be complex and vague, with no identifiable trigger
Examination and Investigations	These may provide little information; pain levels may not be reflected in the results
Diagnosis	Diagnosis does not necessarily follow. A patient may spend a lot of time and energy attempting to identify one.
Treatment	There may be no clear course or pathway to follow as regards treatment. It may only have minimal or short term effect.
Prognosis / Cure	These are often elusive concepts in long term pain

Waddell (1998) stresses the need for patients and health professionals to separate pain from disability, especially in the case of back pain. He argues that psychological and social factors are fundamental in the development of disability due to pain. Individuals who are treated using a purely medical model are passive recipients, may absolve themselves of responsibility for their health, and adopt a rest for recovery approach, which as previously discussed is counterproductive. The biopsychosocial model takes in to account the biological or physical being; psychological processes, attitudes and beliefs; and social influences upon the individual. Using this model would consider the factors outlined below:

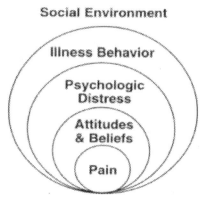

Reproduced by kind permission of Shaheen Emmanuelk Lakhan, Global Initiative Foundation, USA.

Figure 1. The Biopsychosocial model (Waddell 1998).

- *Biological:* The characteristics of pain (sensation and type, mechanical and/or neurological presentation, duration and intensity), any serious pathologies or red flags, general physical condition of the patient, other health problems or contributory factors (e.g. obesity), an objective examination of function, including standardised measures where appropriate (e.g. a 5 minute walk test).
- *Psychological:* The pain experience (emotional factors, beliefs about pain and illness and level of distress) often collectively called yellow flags, expectations of treatment, coping mechanisms, fear avoidance, safety behaviours and potential capacity for change.
- *Social:* Include culture, family pressures and influences, education, societal expectation, involvement in litigation particularly where compensation is an issue and other lifestyle factors. Commonly referred to as blue or black flags, and work related issues both personal an organizational

The biopsychosocial approach broadens the scope for understanding and treating long-term pain. In the late 1970's American Psychiatrist George Engel cited the limitations of the prevailing biomedical approach in understanding illness, and acknowledging mind body duality, he writes *"the dominant model of disease today is biomedical, and it leaves no room within its framework for the social, psychological, and behavioural dimensions of illness. A biopsychosocial model is proposed that provides a blueprint for research, a framework for teaching, and a design for action in the real world of health care".* Engel, 1977 as cited in Lindau, et al. (2003).

BIOLOGICAL ASPECT OF THE BIOPSYCHOSOCIAL MODEL

For hundreds of years, it was assumed that the amount of pain an individual was experiencing was related to the degree of damage in the tissues. Pain was thought to relate to the severity of the injury. If the patient did not recover, it was believed to indicate that there was underlying psychopathology. This assumption was challenged when a seminal paper was published in 1965 expounding the Pain Gate theory (Melzack & Wall, 1965). It was revealed that impulses in pain nerves can be reduced by activity in touch nerve fibres, and this is why rubbing, touch or movement actually reduce the pain experience. This was termed "the Pain Gate". Also described was the mechanism by which nerve impulses from the brain can reduce pain, which is why thinking of something else (distraction) is also helpful. In subsequent years this theory has been validated and expanded, and the management of persistent pain subsequently changed. It is now widely accepted that the perception of pain can be influenced from the brain or the periphery. Activity in the brain can modulate the pain that an individual feels, and various factors can affect the degree of pain experienced. In simple terms, the gate can be opened further and increase pain, and be helped to close, decreasing pain levels.

BIOLOGICAL BARRIERS TO EXERCISE

For many conditions a certain amount of rest may be beneficial and therefore rest is often recommended for the treatment of long-term pain. If medical advice reinforced this strategy, then increasing amounts of disability and deconditioning would prevail. In their review of exercise for osteoarthritis of the hip and knee, Fransen, et al. (2002) found that self-reported pain was lower and physical functioning better in patients who exercised than those who did not. Exercise is beneficial for coronary heart disease, hypertension, non-insulin dependent diabetes, pulmonary disease, inflammatory arthropathies, and to maintain bone mineral density (Hussey & Wilson, 2003). Despite well-documented benefits of exercise, individuals still present barriers to undertaking regular activities, which are biological in origin.

A) Pain

If an individual is in pain, they may be reluctant to exercise for fear of making the pain worse and for causing more damage. It is therefore necessary to give analgesic advice to maximise pain relief, and offer information about pacing activity levels to ensure they do not 'overdo' chosen activities.

B) Scar Tissue

The presence of tight scar tissue, shortening of structures due to lack of use, as well as muscle weakness, will restrict normal movement and activities, and it becomes simpler to avoid them. Sometimes individuals react to pain with increases in muscle tension and adopting abnormal postures, which lead to further deconditioning. They also prevent normal relaxed movements of parts of the body. For instance, normal, relaxed arm swing during walking may be inhibited.

C) Information About Diagnosis

If patients have incomplete information about their pathology, they may become wary about exercise. Simplified explanations like "trapped nerves", "slipped discs" and "wear and tear" do not explain the pain and dysfunction experienced by these patients. They may have been through many ineffective treatments and received different and perhaps conflicting information about the cause of their condition. Information is required about the capacity of the body for healing, an explanation about their condition, and the opportunity to correct any misunderstandings. If a patient thinks that activity may make their pain worse, they are less likely to undertake it.

Case study: Mr A

Mr A. went to his General Practitioner reporting a few weeks of mechanical low back pain. He was given analgesia and reassurance, and advised to remain active, pacing activities to cope with future exacerbations of pain. He became confident in managing his pain, gradually improving his fitness and strength and returning to his former activity levels.

Mr B, having a similar clinical history received similar initial advice and intervention. He believed his pain was a sign of serious harm, and became anxious and guarded, avoiding moving his back. He believed he had inherited a back problem from his father who suffered for many years and was diagnosed with a "slipped disc". He felt unable to return to work, subsequently lost his job, and began claiming state benefits. He became disabled by his pain, his relationships suffered, and he developed depression.

These case studies illustrate that two individuals with similar physical complaints can receive the same initial advice and yet have dramatically different outcomes. The psychological aspect of the model is now considered, which establishes a firm link between the physical, emotional, cognitive and behavioural elements of the individual.

PSYCHOLOGICAL ASPECT OF THE
BIOPSYCHOSOCIAL MODEL

Engel (1977), applied principles from general systems theory, developed by Buckley (1967) proposing that change in any area of the mind or body triggers change in other areas. The psychological aspect of the bio-psychosocial model is grounded in Cognitive Behavioural theory, encompassing cognitive, emotional, physical and behavioural patterns. Therapists aim to facilitate improvement through a process of modification within these elements.

Developed in America in the 1960's by psychotherapist Aaron T Beck; and initially used in the treatment of anxiety and depression, Cognitive Behavioural Therapy (CBT) is now the favoured approach for the treatment of a growing number of long-term conditions, where a pure biomedical approach has been insufficient in attending to psychosocial aspects of the condition. CBT has been the focus of research papers over the last 30 years, aiming to assess its clinical effectiveness in many areas. There is a significant body of evidence which supports the use of CBT in the treatment of long term low back pain (Butler, et al., 2006; Linton & Van Tulder 2001; Vlaeyen et al, 2001); identifying and evaluating pain beliefs, catastrophising and levels of distress (Elfving, et al., 2007; McCracken, et al., 2004; Vlaeyen, et al., 2001); lowering fear avoidance behaviours (Boersma, et al., 2004); reducing pain and restoring function (Kavanagh, 1995; Morley, et al., 1999); and improving patients perceptions of disability (Walsh, et al., 2002). The cognitive model is presented below in figure 2.

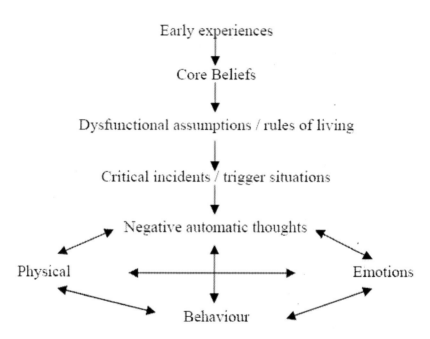

Figure 2. Modified example of cognitive model of emotional dysfunction as described by Beck (1995).

The diagram illustrates the cognitive model as developed Beck (1976). He asserts that early life experiences form individual core beliefs. These beliefs lead to the development of rules by which life should be led. Individuals' core beliefs and rules manifest in everyday discourse through thoughts that govern behaviour and emotions. There is an interdependent relationship between thoughts, emotions, behaviour and the body, which can become cyclical and self-maintaining. Incidents or events during life may periodically trigger individuals to question the validity and relevance of rules and beliefs. In pain management the Cognitive Behavioural approach has been adopted because it facilitates the discovery of unhelpful thinking styles, which maintain dysfunctional behaviour patterns, and impact on mood and the body. This is especially relevant when considering exercise and activity, with patients living with long term painful conditions.

PSYCHOLOGICAL BARRIERS TO EXERCISE

This chapter will now focus on the fundamental role of beliefs, thoughts, motivation and mood; and the potentially negative impact upon exercise and activity levels when encountered by patients with persistent pain.

A) Beliefs About Pain

Many authors have focussed on fear avoidance and catastrophic beliefs about pain. Boersma, et al. (2004), emphasises the damaging role of a catastrophic thinking style following pain experience, largely fuelled by the belief that hurt means harm. Fear of re-injury, the expectation of further pain and previous experiences of pain as a result of movement, contribute to a rise in anxiety levels. These factors frequently lead to activity avoidance and result in patients moving less and attending more to the pain experience.

Other authors describe pain related fear as a significant predictor of future disability, even those involving acute pain experiences (Fritz & George, 2002).

In practice what is seen is patients adopting a range of behaviours to manage their rising anxiety levels and protect themselves against the perceived risk. These are described by Salkovskis (1996) as safety behaviours and involve either avoidance and escape or a plan to manage the situation if it arises. Each of these behaviours has the end result of maintaining the fear related belief. The example below illustrates fear avoidance in a cognitive formulation, and the subsequent maladaptive or safety behaviour. Exploring this with and presenting a formulation to the patient facilitates greater understanding of the role of beliefs and 'safety behaviours', which contribute to the reduction of activities over time and feelings of heightened anxiety associated with activity.

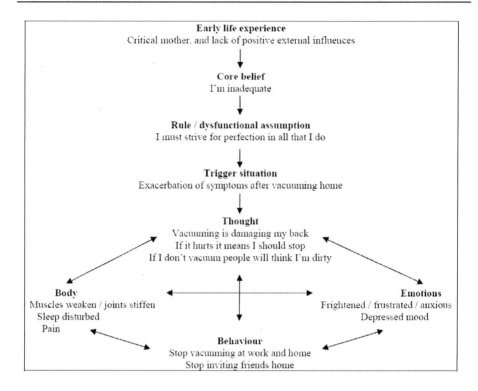

Figure 3. An example of a cognitive formulation.

In this case study Mrs S is initially reducing housework as a result of the belief that the pain she experiences is related to an injury. Pain is interpreted as a warning, and Mrs S believes that in order to protect herself she should not undertake heavier chores around the home. Her experience in the past when she has vacuumed has produced pain. This has an immediate affect on her mood, and in time, her body, leading to further unhelpful thoughts and feelings and maladaptive safety seeking behaviour patterns which mean she avoids tasks and risks becoming socially isolated.

B) Thinking Errors and Imagery

Thoughts follow patterns of which some are learned and some develop. All are shaped by experience. Beck (1964) describes thought patterns as *"automatic...a stream of thinking that coexists with a more manifest stream of thought"*. Not all thought patterns and habits are helpful, particularly those relating to long term pain and activity. Some common thinking errors or cognitive distortions are identified in the table below, with examples of how they are expressed by patients living with long term painful conditions (Beck, 1995).

Table 2. Examples of dysfunctional thoughts / thinking styles

---

All or nothing thinking (often referred to as black and white thinking)
"If I can't do all the gardening there's no point doing any at all"

Catastrophising or fortune telling
"If my pain never gets better, I'll end up in a wheelchair"

Disqualifying the positive
"I did manage to wash the car at the weekend, but it doesn't mean I'm cured"

Emotional reasoning, an over reliance on emotional responses, discounting factual evidence to the contrary
"I know I do most things around the house, but I still feel like a failure"

Labelling, having fixed ideas about identity
"I'm useless, old before my time"

Magnification / minimisation. Tendency to exaggerate negative aspects of events or situations, and minimise positive ones.
"Just being able to mow the lawn in sections proves how inadequate I really am."

Mental filtering or focussing on negative details, rather than the wider situation
"I have done too much housework today (even though during the rest of the week, chores were paced really well), means I can't pace myself"
Mind reading or jumping to conclusions based on what others *might* be thinking
" They don't believe I'm in pain, because they can't see it"

Over generalisation or sweeping statements
"Because I found exercises in the gym hard today, I don't think I should do them again"

Personalisation: Negative responses from others are taken to heart
"My friend walked past me in the supermarket, she must be avoiding me because she's bored of me talking about my pain"

'Should' and 'must' statements, about falling short of expectations
"I should be able to clean my house every week, otherwise people will think I'm dirty"

The previous table highlights common thinking styles expressed by patients suffering from long term pain. Together with current social and environmental triggers, and past experiences of both exercise and pain, these negatively biased and often automatic thoughts provide information about existing barriers to improvement, and useful insights in to psychological functioning and directions for treatment.

In addition to this Beck (1995) emphasises the importance of recognising that thoughts can take other sensory forms, such as images. These can be powerful influences on behaviour and therefore barriers to exercise, for example the image of a crumbling spine, becoming wheelchair bound, or in the extreme, death. Encouraging patients to identify these images can be a key factor in enabling them to overcome the associated anxiety and related behaviours.

The case study below illustrates an unhelpful thinking style in practice.

This pattern is often referred to as the 'boom bust' approach to activity outlined by Surawy (1995) for Chronic Fatigue Syndrome. The table above uses this model adapted by Farr (2006) for use in long term pain. It is another cycle where the end result is reduced activity levels. As previously noted, one of the aims of the Pain Management approach is to identify and address these thoughts, feelings and behaviours by providing alternative evidence and experience in order to facilitate effective rehabilitation.

Case study: Mrs J

Mrs J has widespread body pain. She finds it increasingly difficult to manage her housework. She is determined to continue and tends to over do activities, causing exacerbations of pain.

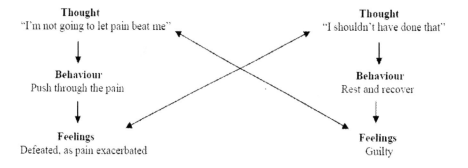

Figure 4. The 'boom / bust' approach to managing pain.

C) Motivation and Mood

Alterations in mood and subsequent motivation levels towards exercise and activity are common barriers to becoming more active. Common qualities associated with low motivation are anxiety, depression and fatigue. Exercise is beneficial for the treatment of low mood as it stimulates the release of endorphins and other chemicals that boost the mood. It is also beneficial in countering the effects of the stress response and is known to be energising.

An understanding of motivation is vital in understanding behaviour. Grahn, et al. (2001) looked at motivation and personal resources such as locus of control, self-focus, body awareness and coping ability and found a relationship between motivation for change and personal resources. Bandura (1986) discovered that social reinforcement enhances behaviour change. Marcus (2003) suggest rewards for initiating new behaviours are important particularly in the case of exercise and physical activity, as health benefits may not be immediately apparent, and intrinsic rewards such as feelings of accomplishment and weight loss may take time to occur. In addition to this they recommend developing a support network around exercise to embed new healthier habits, and emphasise the need to select enjoyable activities.

SOCIAL ASPECTS OF THE BIOPSYCHOSOCIAL MODEL

There are many social influences, which affect an individual's reactions and subsequent treatment of pain. Patients' family and friends may bias beliefs and thoughts about the nature of the pain. An example of this is a lady attending an assessment who had been told by her husband to rest her painful back as he had a colleague at work who had been given similar advice by his Doctor. Every time the lady tried to engage in activities around the house her husband stopped her. This was discussed at the appointment and a planned programme of paced activity was introduced. The ladies husband was also educated both verbally and with written information.

Social support is particularly important in times of illness or crisis (Waddell, 2004). If a patient has effective social support, this can improve their rehabilitation. However, many people find that they become a full or part time carer for their family member with pain and this has an impact upon roles within the family and altered dynamics. This can often lead to resentment, social isolation and dysfunctional relationships, which will affect prognosis.

Having highlighted some of the social influences upon the biopsychosocial model, this chapter will now examine the perceived social barriers to exercise and activity.

SOCIAL BARRIERS TO EXERCISE

This section will examine social barriers which can affect an individual's ability to maintain an exercise regime if suffering from long-term pain.

A) Cost

Despite the belief that exercise has to be an expensive hobby, the evidence actually contradicts this idea. Home Exercise Programme's (HEP's) are often prescribed for people who are undertaking a period of rehabilitation. These can be practised at home everyday and do not have cost implications. Walking, jogging and stretching can also be carried out within the community without the need to visit a gym.

The case study below highlights a concern raised by a patient, which is typical of many people receiving treatment for long term pain. Activities such as gardening and housework can incorporate stretching and strengthening exercises into a daily routine with good effect.

Case study: Mr H

Mr H is 35-year-old gentlemen attending a Pain Management Programme for back and neck pain. He reports that he is unable to afford to use his local leisure centre as he receives a low income and has 3 children to support.

In this instance, Mr H presented cost as an obstacle to continuing a programme of exercise. A plan was devised with him that involved him walking regularly, borrowing a friend's exercise bike, and daily stretches. A recommendation was also made to his G.P for him to be referred to a Prescription for Health scheme, which was free and allowed him to attend supervised sessions at his local Gymnasium. Harrison, et al, (2005) observe that there has been a rapid expansion in exercise referral schemes across the UK. They postulate that this is due to a population who have a sedentary lifestyle and poor existing support for people who want to undertake regular activity. This case study highlights the need for improved access to affordable exercise schemes for people on a low income who are motivated to improve their pain and general health. The rising socioeconomic cost of back pain could only serve to be reduced by a sustained investment in affordable, accessible projects in the community.

B) Work

Work can often be presented as a barrier to undertaking regular activity or exercise and is often cited as a contributory factor in the onset of back pain. Lack of time at the end of the working day is often presented as a barrier. Long term pain, especially low back has been traditionally associated with prolonged periods of sick leave in the United Kingdom. Guidelines regarding work and pain have changed over the last two decades with individual's now being advised to stay at work wherever possible in order to remain as active as possible (RCGP, 1996) Commencing a programme of exercise whilst employed requires planning and prioritisation in order to succeed.

This case study demonstrates that a collection of interventions may be required to improve an individual's ability to manage their pain in the workplace and subsequently at home. It also illustrates that low back pain does not primarily affect people with 'heavy' jobs that have traditionally been associated with incidences of pain and repeated absences from work.

Waddell (1998) concludes that back pain in particular is work related in so far as it affects people of working age, and that may impact on their ability to be employed. He also notes that being at work is important for long term back pain management as long as the right advice is given for its immediate and future management.

Case study: Miss F.

Miss F is a 28-year-old administrative assistant in a local health centre. The majority of her work involves sitting at a desk using a P.C and light office duties. She attended an assessment appointment complaining of a 3 year history of low back and neck pain following a whiplash injury. She regularly attends the gym but finds that her pain is worsened during her working day. In this particular instance, the following plan was agreed

---

between Miss F and the Practitioner carrying out the assessment:

1. Miss F will continue to attend the gym and concentrate on cardiovascular exercise. She was educated about how to escalate her activity levels without increasing her pain.
2. An additional Home Exercise Programme of stretches was given to Miss F. These could be undertaken at home or in the workplace.
3. Miss F was advised to take Paracetamol and Ibuprofen regularly at work and monitor analgesic effect.
4. Pacing advice was given regarding the amount of time Miss F was spending at her desk. She was advised to try and move around or stretch every 20 minutes if practical and alternate her tasks. This would ease some of the stiffness in her spine, which may have been exacerbating her pain.

A letter was sent to Miss F's employer detailing the advice that had been given at assessment. The employer was also informed of Miss F's intention to attend a 7-week treatment programme. A primary aim of this treatment would be for Miss F to improve her overall physical function and be taught self-management strategies that would enable her to remain in a job she enjoyed.

C) Social Support

The final barrier that is often cited by people who struggle to remain active is a lack of social support. This could be from family, friends or work colleagues and the evidence for this remains predominantly anecdotal.

Case study: Mr J

Mr J was a 50 year old gentleman who attended a treatment programme for low back and bilateral knee pain. This had been diagnosed as musculoskeletal in origin. He had stopped exercising 8 years ago because it was exacerbating his pain and his family were unsupportive and not at all keen for him to re-start. This was based largely on their belief that exercise or activity would lead to further problems with his back and knees.

This case study is representative of many people who report poor social support as a reason not to engage in regular activity. In a situation like this, it is paramount that the practitioner and the individual concerned discuss and implement a management plan that is realistic and can be shared with family members. In this instance, the following plan was agreed:

1. Mr J was educated about the benefits of regular activity for both his physical and mental health. This involved teaching him how to establish a goal that he felt was realistic and could escalate in a paced manner.
2. The importance of discussing this goal with his family was discussed. Mr J planned to ask his partner to participate in his goal which was to re-commence swimming.
3. Analgesic advice was given to maximise the effectiveness of Mr J's painkillers. This would allow him to swim more comfortably.
4. A recommendation was made to Mr J's G.P that he would be referred to the Prescription for Health scheme. This would enable him to continue working towards his goal in a supportive environment with qualified coaches.
5. Individual keyworking time was given to Mr J to examine ways in which he might be able to improve his communication style in order to gain support from his family, friends and colleagues.

This section of the chapter has focused on the biopsychosocial model, examining its components in detail. Reference has been made to carious barriers to exercise that can exist, and case studies have been used to provide examples as to how these barriers can be challenged and overcome in clinical practice. The last section of the chapter will consider implications for practice and finish with concluding remarks and recommendations.

IMPLICATIONS IN PRACTICE

This chapter has highlighted the importance of adopting a biopsychosocial approach when introducing exercise to patients with long term pain. The complexities involved in rehabilitating an individual diagnosed with persistent pain demands the skills of an experienced interdisciplinary team. Clark (2000) believes that such teams consist of *'professionals from different backgrounds working together in an integrated way with joint goals which are continuously reviewed'*. Many authors who provide expertise in this field reinforce this belief. Block (2007) adds that the foundation of interdisciplinary pain management is to help patients view their pain outside the medical model and be taught to manage it with sufficient coping strategies This approach contrasts with a multidisciplinary approach which involves the efforts of individuals from a number of disciplines working under a leader with little or no overlap (Melvin, 1980). Almost two decades later, Main and Spanswick (2000) noted that there are problems involved with employing a multidisciplinary team to manage people with pain. They observe that there may be ineffective communication, which ultimately can lead to a fragmented and inconsistent approach. This could prove to be detrimental to the assessment and treatment of individuals with long term pain who demand an experienced, united team who share common goals and beliefs about treatment. The benefits of working and treating people within an interdisciplinary team are highlighted in the case study below:

Pain Management Programmes in the UK should be adopting the biopsychosocial model within a cognitive behavioural framework and the benefits of the model should be demonstrated to patients receiving treatment as early as possible. This will allow the individual to benefit from a demedicalised approach which will address and encompass every aspect of their pain.

Case study: Mr D

Mr D attended for an appointment with an interdisciplinary pain management team. He had been referred by his G.P with a 4-year history of musculoskeletal pain in his lower back and neck. His assessment was undertaken by an Occupational Therapist who was able to complete a full neurological examination and exclude red flags. The Practitioner was able to prescribe a Home Exercise Programme based on her clinical findings and make basic recommendations about how to take analgesia as effectively as possible. The generic approach to both assessment and subsequent management ensured that Mr D received appropriate, timely treatment delivered in a clear consistent manner.

CONCLUSION

This chapter has examined the shift from the prescription of 'bed rest' adopting a passive medical model to a predominantly active rehabilitation for long term pain. The authors have highlighted the significance of the biopsychosocial model in facilitating a self-management approach.

The success of a biopsychosocial model for treating persistent pain can be determined by many factors, but the majority of studies conclude that the use of exercise or activity is borne out of the ineffectiveness of the medical model to treat many long term pain sufferers. These findings lead the authors to conclude that there is increasing dissatisfaction with the medical model in treating pain, which persists, and a move towards assessment and treatment underpinned by psychosocial components.

Specific, staged exercises have previously been a pivotal component of Pain Management Programmes and many papers have attempted unsuccessfully to ultimately discover the effectiveness of these, and pinpoint exacting prescriptions relating to particular diagnoses. General exercise and activity for the treatment of persistent low back pain was recommended by the CSAG report (CSAG,1994), but given the results of recent studies (Hayden, et al., 2007; Karjalainen, et al., 1999), the effectiveness of this in isolation too, is now being questioned.

An integral part of a biopsychosocial approach to pain management is to identify barriers to increasing activity and exercise by individuals with pain. This may require specific cognitive behavioural interventions that enable patients to address these issues and experiment with new coping strategies.

In light of the evidence and discussion within this chapter, the authors make the following recommendations:

- Generalised exercises / activity rather than rigid specific styles should be encouraged. This is more likely to achieve concordance with the patient.
- Exercise and activity should be applied as part of a package of treatment rather than in isolation, addressing all aspects of pain management. This is most effectively delivered through the interdisciplinary team.
- Greater education in preventative strategies; exercise and activity promotion being just one example.

It is now widely acknowledged that increased exercise can reduce the deleterious effects of deconditioning but is most effective when used as part of a 'toolkit' or package of treatment that includes paced activity, medication advice and relaxation training. This approach should be led by an interdisciplinary team, and now forms the basis of contemporary Pain Management Programmes in the UK.

REFERENCES

Bandura, A. (1986). *Social Foundations of thought and action.: A social cognitive theory.* Englewood Cliffs, NJ: Prentice Hall.

Beck, J. (1995). *Cognitive Therapy: Basics and Beyond.* New York: Guildford Press: New York.

Beck, A.T. (1964). Thinking and Depression: 2: Theory and Therapy. *Archives of General Psychiatry.* 10, 561-71.

Boersma, K., Linton, S., Overmeer, T., Jansson, m., Vlaeyen, J., de Jong, J. (2004). Lowering fear-avoidance and enhancing function through exposure in vivo. A multiple baseline study across six patients with back pain. *Pain*, 108, 8-16.

Block, A.R. (2007). *Interdisciplinary Chronic Pain Management vs. Back Surgery: Which is right for you?* Retrieved 22 April, 2009, from www.spine-health.com.

British Heart Foundation (2003) *You and your healthy heart.* BHF. London.

British Pain Society. (2007). *Recommended guidelines for Pain Management Programme's for adults.* British Pain Society.

Buckley, W. (1967). *Sociology and modern systems theory.* Englewood Cliffs: New Jersey.

Busch, A.J., Barber, K.A., Overend, T.J., Peloso, P.M. & Schachter, C.L. (2007). Exercise for treating fibromyalgia syndrome' *Update of Cochrane Database Systematic Review,* 4, CD003786.

Butler, A.C., Chapman, J.E., Forman, E.M., & Beck, A.T. (2006). The empirical status of CBT. A review of meta-analyses. *Clinical Psychology Review.* 26(1), 17-31.

Clark, T.S. (2000). Interdisciplinary treatment for chronic pain: is it worth the money? *Baylor University Medical Center Proceedings,* 13(3), 240-243.

Clinical Standards Advisory Group. (1994). *Clinical Standards Advisory Group: Services for patients with pain.* The Stationery Office, UK.

Elfving, B., Andersson, T., & Grooten, W.J. (2007). Low levels of physical activity in back pain patients are associated with high levels of fear-avoidance beliefs and catastrophising. *Physiotherapy Research International*, 12(1), 14-24.

Engel, G.L. (1977). The need for a new medical model: A challenge for biomedicine. *Science,* 196(4286), 129-136.

European guidelines for the management of chronic non-specific low back pain. (2004). Retrieved 4th September, 2008, from www.backpaineurope.org.

Farr, A. (2006). *A review of cognitive factors associated with chronic low back pain-an initial model and possible interventions.* Unpublished MSc dissertation.

Fordyce, W.E. (1976). *Behavioural methods for chronic pain and illness.* Mosby: St Louis.

Fransen, M., McConnel, S., & Bell, M. (2002). Therapeutic exercise for people with osteoarthritis of the hip or knee: a systematic review. *Journal of Rheumatology,* 29, 1737-1745.

Fritz, J., & George, S. (2002). Identifying psychosocial variables in patients with acute work-related low back pain: the importance of fear-avoidance beliefs. *Physical Therapy,* 82, 973-83.

Frost, H., Klaber Moffet, J.A., Moser, J.S. & Fairbank, J.C.T. (1995). Randomised controlled trial for evaluation of fitness programme for patients with chronic low back pain. *BMJ,* 10,(21), 151-154.

Grahn E.B.M., Stigmar, G.K.E., & Ekdahl, C.S. (2001). Motivation for change and personal resources in patients with prolonged musculoskeletal disorders. *Journal of Bodywork And Movement Therapies,* 5(3), 160-172.

Guzman, J., Esmail, R., Karjalainen, K., Malmivaara, A., Irvin, E. & Bombardier, C. (2001) Multidisciplinary rehabilitation for chronic low back pain: systematic review. *BMJ,* 322, 1511-1516.

Harrison, R.A., McNair, F., & Dugdill, L. (2005). Access to exercise referral schemes- a population based analysis. *Journal of Public Health,* 27(4), 326-330.

Hartigan, C., Rainvillw, J., Sobel, J.B., & Hipona, M. (2000). Long-term exercise adherence after intensive rehabilitation for chronic low back pain, *Medicine & Science in Sports & Exercise,* 32(3),551-557.

Hayden, J.A., van Tulder, M.W., Malmivaara, A., & Koes, B.W. (2007). Exercise therapy for treatment of non-specific low back pain (Review). *Cochrane Library,* 4.

Hides, J.A, Jull, G.A., & Richardson, C.A. (2001). Long-Term Effects of Specific Stabilising Exercises for First-Episode Low Back Pain. *Spine,* 26(11), 243-248.

Hussey, J., & Wilson, F. (2003). Measurement of Activity is an Important Part of Physiotherapy Assessment. *Physiotherapy,* 89(10),585-593.

IASP Pain Terminology. (2001). International Association for the study of pain. Retrieved 4th September, 2008, from http://www.iasp.pain.org/terms-p.html.2001.

Indahl, A., Velund, L., & Reileraas, O. (1995). Good prognosis for low back pain when left untampered. A randomized clinical trial. *Spine,* 20, 473-477.

Karjalainen, K., Malmivaara, A., van Tulder, M., Roine, R., Jauhaiinen, M., Hurri, H., & Koes, B. (1999). Multidisciplinary rehabilitation for fibromyalgia and musculoskeletal pain in working age adults. *Cochrane Database of Systematic Reviews,* 3. Art. No: CD001984. DOI: 1002/14651858. CD001984.

Kavanagh, J.(1995). Management of chronic pain using the Cognitive-behavioural approach. *British Journal of Occupational Therapy,* 2(8), 413-418.

Klaber Moffett, J., Torgeson, D., Bell-Syer, S., Jackson, D., Llwelyn-Phillips, H., Farrin, A., & Barber, J. (1999). Randomised controlled trial of exercise for low back pain: clinical outcomes, costs, and preferences. *BMJ,* 319, 279-283.

Liddle, S.D., Baxter, G.D., & Gracey, J.H. (2004). Exercise and chronic low back pain: what works? *Pain,* 107(1-2), 176-190.

Lindau, S.T., Laumann, E., Levinson, W., & Waite, L. (2003). Synthesis of scientific disciplines in Pursuit of health. The interactive_Biopsychosocial model. *Perspectives in Biological Medicine,* 46(3), 74-86.

Linton, S J. (2000). A systematic review of psychological risk factors for back and neck pain. *Spine,* 25, 1148-1156.

Linton, S J., & Andersson, T. (2000). Can chronic disability be prevented? A randomized trial of a cognitive-behaviour intervention and two forms of information for patients with spinal pain. *Spine,* 25, 2825 – 2833.

Linton, S J. Van Tulder, M W. (2001) Preventative Interventions for Back and Neck Pain Problems: What's the Evidence? *Spine.* 26 (7) 778-787

Long, A. Donelson, R. Fung, T (2004) Does it matter which exercise? A Randomised Controlled Trial of Exercise for Low back Pain. *Spine.* 29 2593-2602

Main, C.J., & Spanswick, C.C. (2000). *Pain Management: an Interdisciplinary Approach.* Churchill Livingstone: Edinburgh.

Main, C.J. Williams A, C de C (2002). ABC of physiological medicine: Muskuloskeletal Pain. *BMJ.* 325 534-537

Malmivaara, A., Hakkinen, U., Aro, R., Heinrichs, M., Koskenniemi, L., Kuosma, E., Lappi, S., Paloheimo, R., Servo, C., Vaaranen, S., & Hernberg, S. (1995). The treatment of acute low back pain- bed rest, exercises or ordinary activity? *New England Journal of Medicine,* 332, 351-355.

Marcus, B.H., & Forsyth, L.H. (2003). *Motivating people to be physically active.* Human Kinetics: USA.

May, S & Johnson R (2008) Stabilisation exercises for low back pain: a systematic review. *Physiotherapy.* 94(3) 179-189.

Mayer, T.G. & Gatchel, R.J. (1988). *Functional restoration for spinal disorders: the sports medicine approach. Lea and Febiger:* Philadelphia.

McCarthy, C. (2005). There is no panacea for low back pain. *Physiotherapy*, 91(1), 2-3.

McCracken, L M. et al (2002). Cognitive behavioural therapy for chronic pain: an overview with specific reference to fear and avoidance. In G.J.G, Asmundson., J., Vlaeyen., & G., Crombez. (Eds.), *Understanding and treating fear of pain*, (pp 293-313) University Press: Oxford.

McKenzie, R. (2006). *Treat your own back (6th Edition)*. Spinal Publications: New Zealand.

Melvin, J.L. (1980). Interdisciplinary and multidisciplinary activities and the ACRM. *Archives of Physical Medicine and Rehabilitation.*61, 379-380.

Melzack, R., & Wall, P.D. (1965). Pain mechanisms: A new theory. *Science*, 150, 971-79

Melzack, R. (1993). Pain: Past, Present and Future. *Canadian Journal of Experimental Psychology*, 47, 615-619.

Morley, S., Ecclesto, C., & Williams, A. (1999). Systematic review and meta analysis of randomised controlled trials of cognitive behaviour therapy for chronic pain in adults, excluding headache. *Pain*, 80, 1-13.

Moss-Morris, R. Humphrey,K Johnson, M H. Petrie, K J (2007) Patients perceptions of their pain condition across a multidisciplinary pain management programme: Do they change and if so does it mater? *The Clinical Journal of Pain*. 23 (7) 558-564

O'Sullivan, P.B., Twomey, L.T., & Allison, G.T. (1997). Evaluation of specific stabilising exercise in the Treatment of chronic low back pain with radiologic diagnosis of Spondylolysis or Spondylolitheses. *Spine,*22(4), 2959-2967.

O'Sullivan, P.B. (2000). Lumbar segmental 'instability': clinical presentation and specific stabilising exercise management, *Manual Therapy*, 5(1), 2-12.

Peterson, T., Kristian, L., & Soren, J. (2007). One-year follow up comparison of the effectiveness of McKenzie treatment and strengthening training for patients with chronic low back pain: outcome and prognostic factors. *Spine*, 15(26), 2948-2956.

Press, V., Freestone, I., & George, C.F. (2003). Physical activity: The evidence of benefit in prevention of coronary heart disease. *QJMed*, 96,:245-251.

Rasmussen-Barr, E., Nilsson-Wikmar, L., & Arvidsson, I. (2003). Stabilizing training compared with manual treatment in sub-acute and chronic low-back pain. *Manual Therapy*, 8(4), 233-241.

Royal College of General Practitioners. (1996): *Clinical Guidelines for the management of acute low back pain*. ISBN number 0850842298. RCGP: London.

Salkovskis P.M. (ed). (1996). *Frontiers of Cognitive behavioural Therapy.* Guildford press: New York.

Smorawinski, J et al (2001). Effects of 3-day bed rest on physiological responses to graded exercise in athletes and sedentary men. *Journal of Applied Physiology,* 91 (1), 249-257.

Standaert, C.J. & Herring, S.A. (2007). Expert opinion and controversies in musculoskeletal and sports medicine: core stabilisation as a treatment for low back pain. *Archives of Physical Medicine and Rehabilitation,* 88(12),1134-1136.

Surway, C., Hackmann, A., Hawton, K., & Sharpe, M. (1995). Cognitive model of chronic fatigue syndrome. *Behaviour Research and Therapy,* 33, 535-544.

Taylor, R. (2002). Exercise based rehabilitation for patients with coronary heart disease. A systematic review and meta analysis of RCT. *American Journal of Medicine,* 116(10), 682-692.

Tulder, M., van Malmivaara, A., Hayden, J., & Koes, B. (2007). Statistical Significance versus Clinical Importance: Trials on exercise Therapy for Chronic Low Back Pain as Example. *Spine,* 32(16),1785-1790.

Vlaeyen, J.W.S., de Jong, J., Geiten, M., Heuts, P.H.T.G., & van Breukelen, G. (2001). Graded exposure in vivo in the treatment of pain-related fear: a replicated single case experimental design in four patients with chronic low back pain. *Behaviour Research and Therapy,* 39, 151-166.

Waddell, G. (1998). *The Back Pain Revolution.* Churchill Livingstone: London.

Waddell, G. & Watson, P. (2004). Rehabilitation 2nd Edition. In G. Waddell. (Ed.), *The Back Pain Revolution* (pp371-400), Churchill Livingstone: Edinburgh.

Walsh, D.A. & Radcliffe, J.C. (2002). Pain beliefs and perceived physical disability of patients with chronic low back pain. *Pain,* 97, 23-31.

Watson, P. (2000). Clinical content of interdisciplinary pain management programmes: Part 3 Physical activities programme content. In C.J. Main., & C.C. Spanswick. (Eds), In *Pain Management: an Interdisciplinary Approach* (pp285-301), Churchill Livingstone: Edinburgh.

Williams, A.C., Richardson, P.H., Nicholas, M.K., Pither, C.E., Harding, V.R., Ridout, K.L., Ralphs, J.A., Richardson, H., Justins, D.M., & Chamberlain, J.H. (1996). Inpatient versus outpatient pain management: results of a randomised control trial. *Pain,* 66(1), 13-22.

In: Physical Activity in Rehabilitation and Recovery   ISBN: 978-1-60876-400-6
Editor: Holly Blake   © 2010 Nova Science Publishers, Inc.

Chapter 5

PHYSICAL ACTIVITY IN TRAUMATIC BRAIN INJURY REHABILITATION

*Holly Blake**

Faculty of Medicine and Health Sciences, University of Nottingham, UK.

ABSTRACT

Traumatic brain injury (TBI) can result in a range of physical, cognitive, emotional and behavioural problems. Exercise is increasingly advocated in brain injury rehabilitation since individuals with long-term conditions are at particular risk of deconditioning and secondary disease or impairment as a result of inactivity. Maintaining an active lifestyle can help brain injured individuals to regain confidence and independence, and further, exercise has been associated with reductions in physical and cognitive impairments, fatigue and depression, which often accompany TBI. This chapter identifies some key arguments for promoting exercise in TBI, and provides an overview of the research evidence evaluating exercise intervention in this population identifies some major limitations of existing work in this field and provides suggestions for further investigation. A case study is presented which shows the introduction of an alternative form of exercise intervention into the community day centre setting.

* Tel: +44 (0)115 8231049; Fax: +44 (0)115 8230999; Email: Holly.Blake@nottingham.ac.uk

INTRODUCTION

Defining Traumatic Brain Injury

Traumatic brain injury (TBI) is also called 'acquired brain injury' or more simply 'head injury'. It is a leading cause of death and long-term disability in Europe, and has been estimated to result in 1.4 million accident and emergency department admissions in the UK alone, each year (Moulton & Yates, 1999). This figure is likely to be an underestimate since it is thought that only a quarter of all TBI cases are actually assessed and treated in hospital (Sosin, Sniezek, & Thurman, 1996). A brain injury can be defined as a 'craniocerebral injury that results from initial sudden forces levied to the head and secondary brain damage (e.g. raised intracranial pressure, intracranial demotoma) which leaves residual disabilities' (Zoerink & Lauener, 1991). The brain insult, resulting from external force, can result in a diminished or altered state of consciousness and this can result in the diverse consequences of TBI, which range from physical disabilities to cognitive, behavioural, emotional and social deficits. These may be, mild, moderate or severe, depending on the extent of damage done to the brain. Impairments can be temporary or long-term, causing partial or total functional disability or psychosocial maladjustment.

Causes and Consequences

Causes of brain injury are wide ranging and may include near-drowning, airway obstructions, electrical shock, vascular disruptions, infections, diseases or tumours, toxic exposure. However, the vast majority of traumatic brain injuries are caused by motor vehicle accidents and most frequently occur in young males aged 15-24. Psychomotor impairments may include slowness or confusion in the planning and sequencing of movements (ataxia/apraxia), muscle spasticity, contractures, fatigue and balance impairment (Basford, et al., 2003; Lepore, 1987). Sensory impairments including vision and hearing loss may also manifest (Poretta, 2000). These impairments can affect activities of daily living and engagement with premorbid activities (Masanic & Bailey, 1998; Quinn and Sullivan, 2000). Motor performance symptoms affecting static and dynamic balance, agility and rhythm co-ordination may be observed even in patients who appear physically well-recovered (Rinne, et al., 2006).

There may be cognitive deficits including short and/or long term memory loss, poor concentration, communication disorders related to speech, writing and reading, and difficulties with logical reasoning, organisation skills and orientation (Lepore, 1987).

Emotional, behavioural and social impairments are diverse and may include low self-esteem, lack of motivation and a difficulty in relating to other people. These may also include impulsive behaviour, impatience, being dependent on others, irritability, apathy, inability to learn from experiences, personality changes, short temper, and a lack of awareness of physical and/or mental limitations (Lepore, 1987). Disturbances in behaviour and emotion experienced as a result of brain injury may impact on mood and self-esteem, causing problems with engagement and participation in a social environment.

For these reasons, TBI is a complicated injury, with a very broad spectrum of disabilities and symptoms, and is therefore associated with significant financial burden (Chesnut, et al., 1999; Max, Mackenzie, & Rice, 1991). The resulting impairments and prognosis are very much dependent on the severity and location of the injury, age and general health of the patient.

Rehabilitation and TBI

Patients with moderate or severe injuries undergo rehabilitation including individually tailored treatment programmes, which may include occupational therapy, physical therapy, speech therapy, psychology, and social support. Therapeutic activity is essential in clinical neurorehabilitation following TBI and rehabilitation programmes can have encouraging outcomes. Programmes focusing on cognitive and perceptual remediation, problem-solving, personal counselling, physical exercise and relaxation, social skills and prevocational training have all shown positive outcomes for cognitive function whilst in the chronic stage (average postcoma interval, 59 months) (Sherzer, 1986).

Physical Exercise in TBI

Much of the exercise research in TBI focuses on the benefits of aerobic exercise such as cycling, running or swimming. Other forms of exercise such as yoga, Tai Chi, walking, weight training, bowling, golf and other non-aerobic activities may be beneficial in terms of relaxation, muscular strength, improved concentration and psychological outcomes.

Disability in patients with brain injury may be a result of neurological damage; indeed, experimental studies with animals have investigated early rehabilitation models and the relationship between neurotransmitter effects, brain impairment, behavioural outcome and functional recovery (Goldstein, 2006; Lippert-Grüner, et al., 2007). However, disability may also be a result of secondary problems resulting from immobility, such as altered muscle function or reduced aerobic capacity (Bateman, et al., 2001), which have been shown to reduce fitness in other patient groups including in arthritis (Harkcom, Lampman, Banwell, & Castor, 1985), multiple sclerosis (Petajan, 1986) and stroke (Macko, et al., 1997). It is well-known that sedentary lifestyles have negative effects on health and increase the risk of chronic disease in the general, healthy population. Physical disability may increase this risk even further. Research has shown that patients with TBI, specifically, are significantly more deconditioned than sedentary people without a disability (Mossberg, et al., 2007) and may thus be at even greater risk for cardiovascular disease, diabetes and other preventable diseases although this is yet to be determined in longitudinal studies. Promoting physical activity is therefore important in the prevention and management of secondary health issues in this client group.

Exercise programmes for brain injury are not a new concept and have been identified as an important part of rehabilitation since the 1950s (Torp, 1956). However, the majority of published research in this field concentrates on interventions for rehabilitation, which are targeted at a specific disability, such as physical therapy interventions to improve gait, ambulation or sitting balance, or to restore cognitive or motor function. Exercise is known to provide physiological benefits for brain injury, and newer restorative activity-based therapies (ABTs) such as constraint-induced therapy, virtual reality, robotic therapy and treadmill training techniques are being developed and have been used for rehabilitation purposes with mixed findings (Dromerick, Lum, & Hidler, 2006). A detailed review of rehabilitation treatment strategies, which include exercise intervention, is provided by Marshall, et al. (2007).

Research in the 1990s showed that aerobic exercise may help to decrease some of the difficulties experienced by people with TBI, including health problems, cognitive challenges and depression. The positive benefits of exercise were identified in the late 1990s, when Gordon, et al. (1998) demonstrated improvements in general health and mood status with physical exercise. In this retrospective community study, 240 individuals with TBI (64 exercisers and 176 non-exercisers), and 139 individuals without a disability (66 exercisers and 73 non-exercisers) were assessed on scales measuring disability and handicap. Whilst there were no observable differences between exercisers and non-exercisers on measures of disability and handicap, this study showed that TBI exercisers were less depressed than non-exercising individuals with TBI, and further, they reported fewer symptoms and had better self-reported health status than non-exercising individuals. In this study, individuals with TBI who exercised reported fewer physical, emotional and cognitive complaints and symptoms, including sleep problems, irritability, forgetting and being disorganised. By contrast, the non-exercising individuals with TBI reported more of these symptoms. Exercisers with TBI were also less depressed and more often engaged in school, work or community activities than non-exercisers with TBI. Finally, the study showed that exercisers had more severe brain injuries than the non-exercisers. Although this study did not account for health and lifestyle prior to the brain injury, and is limited by retrospective methodology and non-randomised design, it may suggest that a severe injury does not prevent patients from engaging in exercise.

Brain Health and Plasticity

In addition to the published literature evaluating the effects of exercise on general health, cardiorespiratory fitness and wellbeing, there is a body of evidence, which argues for a link between exercise and brain health, based on animal models of TBI and stroke. It has been argued that a pattern of exercise before brain injury can promote a defense against cell death from TBI. It is also becoming increasingly clear that behavioural stimulation and exercise post-TBI can have a positive impact on brain health and plasticity, reactivating the mechanism of healing. It has been suggested that physical activity be employed as a tool to improve neural function both in healthy adults and in patients suffering from neurological damage (Achiron & Kalron, 2008). Exercise activates molecular and cellular cascades that support and maintain brain plasticity (Cotman & Berchtold, 2002).

Studies based on animal models have shown that voluntary exercise can increase levels of brain-derived neurotrophic factor (BDNF) and other growth factors, stimulate neurogenesis, increase resistance to brain insult and improve learning and general mental performance (Cotman & Berchtold, 2002). Specifically, clinical studies have shown that exercise increases brain volume in areas implicated in executive processing. With regards intensity of exercise required to optimise neurotrophins, studies have suggested that moderation is important, with sustained increases in neurotrophin levels occurring with prolonged low intensity exercise (Ploughman, 2008). By contrast, animal models have suggested that high intensity exercise immediately after TBI can be damaging since it is associated with elevated levels of the stress hormone, corticosterone.

It has therefore been suggested that moderate intensity physical activity is critical particularly for young people with physical disabilities (Ploughman, 2008).

Psychological Benefits of Exercise in TBI

Traumatic brain injury can be associated with negative psychological outcomes. A study of psychiatric illnesses following TBI found that 34% of those patients with mild TBI had a high initial and ongoing risk of persistent psychiatric illness (Fann, et al., 2004). Depression and anxiety are common sequalae of TBI. Patients who are depressed will typically experience a loss of pleasure in activities they previously found enjoyable, have feelings of sadness and worthlessness, difficulty concentrating and altered appetite and patterns of sleep. A large proportion of TBI patients experience depression and it is estimated that the number of TBI patients experiencing major depression is ten times the incidence usually found in the general population (Hibbard, et al., 1998).

Many TBI patients suffer from anxiety disorders after their brain injury. These may include post-traumatic stress disorders, in which patients experience 'flashbacks' of the incident or event which caused their brain injury, or phobias, in which the patients experiences great fear centred on a specific situation (e.g. being in a car or on an aeroplane). It has been estimated that these occur after traumatic brain injury at twice the incidence usually found in the general population (Hibbard, et al., 1998).

Emotional disturbances in TBI are frequently treated with medications or psychotherapy. However, exercise at an appropriate level for the patient is increasingly proposed as an alternative and sustainable treatment for psychological conditions after TBI. Aerobic exercise is known to assist with tension and fatigue, and help to increase energy levels and improve self-esteem.

Health Risk Screening Prior to Exercise Intervention

It is beyond the scope of this chapter to discuss in detail the health risk factors to be screened before exercise in the TBI population. However, a proper medical referral or health evaluation screening is essential before an exercise regime is implemented. Researchers in Canada used a modified Delphi technique to obtain group consensus on the health risk factors that need to be verified before starting an exercise programme or intervention with TBI patients. The study included expert opinions from 31 rehabilitation professionals (RPs) from nine rehabilitation centres throughout the province of Québec (Vitale, et al., 1996). A total of 87 items were generated, which the authors grouped into 27 health risk factors, and each RP rated each for importance on a five point likert-type scale. Factors that were considered important by at least 50% of RPs included angina pectoris, aortic stenosis, exertional syncope, musculoskeletal sequelae, which are exacerbated by exercise, outward aggressivity, pulmonary embolism, uncontrolled epilepsy (seizures), and ventricular arrhythmias. Such factors may be considered in the development of exercise intervention as part of a tailored rehabilitation programme.

Review of Outcomes of Exercise Intervention

The benefits of physical activity for physical and psychological health are well-documented (Biddle, 2001; Brooks, Fahey, & White, 2001) and increasing activity levels has become an important public health priority internationally. The benefits of exercise and the need to increase population physical activity are certainly recognised and advocated in UK government policy documents (Department of Health (DH), 2004).

In traumatic brain injury specifically, the structure and routine often associated with exercise regimens can be beneficial and impact positively on psychosocial outcomes for people with TBI. For example, it has been suggested that the well-established positive effects of structured exercise intervention on social support, psychological well-being and feelings of autonomy may assist in long-term rehabilitation following brain injury (Driver, 2004).

Despite this knowledge from the research literature, in practice, British investigations into community and support services for long-term care for brain injury revealed a paucity of services for physical and psychological adjustment, which contributed to the development of the UK government National Service Framework for Long-Term Conditions (DH, 2008). Although there is published evidence suggesting that exercise is important for targeted rehabilitation, there is a dearth of quality research evidence investigating the outcomes of general exercise programmes for fitness or health benefit in clients after TBI. Yet therapists can play a key role in promoting healthy lifestyles and encouraging exercise that is individually tailored to the physical condition and abilities of each person. Physical therapists aim to increase flexibility, improve strength, improve cardiorespiratory endurance, improve muscular endurance and improve range of motion. By developing an individual exercise regime, the therapist can help to improve physical conditioning and recommend the nature and type of activities to be undertaken, whilst providing support and guidance for the afflicted individual. Muscle stretching and gentle exercise may be important in reducing or avoiding spasticity and research has shown that exercise intervention may indeed be effective without increasing spasticity in TBI (e.g. Bateman, et al., 2001).

The literature on general exercise interventions in TBI is limited with few large-scale randomised trials, therefore a discussion of a range of evidence in this field is presented. This highlights areas for further research and helps to identify future directions in this field, including alternative strategies for exercise intervention.

Review Methods

A literature search was undertaken of exercise interventions with adults with TBI. This was not a systematic review of the published evidence, although provides a general overview of the outcomes of key exercise interventions in TBI. These studies included only general exercise or fitness interventions targeted at either wellbeing or specific fitness parameters, including aerobic conditioning, strength and power, flexibility or muscle endurance. These studies included both physical and psychosocial outcomes. Interventions focused on targeted rehabilitation of a specific disability were not included, and these include Virtual Reality or ABT studies, which may have a different rationale than physiological. Published research between 1990–2008 was considered, with an increasing number of studies published in more recent years reflecting developments in policy and practice in the rehabilitation of individuals with long-term conditions. The review included only studies where participants were adults with acquired TBI in any setting, using exercise as the sole component, the main component or a partial component of intervention. Review articles were included. Key search terms were: physical activity, exercise, traumatic brain injury, TBI, disabilities, rehabilitation, entered into MEDLINE and CINAHL (nursing and allied health).

REVIEW FINDINGS

Physical Conditioning

Early research centred around physical conditioning suggested that there may be a role for physical activity in the development of physical work capacity, by incorporating physical conditioning within a rehabilitation programme for people with brain injury (Sullivan, Richer, & Laurent, 1990). Early studies with late brain-injured patients also showed improvements in fitness although lacked standardized measures for outcomes and lacked a control comparison group (Hunter et al, 1990; Jankowski & Sullivan, 1990). For example, Jankowski and Sullivan (1990) assessed the value of exercise training in 14 sedentary adults with TBI. Participants in this study performed a supervised circuit training program three times per week for 16 consecutive weeks. The program was designed to include equal volumes of both aerobic and neuromuscular training to increase the subjects' oxidative capacity and improve their locomotor efficiency. The researchers measured height, weight, blood pressure, skinfold thickness, grip strength, abdominal muscular endurance, and submaximal and peak rates of oxygen consumption before and after the intervention and the index of physiological fatigue was calculated. TBI patients manifested subnormal oxidative capacities and above-average oxygen costs locomotion. These authors found a beneficial effect of exercise intervention on oxidative capacity and abdominal muscular endurance but no improvement in the oxygen cost of walking. Despite the small sample size, this work does suggest that moderate and prolonged muscular and aerobic physical activity may be beneficial in the rehabilitation of patients with TBI (Jankowski & Sullivan, 1990).

Bhambhani, Rowland, & Farag (2005) found mixed findings in an evaluation of a 12-week circuit-training programme designed to enhance muscular strength, endurance and aerobic fitness in moderate to severe brain injured inpatients (n=14) in a community rehabilitation hospital(time since injury = 17.2+/-17 months). The authors looked at changes in peak cardiorespiratory function and body composition in a time-series design consisting of 32 1-hour sessions. Although body composition did not alter significantly, peak cardiorespiratory responses improved but required more than 6 weeks of training. Although this study may have implications for maintaining functional independence of TBI patients following discharge, the study needs to be replicated with a larger sample.

Some research has focused on improving specific functions and components of fitness with physical exercise. Often these interventions are focused on rehabilitation of injury or regaining specific motor functions rather than assessing outcomes of exercise on general health and well-being. These studies include neuromuscular training (Jankowski & Sullivan, 1990), arm ability training (Platz, Winter, & Muller, 2001), and balance and coordination training (Dault & Dugas, 2002). For example, Dault and Dugas (2002) focused on the impact of aerobic exercise specifically on balance and coordination in patients with TBI. Whilst the intervention here was aerobic exercise, the outcomes measured were not aerobic fitness but rather the effects of aerobic intervention on specific TBI impairments. These researchers evaluated the effectiveness of an aerobic dancing training programme designed to reduce postural imbalance and coordination deficits in these patients. These researchers compared outcomes of aerobic dancing (Slide and Step Programme – specific training/ST) with traditional muscular training (TMT). In this study aerobic dancing training improved both coordination and postural sway compared with muscular-based training.

Aerobic Fitness

Aerobic fitness has also been targeted in exercise interventions reported in the literature (Bateman. et al., 2001; Hunter, Tomberlin, & Kirkikis, 1990; Lapier, Sirotnak, & Alexander, 1998; Santiago, Coyle, & Kinney, 1993). In a randomized controlled trial (n=157), Bateman, et al. (2001) examined the impact of a 3-month cycle ergonometer aerobic training intervention with brain injured inpatients early after injury, compared with a control group taking relaxation classes. Outcomes included physical function and psychological measures, taken pre- and post-intervention and 3months later. The exercise training group exhibited better exercise capacity with an improvement to cardiovascular fitness, when compared to controls. However, this improvement was not also evident in functional independence, mobility or psychological function either post-intervention or at follow-up. Findings were consistent with an earlier study of exercise participation in chronic brain injury (Gordon, et al., 1998). This work showed that exercise participation for brain injured individuals is feasible, as there was no evidence of increased spasticity or greater occurrence of spasticity in those who participated. The sample size was larger than many of the exercise interventions reported in the literature and included assessment of functional and psychological outcomes. However, results suggested that although aerobic activity such as cycling may improve fitness, it may not be enough to affect change in psychological outcome. It may be that a different form of exercise intervention is required to improve social or psychological outcomes, which are important aspects of quality of life after brain injury.

Early Intervention

Studies targeting intervention early after brain injury are limited. Research evidence has showed that brain-injured patients with a range of disabilities are able to participate in an aerobic exercise programme during early inpatient rehabilitation (Jackson, et al., 2001). In this intervention, patients in one of four neurological inpatient units cycled for up to 30 minutes three times weekly for

24–36 sessions over 12 weeks. Ninety patients started the intervention and 55 of these completed 24 sessions. The researchers measured mean cycling time and the number of sessions required to reach a 30 minute cycling time. The study showed that participation in exercise is plausible early in rehabilitation, although patients vary in the length of time it takes them to achieve an adequate intensity of aerobic exercise.

Exercise in the Community and Aquatic Interventions

Although early intervention in acute or rehabilitation facilities is important, many patients with brain injuries live out in the community, adjusting to a range of physical, behavioural, cognitive and emotional impairments. Community facilities are therefore central in assisting with this adjustment and improving quality of life for brain injured individuals. Participants in exercise studies are often recruited from hospital or residential care facilities and training is often conducted in a laboratory environment rather than a community setting (e.g. Bateman, et al., 2001; Jackson, et al., 2001).

Studies incorporating exercise programmes for brain injured patients in the community are few, although these have shown promising findings, particularly aquatic interventions. Aquatic recreation therapy is ideal as part of a lifetime physical activity and recreation program after brain injury. Exercise in water allows brain injured individuals to attempt patterns of movement without fear of falling or weakness, which can be common barriers to engaging in physical activity (Driver, O'Connor, Lox, & Reese, 2003). Completing physical movements in water also aids in strengthening of postural muscles and improving stability, which can be particularly important for individuals with brain injury in whom balance may be compromised (Hrenko, Rees, Lox, & O'Connor, 2003). Aquatic rehabilitation programmes, and indeed any form of exercise intervention, need to be tailored according to the level of physical and cognitive functioning exhibited by the individual, and the reader is referred to (Lepore, 1987) for further practical guidance.

In a randomized controlled trial ($n=16$), Driver, O'Connor, Lox, & Rees (2004) evaluated the outcome of an 8-week aquatic exercise intervention on cardiovascular endurance, body composition, muscular strength, endurance and flexibility. Eight participants were assigned to the aquatic exercise group and eight participants were assigned to a control group. Outcomes were assessed pre- and post- intervention. The authors found that physical fitness increased in the intervention group, which in turn impacted on functional capacity of individuals who participated, and resulted in an increased ability to complete activities of daily living. These benefits were not observed in the control group. Although the sample size was small, this study showed that aquatic exercise may therefore improve fitness in individuals with brain injury living in the community, and also positively impact on both primary and secondary outcomes of brain injury by improving physical skills required for daily living and increasing participant's sense of autonomy. Exercise interventions in brain injured patients living in the community are therefore promising although further research is needed to evaluate different forms of exercise with standardized measures, and longer follow-up periods. In this type of intervention, the therapist's role would be crucial in encouraging adherence to an exercise regime, recommending individual programmes, and offering advice, information and support.

Psychological Outcomes of Exercise Intervention

Therapeutic physical activity has a crucial role in the psychological rehabilitation of brain injured patients. Aquatic interventions may have a positive influence on psychological outcomes for the brain injured patient. It has been suggested that this form of exercise helps individuals to understand their bodies, a concept which holds particular relevance for individuals with brain injury who often lack feeling and awareness of what their body is doing (Lepore, et al., 1998). Furthermore, there are known therapeutic effects of water-based exercise including muscle relaxation, increased range and motion of joints, improvements in muscular strength and endurance and relief of pain and muscle spasms. These factors may all contribute to increased self-awareness, self-efficacy or self-esteem and an overall increase in enjoyment of life for individuals with TBI as they become able to complete tasks on their own (Lepore, et al., 1998).

Tai Chi Chuan (TCC), an ancient form of Chinese martial arts, has been used as an effective intervention for patients with brain injury and has shown to have a positive influence on patient mood (Gemmell & Leathem, 2006; Shapira, et al., 2001). For example, Shapira and colleagues present three case reports of patients with severe head injury who had undergone TCC therapy, and found reductions in mental stress and frustration. Although these subjective findings are reported in the context of assisting rehabilitation, TCC has implications for engaging TBI patients in the community with group exercise activities for general benefits to health and well-being. However, TCC requires complex and precise movements that, with normal coordination abilities, can take many years to master. In comparison, Qigong, an ancient form of Chinese therapeutic exercise uses more simplified movements to facilitate balance and awareness of mind and body. This method has been employed with older adults to increase coordination and flexibility for the prevention of falls (Dupoy, Borfiga, & Richardson, 2002) and is currently used in practice at TBI community day centres (see Figure 1). It is proposed that Qigong may be a suitable method of exercise intervention for individuals with brain injuries since it involves less complex movement and is therefore accessible to a wider brain injured population over a set intervention period.

In the UK, a single centre pilot randomised controlled trial (n=20) compared an eight week Tai Chi Chuan Qigong intervention with non-exercise based social and leisure activities (Blake & Batson, 2009). Tai Chi Chuan Qigong ('Qigong') has many potential health benefits including increased relaxation, flexibility, balance, coordination, strengthening and posture. It is a low intensity physical activity, and unlike many types of exercise, is accessible to people of all ages and physical conditions. Since this exercise form is not strenuous it carries no potentially harmful side effects. A certified instructor with seven years experience in working with individuals with brain injury in the local area conducted the Qigong sessions at a community day centre, and these sessions included a combination of both hard and soft martial arts techniques called 'Neigong'. Each session started with chair based stretching and warm-up followed by work in self-hand massage reflexology. The original 'Shibashi', an 18-style form of Qigong, was adapted for seated instruction for individuals with a range of physical impairments. The Shibashi Qigong programme combines traditional Qigong breathing and movements with the Tai Chi Yang form. All eighteen postures were covered by week eight of the intervention.

Outcome was assessed at baseline and post-intervention using the General Health Questionnaire-12, the Physical Self-Description Questionnaire and the Social Support for Exercise Habits Scale, to measure perceived mood, self-esteem, flexibility, coordination, physical activity and social support. In this study, the intervention and control groups were comparable at baseline. After the intervention, mood was significantly improved in the exercise group when compared with controls. Improvements in self-esteem and mood across the study period were also evident in the exercise group only. There were no significant differences in physical functioning between groups. This study provides preliminary evidence that a brief Qigong exercise intervention programme may improve mood and self-esteem for individuals with TBI (Blake & Batson, 2009). However, in view of the small sample size and short follow-up period, these findings need to be tested in a large-scale randomised trial, to confirm the findings but also to ascertain whether some participants benefited more than others, and if so, why.

The need to provide interventions for people with long-term conditions and disabilities, which focus on quality of life and prevention of secondary health complications, is now recognised. As a result, ccommunity-based rehabilitation centres (e.g. those run by 'Headway' in the UK) are focusing more on increasing independence in people with TBI and decreasing further injury or disability through engagement in exercise activities to promote strength building, flexibility, coordination, and self-reliance. A case study is presented below which demonstrates the practical implications of a single small-scale research study on a rehabilitation service in the UK (Figure 1).

Case Study – Headway House, UK
Community Day Centre, Brain Injury Rehabilitation

Headway is a registered charity which operates several community day centres around the UK. Headway House in Nottingham is a day centre for individuals with brain injury located just 15 minutes outside the city centre. There are presently 50 members from the community who regularly visit the centre with an average of 10 to 15 members attending per day. In 2008, as part of a pilot randomised controlled trial research study in conjunction with the University of Nottingham (UK), registered members were invited to take part in a study investigating the outcomes of a Tai Chi/Qigong exercise intervention. Participants randomised to the exercise group received one hour per week of seated Qigong exercise instruction. Participants in the comparison group engaged in one hour per week of usual social and leisure activities offered at the centre. Participants completed questionnaires before and after to assess self-reported physical function and psychological outcomes. It was observed that mood and self-esteem were improved in the group who received the exercise intervention.

In addition to the positive outcomes of the research study, it was noted that the weekly exercise sessions had been integrated successfully into Headway's existing programme of activities and were well-received by those individuals with TBI who took part, and their families. Exercise classes in various forms had been available at the centre periodically in previous years although this was the first time that Tai Chi/Qigong had been offered at one of the centres. On the basis of this pilot intervention, the exercise classes were continued after the study ended and made available to all members of the centre, thus improving the local community services available to individuals with brain injury at that time. This intervention helped to address the public health priority of increasing physical activity levels in the population, particularly for those with long-term conditions.

Figure 1. Brain Injury Rehabilitation Case Study

CONCLUSION

Exercise and rehabilitation go hand in hand. Despite the limitations of the published literature, there is an emerging body of evidence to suggest that physical exercise is beneficial for individuals with TBI due to positive effects on physical and cognitive function, psychological health and psychosocial outcomes. As the importance of exercise is increasingly recognised in practice in the development of rehabilitation programmes, so the need for more well-designed research studies increases. In general, successful exercise programmes need to incorporate a combination of strength training, cardiovascular exercise and flexibility conditioning. The individual with brain injury has the same fitness needs as those of a non-injured person, however, exercise must be carefully tailored to the specific needs of each individual based on their physical and cognitive abilities, overall health profile and specific preferences for activities. Despite acknowledging the need for individual tailoring, there is still a need for further research to ascertain more about the type of exercise, the intensity and duration of intervention which will be of most benefit overall to people with TBI.

The UK National Service Framework for Long-Term Conditions (DH, 2008) has ensured government support in Britain for the improvement of services for people with brain injury. However, although evidence is now emerging, there is still a paucity of literature on the outcomes of exercise or physical activity programmes in TBI for fitness, general health and psychosocial reasons, rather than for physical therapy of specific motor impairment. There are government initiatives, which have raised national awareness of the benefits of promoting physical activity for health in Britain (e.g. 'Choosing Health' White Paper, DH, 2004). However, only recently has there been a focus on the impact of 'exercise for health' programmes for people with chronic disabilities. As a result, health promotion programmes are now developing which aim to improve patient quality of life and reduce occurrence of negative effects of secondary health conditions resulting from a sedentary lifestyle (Powell & Blair, 1994; Rimmer, 1999).

In addition, community-based support centres are focusing more on increasing and maintaining independence and reducing further disability through engagement in exercise activities to improve physical and psychological outcomes and promote self-reliance. The research evidence suggests that exercise interventions may be feasible early after brain injury (Jackson, et al., 2001), however, many patients are left living in the community for many years with long-term chronic disabilities and impairments. Intervention is required which would be appropriate for long-term rehabilitation of those left living in the community with the after-effects of TBI, and that which would help such individuals to further participation in physical activity.

Exercise Interventions: An Evaluation

Exercise interventions in brain injury are steadily emerging and a recent Cochrane review identified a small number of randomised trials reporting mixed outcomes of cardiorespitory fitness training (Hassett, Moseley, Tate, & Harmer, 2008). Aerobic studies are often in hospital or rehabilitation inpatient settings, focused on moderate to severe injury or lacking randomisation of participants. Psychological outcomes of interventions for people with traumatic brain injury, living in the community, are less available, although community-based aquatics programs based on small numbers of participants have shown increases in both functional capacity and physical self-esteem. Conventional forms of exercise such as water or gym-based activities have shown promise although may not suit all, yet little is known about less conventional forms of physical activity.

Tai Chi Chuan ('Tai Chi') is gaining popularity in the Western world and has demonstrated potential for both physiological and psychological benefits in those with chronic conditions. However, this ancient Chinese fitness and martial arts form can take several years to master for full benefit. Tai Chi Qigong ('Qigong') is a Chinese mindful exercise, based on similar principles, but is a simpler form requiring less physical and cognitive demands and is therefore proposed as suitable for individuals with traumatic brain injury at varying levels of function. It requires no equipment, can be practiced in the home and can be learned over a shorter period of time than Tai Chi, potentially giving participants a more immediate sense of independence, self-esteem and mastery of postures involved. The core components include concentration, relaxation, mind exercises, breathing exercises, body posture and movement. Qigong may serve to reduce self-perceived functional limitation and has a proposed anti-depressant effect (Tsang & Fung, 2008).

Tai Chi and Qigong are suggested to improve indicators of health-related quality of life and psychological health in chronic illness (Tsang & Fung, 2008; Wang, Collet, & Lau, 200). Confidence to exercise, coordination and flexibility have all improved with Tai Chi in an older population (Dupoy, et al., 2002). A community Tai Chi intervention in individuals with traumatic brain injury demonstrated improvements in mood, but not self-esteem (Gemmell & Leather, 2006), although the effects of either Tai Chi or Qigong in neurological samples is still unclear and at present evidence is based mostly on nonrandomised studies

(Dupoy, et al., 2002; Mills, Allen, & Morgan, 2000). Introducing Qigong exercise sessions within community day centre activities may help in making exercise more accessible to this group and set exercise within a social context (see Figure 1) since social support is known to influence physical activity participation (Driver, 2005) and Qigong has been shown to improve psychological outcomes in TBI although this is based on a small pilot randomised sample, is therefore inconclusive and warrants further investigation (Blake & Batson, 2009). Nevertheless, exercise interventions, which have potential to improve psychological outcomes, may therefore also help to support social integration and readjustment in TBI.

Limitations of the Evidence Base

Existing research studies are difficult to compare, as they are limited in number and often measure different outcomes. Some studies are laboratory based, others collect data in hospital or rehabilitation settings and others are based in the community. Many studies collect only self-report measures whereas supplementing these with objective, performance-based outcome measures would improve accuracy of data collection. Many exercise intervention studies exclude participants with moderate to severe cognitive impairment, however, by doing so they exclude a large proportion of the brain injured population. Conversely, those studies which collect questionnaire data but do not screen potential participants on neuropsychological measures means that it is difficult to ascertain to what extent participant responses may have been affected by limited awareness of their thoughts, feelings and behaviour, or difficulties in aggregating the occurrence of behaviours across times and situations. Furthermore, it may be that some participants benefit more than others from different forms of exercise intervention and whether this is the case, and the reasons for this are still unclear, with available studies either not considering this outcome or having samples too small to draw conclusions.

The primary outcomes of many exercise intervention studies are changes in physical fitness, time taken to engage in activity or body composition. Few studies have also included psychosocial outcomes of exercise intervention and those that have often concentrate on mood state as the key outcome, but tend not to consider other factors such as self-esteem or the potential social support benefits of participation. However, psychosocial outcomes are important, since engaging in activity with others is beneficial to mental health and it is well-documented that psychological factors such as depression can hinder recovery from illness (Jorge, et al., 2004). Furthermore, it has been suggested that the type and source of social support changes after brain injury (Driver, 2005) and that in this patient group, social influence from family, friends and caregivers is important and can impact on physical activity participation (Driver, 2007). Attendance at exercise interventions is variable and further research is needed to identify the determinants and barriers to exercise participation in TBI..

In addition to the potential influence of the caregiver on the patient and their willingness to participate in exercise programmes, few studies have explored the actual impact of exercise intervention on caring for adults with brain injury. Caregivers of any individual with chronic disability may be under considerable stress and at risk of depression and exercise intervention for patients with TBI could provide much needed respite. Furthermore, studies and reviews conducted with carers of brain injury and other neurological patients suggest that carer strain is common and carers are at risk of low mood (Blake, 2008; Blake and Lincoln, 2000; Blake, Lincoln, & Clarke, 2003; Watanabe, et al, 2000), which is important as mood of the carer can also negatively impact on patient recovery from illness. Future research should consider the impact of exercise intervention for the primary caregiver, and rehabilitation centres may consider incorporating caregivers within Qigong sessions to maximize the benefits and increase likelihood of home practice for both the person with TBI and their caregiver, outside of supervised session time. Finally, whilst exercise interventions for people with TBI are on the increase in practice, the cost-effectiveness of engaging in alternative forms of physical activity has not yet been assessed, but needs to be determined to inform future service development.

This chapter is by no means an exhaustive review although does provide an overview of previous and current interventions, future developments and most importantly, highlights the need for more research on the impact of exercise interventions on both physical and psychosocial outcomes in people with TBI.

KEY POINTS

1. Physical activity must be considered as part of the treatment plan for patients with TBI and exercise programmes now have a key role in rehabilitation practice

2. Research based on animal models has shown that exercise improves the ability of the brain to repair itself and can therefore help the body recover physical and cognitive function

3. Evidence for the effectiveness of exercise interventions in TBI is limited and research studies have many methodological weaknesses

4. However, the evidence is promising for a positive effect of exercise in various modalities on physical conditioning, and psychosocial outcomes.

5. More research is needed to clarify the type and intensity of exercise of most benefit, and the cost-effectiveness of exercise interventions in service delivery.

REFERENCES

Achiron, A., & Kalron, A. (2008). Physical activity: positive impact on brain plasticity. *Harefuah 147(3)*, 252-255, 276.

Basford, J., Chou, L., Kaufman, K., Brey, R., Walker, A., & Malec, A. (2003). An assessment of gait and balance deficits after traumatic brain injury. *Archives of Physical Medicine and Rehabilitation, 84(3)*, 343–349.

Bateman, A., Culpan, F., Pickering, A., Powell, J., Scott, O., & Greenwood, R (2001). The effect of aerobic training on rehabilitation outcomes after recent severe brain injury: A randomized controlled evaluation. *Archives of Physical Medicine and Rehabilitation, 82*, 174–82.

Bhambhani, Y., Rowland, G., & Farag, M. (2005). Effects of circuit training on body composition and peak cardiorespiratory responses in patients with moderate to severe traumatic brain injury. *Archives of Physical Medicine and Rehabilitation, 82(2)*, 268–76.

Biddle, S., & Mutrie, N. (2001). *Psychology of physical activity.* Routledge: New York.

Blake, H., & Batson, M. (2009). Exercise intervention in brain injury: a pilot randomised study of Tai Chi Qigong. *Clinical Rehabilitation.* In Press.

Blake, H. (2008). Caregiver stress in traumatic brain injury. *International Journal of Therapy and Rehabilitation, 15(5)*, 263-271.

Blake, H., Lincoln, N.B., & Clarke, D.D. (2003). Caregiver strain in spouses of stroke patients. *Clinical Rehabilitation, 17,* 312–317.

Blake, H., & Lincoln, N.B. (2000). Factors associated with strain in co-resident spouses of stroke patients. *Clinical Rehabilitation, 14(3),* 307–314.

Brooks, G., Fahey, T., & White, T. (2001). *Exercise physiology (3rd Edition).*Mayfield Publishing Company: San Diego, CA

Chesnut, R., Carney, N., Maynard, H., Patterson, P., Mann, N., & Helfand, M. (1999). *Evidence Report: Rehabilitation for Traumatic Brain Injury.* Rockville, MD: Agency for Health Care Policy and Research, 1-81.

Cotman, C.W., & Berchtold, N.C. (2002). Exercise: a behavioural intervention to enhance brain health and plasticity. *TRENDS in Neurosciences, 25(6),* 295-301.

Dault, M., & Dugas, C. (2002). Evaluation of a specific balance and coordination programme for individuals with a traumatic brain injury. *Brain Injury, 16,* 231–44.

Department of Health. (2004.) *Choosing Health: Making healthy choices easier.* Retrieved 26 February, 2009, from: http://www.dh.gov.uk/en/Publicationsandstatistics/Publications/PublicationsPolicyAndGuidance/DH_4094550.

Department of Health. (2008). *Long Term Conditions.* Retrieved 25 February, 2009, from: http://www.dh.gov.uk/en/Healthcare/NationalServiceFrameworks/Longtermconditions/index.htm.

Driver, S., O'Connor, J., Lox, C., & Rees, K. (2003). Effects of an aquatics program on psychosocial experiences of individuals with brain injuries: a pilot study. *Journal of Cognitive Rehabilitation, 21(1),* 22-31.

Driver, S., O'Connor, J., Lox, C., & Rees, K. (2004). Evaluation of an aquatics programme on fitness parameters of individuals with a brain injury. *Brain Injury, 18(9),* 847–869.

Driver, S. (2005). Social support and the physical activity behaviours of people with a brain injury. *Brain Injury, 19(3),* 1067–75.

Driver, S., Rees, K., O'Conner, J., & Lox, C. (2006). Aquatics, health-promoting self-care behaviours and adults with brain injuries. *Brain Injury, 20,* 133-141.

Driver, S. (2007). Psychometric properties and analysis of the physical activity Social Influence Scale for adults with traumatic brain injuries. *Adapted Physical Activity Quarterly, 24(2),* 160–170.

Dromerick, A.W., Lum, P.S., & Hidler, J. (2006). Activity-based therapies. *NeuroRx, 3(4),* 428–438.

Dupoy, M., Borfiga, T., & Richardson, M. (2002). Dao Yi Yang Sheng Gong: reducing the risk of falls. *The Journal of the Institute of Ageing and Health, 8,* 17–21.

Durstine, J.L, Painter, P., Franklin, B.A., Morgan, D., Pitetti, K.H, & Roberts, S.O. (2000). Physical Activity for the Chronically Ill and Disabled. *Sports Medicine, 30,* 207-19.

Fann, J.R., Burington, B., Leonetti, A., Jaffe, K., Katon, W.J., & Thompson, R.S. (2004). Psychiatric illness following traumatic brain injury in an adult health maintenance organization population. *Archives of General Psychiatry, 61(1),* 53-61.

Gemmell, C., & Leathem, J. (2006). A study investigating the effects of Tai Chi Chuan: individuals with traumatic brain injury compared to controls. *Brain Injury, 20(2),* 151–156.

Goldstein, L. (2006). Neurotransmitters and motor activity: effects on functional recovery after brain injury. *NeuroRx, 3(4),* 451–457.

Gordon, W.A., Sliwinski, M., Echo, J., McLoughlin, M., Sheerer, M., & Meili, T.E. (1998). The benefits of exercise on individuals with traumatic brain injury: a retrospective study. *Journal of Head Trauma Rehabilitation, 13,* 58–67.

Harkcom, T., Lampman, R., Banwell, B., & Castor, C. (1985). Therapeutic value of graded aerobic exercise training in rheumatoid arthritis. *Arthritis Rheumatism, 28,* 32–39.

Hassett, L., Moseley, A.M., Tate, R., & Harmer, AR. (2008). Fitness training for cardiorespitory conditioning after traumatic brain injury. *Cochrane Database of Systematic Reviews, 2,* Art. No.: CD006123. DOI:10.1002/14651858.CD006123.pub2.

Hibbard, M., Uysal, S., Kepler, K., Bogdany, J., & Silver, J. (1998). Axis I psychopathology in individuals with TBI: a retrospective study. *Journal of Head Trauma Rehabilitation, 13(4),* 24-39.

Hrenko, B.K., Rees, K.S., Lox, C., & O'Connor, J. (2003). *The effects of aquatic and land exercise on activities of daily living among individuals with traumatic brain injury.* Unpublished master's thesis, Southern Illinois University: Edwardsville.

Hunter, M., Tomberlin, J., Kirkikis, C. (1990). Progressive exercise testing in closed head-injured subjects: comparison of exercise apparatus in assessment of a physical conditioning program. *Physical Therapy, 70,* 363–371.

Jackson, D., Turner-Stokes, L., Culpan, J., Bateman, A., Scott, O., Powell, J., & Greenwood, R. (2001). Can brain-injured patients participate in an aerobic exercise programme during early inpatient rehabilitation? *Clinical Rehabilitation, 15(5),* 535–544.

Jankowski, L.W., & Sullivan, S.J. (1990). Aerobic and neuromuscular training: effect on the capacity, efficiency, and fatigability of patients with traumatic brain injuries. *Archives of Physical Medicine and Rehabilitation, 71(7),* 500–504.

Jorge, R.E., Robinson, R.G., Moser, D., Tateno, A., Crespo-Facorro, B., & Arndt, S. (2004). Major depression following traumatic brain injury. *Archives of General Psychiatry, 61(1),* 42-50.

Lapier, T., Sirotnak, N., Alexander, K. (1998). Aerobic exercise for a patient with chronic multisystem impairments. *Physical Therapy, 78,* 417–424.

Lepore, G. (1987). Teaching aquatic activities to persons with head injuries. *National Aquatics Journal,* 8-9.

Lepore, M., Gayle, G.W., & Stevens, S. (1998). *Adapted aquatics programming: A professional guide.* Champaign, IL: Human Kinetics.

Lippert-Grüner, M., Maegele, M., Pokorny, J., Angelov, D.N., Swetkova, O., Wittner, M., & Trojan, S. (2007). Early rehabilitation model shows positive effects on neural degeneration and recovery from neuromotor deficits following traumatic brain injury. *Physiological Research, 56(3),* 359–368.

Macko, R., DeSouza, C., Tretter, L., Silver, K.H., Smith, G.V., Anderson, P.A., Tomoyasu, N., Gorman, P., & Dengel, D.R. (1997). Treadmill aerobic exercise training reduces the energy expenditure and cardiovascular demands of hemiparetic gait in chronic stroke patients. *Stroke, 28,* 326–330.

Marshall, S., Teasell, R., Bayona, N., Lippert, C., Chundamala, J., Villamere, J., Mackie, D., Cullen, N., & Bayley, M. (2007). Motor impairment rehabilitation post acquired brain injury. *Brain Injury, 21(2),* 133–160.

Masanic, C., & Bayley, M. (1998). Interrater reliability of neurologic soft signs in an acquired brain injury population. *Archives of Physical Medicine and Rehabilitation, 79,* 811–815.

Max, W., Mackenzie, E., & Rice, D. (1991). Head Injuries: cost and consequences. *Journal of Head Trauma Rehabilitation, 6,* 76-91.

Mills, N., Allen, J., & Morgan, C. (2000). Does Tai Chi/Qi Gong help patients with Multiple Sclerosis? *Journal of Bodywork and Movement Therapies, 4,* 39-48.

Mossberg, K., Ayala, D., Baker, T., Heard, J., & Masel, B. (2007). Aerobic capacity after traumatic brain injury: comparison with a nondisabled cohort. *Archives of Physical Medicine and Rehabilitation, 88(3),* 315–20.

Moulton, C., & Yates, D. (1999). *Lecture notes on emergency medicine. Head Injury* (2nd Edition). Blackwell Science Ltd: Oxford, UK.

Petajan, J., Gappmaier, E., White, A., Spencer, M., Mino, L., & Hicks, R. (1996). Impact of aerobic training on fitness and quality of life in multiple sclerosis. *Annals of Neurology, 39,* 432–441.

Platz, T., Winter, T., & Muller, N. (2001). Arm ability training for stroke and traumatic brain injury patients with mild arm paresis: a single-blind, randomized, controlled trial. *Archives of Physical Medicine and Rehabilitation, 82,* 961–968.

Ploughman, M. (2008). Exercise is brain food: the effects of physical activity on cognitive function. *Developmental Neurorehabilitation, 11(3),* 236-240.

Poretta, D. (2000). Cerebral Palsy, stroke and traumatic brain injury. In J.P. Winnick (Ed.), *Adapted physical education and sport* (pp. 187-196). Champaign: Human Kinetics.

Powell, K., & Blair, S. (1994). The public health burdens of sedentary living habits: theoretical but realistic estimates. *Medicine and Science in Sports and Exercise, 26,* 851–856.

Quinn, B., & Sullivan, J. (2000). The identification by physiotherapists of the physical problems resulting from a mild traumatic brain injury. *Brain Injury, 14,* 1063–1076.

Rimmer, J. (1999). Health promotion for people with disabilities: the emerging paradigm shift from disability prevention to prevention of secondary conditions. *Physical Therapy, 79(5),* 495–502.

Rinne, M., Pasanen, M., Vartiainen, M., Lehto, T., Sarajuuri, J., & Alaranta, H. (2006). Motor performance in physically well-recovered men with traumatic brain injury. *Journal of Rehabilitation Medicine, 38(4),* 224–229.

Santiago, M., Coyle, C., & Kinney, W. (1993). Aerobic exercise effect on individuals with physical disabilities. *Archives of Physical Medicine and Rehabilitation, 74,* 1192–1198.

Scherzer, B. (1986). Rehabilitation following severe head trauma: results of a three-year program. *Archives of Physical Medicine and Rehabilitation, 67(6),* 366–374.

Shapira, M., Chelouche, M., Yannai, R., Kaner, C., & Szold, A. (2001). Tai Chi Chuan practice as a tool for rehabilitation of severe head trauma: 3 case reports. *Archives of Physical Medicine and Rehabilitation, 82,* 1283–1285.

Sosin, D., Sniezek, J., & Thurman, D. (1996). Incidence of mild and moderate brain injury in the United States, 1991. *Brain Injury, 10,* 47–54.

Sullivan, S., Richer, E., & Laurent, F. (1990). The role of and possibilities for physical conditioning programmes in the rehabilitation of traumatically brain-injured persons. *Brain Injury, 4(4),* 407–414.

Taylor, W., Baranowski, T., & Young, D. (1998). Physical activity interventions in low-income, ethnic minority and populations with a disability. *American Journal of Preventive Medicine, 15,* 334–343.

Torp, M. (1956). An exercise program for the brain-injured. *Physical Therapy Review, 36(10),* 664–675.

Tsang, H.W.H., & Fung, K.M.T. (2008). A review on neurobiological and psychological mechanisms underlying the anti-depressive effect of Qigong exercise. Journal of Health Psychology, 13(7), 857-863.

Van der Ploeg, H., Van der Beek, A., Van der Woude, L., & Mechelen, W.V. (2004). Physical activity for people with a disability: a conceptual model. *Sports Medicine, 34(10),* 639–649.

Vitale, A.E, Sullivan. S.J, Jankowski, L.W., Fleury, J., Lefrancois, C. & Lebouthillier E. (1996). Screening of health risk factors prior to exercise or a fitness evaluation of adults with traumatic brain injury: a consensus by rehabilitation professionals. *Brain Injury, 10(5),* 367-375.

Wang, C., Collet, J.P., & Lau, J. (2004). The effect of Tai Chi on health outcomes in chronic conditions: a systematic review. *Archives of Internal Medicine, 164,* 493-501.

Watanabe, Y., Shiel, A., Asami, T., Taki, K., & Tabuchi, K. (2000). An evaluation of neurobehavioural problems as perceived by family members and levels of family stress 1–3 years following traumatic brain injury in Japan. *Clinical Rehabilitation, 14,* 172–177.

Zoerink, D.D., & Lauener, K. (1991). Effects of a leisure education program on adults with traumatic brain injury. *Therapeutic Recreation Journal, 25(3),* 19-28.

In: Physical Activity in Rehabilitation and Recovery   ISBN: 978-1-60876-400-6
Editor: Holly Blake   © 2010 Nova Science Publishers, Inc.

Chapter 6

AEROBIC AND RESISTANCE EXERCISE IN PATIENTS WITH CONGESTIVE HEART FAILURE

*Pamela Bartlo**

Physical Therapy Department, D'Youville College;
NY 14201; U.S.A.

ABSTRACT

Congestive heart failure (CHF) is a common disease that leads to multiple body system changes. People with CHF experience difficulties with left ventricular function and heart rate control. They also sustain changes at the skeletal muscles that lead to inefficiencies in muscle function. These central and peripheral changes lead to multiple symptoms, the most common of which are decreased exercise tolerance and dyspnoea. Research has focused on exercise for people with CHF and has shown promising results. Both aerobic and resistance exercise have been shown to have positive effects on the cardiovascular system and several peripheral systems. Exercise has been shown to be safe and able to improve the quality of life for people with CHF. Recommendations for exercise prescription, based on the literature, are outlined in this chapter.

---

* Tel: 716-829-8390 ; Fax: 716-829-7680 ; e-mail: bartlop@dyc.edu

INTRODUCTION

Vascular diseases continue to be the leading causes of death in most industrial countries.(World Health Organization, 2008) These disorders include ischemic heart disease and cerebrovascular accidents. In most of these countries heart disease is the leading cause of death with rates varying from 6% of all deaths in France to 30% of all deaths in Russia. In the United States, in adults ages 65-74 years, 60% of males and 40% of females are diagnosed with CHF.(American Heart Association, 2006) In Australia, approximately 1.5-2% of the population is affected by heart failure and approximately 2-2.3% in the UK.(World Health Organization, 2008) CHF is a complex disease process that leads to multiple body system changes. Extensive physiologic research has shown impairments in left ventricular function, autonomic nervous system functions, and peripheral changes.(Beniaminovitz, Lang, LaManca, & Mancini 2002; Braith & Beck, 2008; Delagardelle & Feiereisen, 2005; Freimark et al., 2007; Levinger, Bronks, Cody, Linton, & Davie, 2005; National Institute for Clinical Excellence, 2003; Pu et al., 2001; Wise, 2007)

This chapter will meet the following objectives:

- Explain the physiologic changes that occur due to CHF
- Review the history of exercise in relation to CHF
- Provide a thorough review of the current literature and how it supports aerobic and resistance exercise for people with CHF
- Examine safety of exercise for this population and the impact that exercise has on mortality for people with CHF
- Briefly highlight the possible benefits of exercise on quality of life (QOL) in people with CHF
- Provide recommendations for exercise prescription for people with CHF
- Lastly examine three case studies of people with different stages of CHF.

PHYSIOLOGIC IMPACT OF CHF

Much of the research conducted with people with CHF has involved exercise. These studies have almost all shown that people with CHF have decreased exercise tolerance.(Fletcher et al., 2001; Gademan et al., 2008; Kiilavuori, Sovijarvi, Naveri, Ikonen, & Leinonen, 1996; Williams et al., 2007) Even asymptomatic patients with CHF have maximal exercise capacities between 60-

70% of normal and symptomatic patients are often <50% of normal.(Freimark et al., 2007) Most often this decreased tolerance is reported as dyspnoea and/or fatigue. The decreased exercise tolerance is due to a combination of multiple changes in the central and peripheral systems. (See table 1 for a full list of changes) It is believed that the decreased peripheral muscle oxidative function is the main cause of reduced exercise tolerance.(Williams et al., 2007) Put simply, this means that the muscles in people with CHF need to use anaerobic metabolism at a lower exercise intensity than people without CHF. Therefore, people with CHF will not be able to tolerate as high of levels of exercise as people without CHF due to lactate levels building sooner causing muscle fatigue.

Table 1. System Changes Contributing to a Decreased Exercise Tolerance in Patients with CHF

Central Changes:	Impaired left ventricular function
	Increased sympathetic system activity
	Decreased parasympathetic system activity
	Decreased heart rate (HR) variability
Peripheral Changes:	Muscle Fibre type alteration (specifically decreased type I - slow twitch fibres)
	Skeletal muscle atrophy
	Decreased skeletal muscle blood flow
	Impaired skeletal muscle metabolism – mainly decreased oxidative function

Lower exercise levels in people with CHF are also evident in peak oxygen consumption (VO_2) levels. People with CHF typically have decreased VO_2 levels compared with healthy adults.(Bjarnason-Wehrens et al., 2004; Fletcher et al., 2001; Moffat & Frowfelter, 2007; Rossi, 1992) Rossi even states that VO_2 is the best physiologic parameter to use when defining exercise capacity in people with CHF.(Rossi, 1992) One study found that symptomatic CHF patients had a maximal exercise capacity often <50% of normal.(Freimark et al., 2007) This decrease in exercise capacity also impacts quality of life and functional abilities in people with CHF. People with CHF often report difficulties with mobility, activities of daily living (ADLs), household tasks, work outside the home, and social activities. Many quality of life and functional outcome measures have been developed and are used to classify people with CHF. The most common international classification system is the New York Heart Association (NYHA) Classification of Heart Failure. The NYHA classes are shown in table 2. The NYHA classes can be useful for health care providers to categorize the severity of the patient's CHF. We can also use NYHA classification to show effectiveness of exercise interventions if the patient is able to improve from one classification to a more mild classification.

**Table 2. New York Heart Association (NYHA)
Classification of Heart Failure**

Class I	Patients with no limitation of activities; they suffer no symptoms from ordinary activities.
Class II	Patients with slight, mild limitation of activity; they are comfortable with rest or with mild exertion.
Class III	Patients with marked limitation of activity; they are comfortable only at rest.
Class IV	Patients who should be at complete rest, confined to bed or chair; any physical activity brings on discomfort and symptoms occur at rest.

HISTORY OF EXERCISE IN RELATION TO CHF

Prior to the 1970's, people with CHF were advised not to perform any aerobic or resistance exercise beyond daily functional needs. It was believed by the medical community that the added stress of exercise posed a significant risk of mortality for a person with an already compromised heart. During the 1970's and 1980's, research began to show that at a minimum, low level walking or bicycle ergometry could be beneficial in the management of patients with CHF.(Franciosa, Ziesche, & Wilen, 1979; Mason, Zelis, Longhurst, & Lee 1977; Vatner & Pagani, 1976) Once the research started to show that exercise may not be harmful for people with CHF, numerous studies began to examine a wide array of exercise modes, intensities, frequencies and durations. Most studies have shown that not only is exercise not harmful for people with CHF, but there are actually many benefits.(Austin, Williams, Ross, & Hutchinson, 2008; Bartlo, 2007; Beniaminovitz et al., 2002; Gianuzzi, Temporelli, Corra, & Tavazzi, 2003; Meyer 2001; 2006; Rees, Taylor, Singh, Coats, & Ebrahim, 2004) Due to the overwhelming amount of research showing benefits of exercise, specific guidelines have been developed for both aerobic exercise(Bartlo, 2007; Bjarnason-Wehrens et al., 2004; Fletcher et al., 2001; Pina & Fitzpatrick, 1996; Working Group on Cardiac Rehabilitation & Exercise Physiology and Working Group on Heart Failure of the European Society of Cardiology, 2001) and resistance exercise in individuals with CHF. (Bartlo, 2007; Braith & Beck, 2008; Bjarnason-Wehrens et al., 2004; Delagardelle & Feiereisen, 2005; Fletcher et al., 2001; Kelley, 2000; Meyer, 2001; 2006, Pina & Fitzpatrick, 1996; Working Group on Cardiac Rehabilitation & Exercise Physiology and Working Group on Heart Failure of the European Society of Cardiology, 2001).

In 2001, the American Heart Association issued standards for exercise testing and training,(Fletcher et al., 2001) followed by a similar statement from the German Federation of Cardiovascular Prevention and Rehabilitation in 2004.(Bjarnason-Wehrens et al., 2004) In 2003, the UK National Institute for Clinical Excellence issued guidelines that state, "patients with chronic heart failure should be encouraged to adopt regular aerobic and/or resistive exercise."(National Institute for Clinical Excellence, 2003) These recommendations were determined by bodies of experts reviewing the scientific literature. However, in reviewing research studies completed to date, it is evident that studies have examined different modes, intensity levels, and durations of exercise. The interpretation of these findings is further complicated by the varied inclusion criteria, parameters of exercise, and the heterogeneity of patient populations. Systematic reviews have been completed that also provide a thorough review of the literature that is completed.(Bartlo, 2007; Bjarnason-Wehrens et al., 2004; Delagardelle & Feiereisen 2005; McCartney, 1998; Meyer, 2001; Pu et al., 2001) It is important to realize that in most literature reviews, the rigor and strength of evidence is not graded. However, the review by Bartlo did grade the available research and differentiated between aerobic and resistance exercise.(Bartlo, 2007) There was also one meta-analysis done with progressive resistance exercise, but the only physical parameter examined was blood pressure levels.(Kelley & Kelley, 2000)

CURRENT LITERATURE RESULTS IN RELATION TO EXERCISE FOR PEOPLE WITH CHF

Isometric Exercise

Isometric exercise is a muscle contraction that is held in one position. It is usually held in a middle to end range position. Current literature still does not support the use of isometrics for people with CHF.(Braith & Beck, 2008; Bjarnason-Wehrens et al., 2004; DeTurk & Cahalin, 2004; Meyer, 2001; Volaklis & Tokmakidis, 2005) When a person performs isometric exercise, HR, systolic blood pressure (SBP) and diastolic blood pressure (DBP) all increase, yet stroke volume (SV) remains relatively unchanged. This causes a moderate increase in cardiac output (CO) with little increase in VO_2. Also, blood flow to non-working muscles does not increase due to reflex vasoconstriction(Braith & Beck, 2008) and intramuscular pressure compressing the arterial blood vessels.(Volaklis, & Tokmakidis, 2005) These changes continue to compound as the duration of exercise continues. Thus the myocardium and vascular systems have a significant load placed on them.(Braith & Beck, 2008) Since people with CHF already have a decreased ability to withstand increases in demands on the myocardium and vascular systems, isometric exercise provides too much central stress to offset the peripheral gains.

Contraindications

In subsequent sections of this chapter, there will be numerous benefits given for the use of exercise for people with CHF. However, there are some contraindications to performing exercise for this population.

The list in table 3 was compiled from references reviewed.(Braith & Beck, 2008; Moffat & Frowfelter, 2007; Rossi, 1992; Volaklis, Tokmakidis, 2005; Wise, 2007; Working Group on Cardiac Rehabilitation & Exercise Physiology and Working Group on Heart Failure of the European Society of Cardiology, 2001)

Although the contraindications listed in table 3 may seem daunting, upon review, these are contraindications for exercise in almost all populations. When people with CHF are stable and without further system decompensation, exercise is not contraindicated.

Table 3. Relative and Absolute Contraindications to Use of Exercise in People with CHF

Absolute Contraindications

- Worsening of dyspnoea or exercise tolerance at rest or on exertion during previous 3-5 days
- Significant ischemia at low work rates (< 2 METS)
- Threatening arrhythmias
- Uncontrolled diabetes
- Active pericarditis, myocarditis, endocarditis, thrombophlebitis, or recent embolism
- Acute systemic illness or fever
- Moderate to Severe aortic stenosis
- Obstructive or regurgitant valvular disease requiring surgery
- Unstable angina or myocardial infarction within the previous 3 weeks

Relative Contraindications

- NYHA class IV (some sources list this as an absolute contraindication)
- New onset atrial fibrillation
- Increase in bodyweight within 24 hours greater than 1 kg
- Decrease in SBP with exercise >20 millimetres of mercury
- Significant exercise-induced ischemia (>3mm ST-segment depression)
- Complex arrhythmias which increase in severity/frequency with exercise or exertion
- Severe pulmonary hypertension
- Resting HR > 100 beats per minute

Aerobic Exercise

Aerobic exercise is sustained physical activity that increases the HR and oxygen consumption of the muscles. Done over time, aerobic exercise will improve the function of the cardiovascular and respiratory systems. Aerobic exercise was the earliest form of exercise to be used with people with CHF. Simple bicycle ergometry and treadmill walking programs were instituted and found to be effective. People with CHF that perform aerobic exercise have been shown to have beneficial adaptations of the cardiac and skeletal muscles.(Kulcu, Kurtais, Tur, Gulec, & Seckin, 2007) Aerobic exercise has been shown to improve

VO$_2$ peak, dyspnoea, work capacity or exercise endurance, left ventricular function as measured by ejection fraction (EF), resting HR, sub-maximal exercise HR, and anaerobic threshold level.(Beniaminovitz et al., 2002; Coats et al.,1992; Delagardelle, Feiereisen, Krecke, Essamri, & Beissel, 1999; Franklin, Swain, & Shephard, 2003; Gianuzzi et al., 2003; Hambrecht et al., 2000; Kiilavuori et al., 1996; Rees et al., 2004; Williams et al., 2007) All these changes will lead to improvements in exercise tolerance in people with CHF. This increased exercise tolerance is accomplished by a combination of central and peripheral physiologic changes. It was first believed that aerobic exercise would improve the heart function directly thus improving the physical status of people with CHF. It is now understood that the peripheral changes that occur with exercise are the most beneficial in improving physical status for people with CHF.(Rees et al., 2004) The participants in a study by Beniaminovitz et al. did not show improvements in ventilatory and respiratory muscle function, yet significant gains were seen in VO$_2$, peak VO$_2$, dyspnoea, and exercise performance.(Beniaminovitz et al., 2002) This further demonstrates that peripheral changes may have a greater overall effect on exercise tolerance in people with CHF.

There are a multitude of adaptations that occur in the peripheral systems due to regular exercise. One such change is a decrease in the vasoconstriction of arterioles in skeletal muscles.(Working Group on Cardiac Rehabilitation & Exercise Physiology and Working Group on Heart Failure of the European Society of Cardiology, 2001) These muscles will also improve in their ability to extract oxygen from the blood. Skeletal muscle metabolic function improves, thus allowing active muscles to prolong the time until anaerobic metabolism is needed. Aerobic exercise training will reduce the activity of the sympathetic and renin-angiotensin system.(Working Group on Cardiac Rehabilitation & Exercise Physiology and Working Group on Heart Failure of the European Society of Cardiology, 2001) This is responsible for the improved HR response to exercise that allows greater activity endurance. A study by Freimark et al. demonstrated this improvement in activity endurance. After the subjects completed an eighteen-week exercise programme, they showed highly significant gains in 6-minute walk test (6MWT) results, exercise testing duration, and metabolic equivalents (METs) achieved during exercise testing compared with subjects that did not complete an exercise programme.(Freimark et al., 2007) This is especially significant when coupled with the statistic from Franklin et al. that states that for patients with coronary artery disease (CAD), every 1 MET increase in activity, provides a 10% decrease in mortality.(Franklin et al., 2003) The study by Franklin et al. was completed on patients with CAD and not CHF, but since most patients with CHF start the disease progression with CAD, it is not unreasonable to think that patients with stable CHF may see similar results. Literature support of safety and changes to mortality will be discussed more in depth later in the chapter.

The improvement of exercise/activity tolerance is often the most important change for people living with CHF. They want to be able to perform greater activity with less symptoms. They want to function at as high a level as possible. Regular exercise in people with CHF has been shown to improve NYHA class.(Delagardelle et al., 1999; Gademan et al., 2008; Kiilavuori et al., 1996; Working Group on Cardiac Rehabilitation & Exercise Physiology and Working Group on Heart Failure of the European Society of Cardiology, 2001) These studies have shown on average a one class improvement on the NYHA scale. Although the change in NYHA class number may seem small, when symptoms and patient function are examined, a one class improvement is clinically significant. Since most of the studies were performed on people in NYHA class II and III, these people, on average, were able to improve to a class I or II. It is important to discuss and highlight these functional changes for patients so that they can truly see the benefits of their exercise. A person is more likely to continue with an exercise programme if they are aware of the benefits. The maintenance of functional improvement is vital in the management of CHF. The more active a person with CHF can be, the less quickly the disease progression occurs. Participants in the study by Kiilavouri et al. performed an independent exercise programme upon completion of a supervised program and were thus able to maintain this improved NYHA class six months after the initiation of the study.(Kiilavuori et al., 1996) We need to perform further research to examine this change more closely and exploit it, if in fact; it is reproduced in subsequent studies.

Resistance Exercise

Resistance exercise increases muscle strength and endurance by doing repetitive motions with weights or other resistance to the movement. Resistance exercise was once thought to be deleterious to people with CHF. Concerns were that resistance exercise would increase BP and afterload too much, which would accelerate the left ventricular remodeling phase.(Levinger et al., 2005) Recent studies however, have shown that resistance exercise can improve left ventricular (LV) function, peak lactate levels, VO_2 peak, muscle strength, muscle endurance (due to shift in muscle fibre type and/or improvements in lactate levels), muscle capillary density, and work capacity.(Braith, 1998; Braith & Beck, 2008; Degache et al., 2007; Delagardelle et al., 2002; Karlsdottir et al., 2002; Levinger et al.,

2005; Meyer, 2006; Gianuzzi et al., 2003; Pu 2001; Selig et al., 2004; Volaklis & Tokmakidis, 2005; Williams et al., 2007) A study by Umpierre and Stein demonstrated that resistance exercise for people with acute or chronic CHF does not cause an adverse increase in BP and in fact the exercise intervention may facilitate long-term BP control.(Umpierre & Stein, 2007) It has been found that even in cases where resistance exercise does not improve LV function; it can inhibit the reduction in LV contractile function that typically follows the disease progression of CHF.(Levinger et al., 2005) Most programmes that use resistance exercise also incorporate aerobic exercise too. There are benefits to this as will be discussed in the recommendations section of this chapter. However, for some systems, resistance exercise used alone can be just as beneficial as a combined resistance and aerobic programme. When performed at 30-80% of maximal strength, resistance exercise may cause less stress on the cardiovascular system than submaximal aerobic exercise does.(Levinger et al., 2005) In a review of literature related to CHF and exercise, Meyer found that resistance exercises resulted in lower HR responses and rate-pressure products than bicycle ergometry performed at 70% peak VO_2.(Meyer, 2006) Also, LV ejection fraction and volumes were similar between resistance and aerobic exercise.

It is important to recognize that the focus of resistance exercise is on the peripheral systems. This reminds us that therapeutic interventions do not always need to be directed at the central site of a disease process. Even though the heart is the organ affected most by CHF, it is not the only system that is affected. Through our interventions, we can address the peripheral changes, as well as the central changes that occur with CHF (see table 1 again). The peripheral changes associated with resistance exercise will help manage or improve symptoms associated with CHF, exercise tolerance, and overall functional status. The shift in fibre type and skeletal muscle atrophy seen in people with CHF can be slowed, stopped, or reversed with resistance exercise. Skeletal muscle strength and endurance can be improved from 10-80%.(Braith & Beck, 2008; Selig et al., 2004; Volaklis & Tokmakidis, 2005) Strength and endurance aren't the only peripheral changes that occur with resistance exercise. Skeletal muscle metabolism, fibre type, and capillary density can also improve with exercise and can have a clinically significant benefit to patient presentation. In a study by Williams et al., results showed that mitochondrial ATP production is a strong predictor of aerobic capacity for people with CHF.(Williams et al., 2007) A resistance exercise programme will produce these results in people with CHF. So how we can be sure that these peripheral changes actually improve the status of people with CHF? Studies are examining the relationships between changes due to exercise and the status of people with CHF. Volaklis and Tokmakidis found that improvements in skeletal muscle metabolism and histology were directly associated with 6 MWT results.(Volaklis & Tokmakidis, 2005) Studies like these prove that if our therapeutic interventions can change peripheral systems, there will be a direct effect on the overall presentation of CHF symptoms and function. Skeletal muscle strength and endurance are also very important to use in risk stratification and determination of prognosis of people with CHF. Leg strength has been shown to be a better predictor of long-term outcome in people with CHF than VO_2 peak.(Braith & Beck, 2008)

Alternative Therapeutic Interventions

As discussed already, most of the exercise research on patients with CHF has focused on the use of bicycle ergometers, walking (treadmill or on land), resistance machines or free weights, and general active range of motion exercise. Research has begun to venture toward other methods of exercise for people with CHF. A review of alternative modes of exercise for people with CHF is beyond the scope of this chapter. However, research is presently evaluating the use of aquatic therapy (walking in the water, as well as limb exercises), heat therapy, tai chi, meditation, and stress reduction through deep breathing. These methods may have significant benefits, and may therefore be useful when prescribing exercise for people with CHF. Before initiating any of these interventions however, the clinician should do further literature review on the particular mode, its benefits and risks, and the appropriate intervention parameters.

THE IMPACT OF EXERCISE ON QUALITY OF LIFE FOR PEOPLE WITH CHF

People with CHF have a variety of symptoms associated with the disease. The most common of these are dyspnoea, fatigue, exercise intolerance, decreased strength, and weight gain or oedema.(Beniaminovitz et al., 2002; DeTurk & Cahalin, 2004; Freimark et al., 2007; Rees et al., 2004) These symptoms contribute to a decreased quality of life (QOL) for people with CHF. Many people with CHF report moderate or low levels on QOL measures. Important to note though is that many people with CHF rate QOL as more important to them than life span.(Austin et al., 2008) The medical community has a habit of focusing first on disease management which primarily addresses life span and then secondarily addresses QOL. We need to remind ourselves that although it is necessary to address any life threatening issues first, we should then address QOL issues simultaneously with other CHF disease management issues. Both aerobic and resistance exercise have been shown to improve QOL measures in people with CHF.(Austin et al., 2008; Beniaminovitz et al., 2002; Kulcu et al., 2007; McCartney, 1998; Working Group on Cardiac Rehabilitation & Exercise Physiology and Working Group on Heart Failure of the European Society of Cardiology, 2001) Exercise allows a person to become more tolerant of exertion. They will experience less fatigue and dyspnoea which will allow the person to increase their performance of daily tasks. Increased independence and function improve the person's QOL and feeling of well being.(Working Group on Cardiac Rehabilitation & Exercise Physiology and Working Group on Heart Failure of the European Society of Cardiology, 2001) As expected, the greatest change in QOL is immediately following an exercise programme intervention.(Austin et al., 2008) Unfortunately, most follow-up studies find that the QOL improvements are lost over time if exercise is not maintained. This is yet another reason why it is so important to prescribe an appropriate exercise programme for someone with CHF.

SAFETY OF EXERCISE AND EXERCISE'S EFFECT ON DISEASE PROGRESSION

So far, this chapter has focused on the research supporting the use of exercise to cause positive changes in the central and peripheral systems of people with CHF. Before prescribing any sort of exercise, it is important to know what the risks are and what the expected outcomes are. This allows a risk vs. benefit analysis to be done in order to decide if the intervention should be applied. Exercise in people with CHF NYHA class I-III has been shown to be safe.(Braith, 1998; Freimark et al., 2007; Rees et al., 2004; Working Group on Cardiac Rehabilitation & Exercise Physiology and Working Group on Heart Failure of the European Society of Cardiology, 2001) These studies have shown that exercise in people with CHF does not produce adverse effects or deterioration of the cardiovascular system. A study by Freimark et al. examined outcomes related to exercise versus a control (no exercise) in people with CHF. They actually found a greater number of deaths in the control group (33%) compared to the exercise group (4.5%).(Freimark et al., 2007) Very few studies have closely examined exercise in people with NYHA class IV CHF; therefore, at this time it can not be determined that exercise is safe for this population. Until further research documents safety of exercise for people with NYHA class IV CHF, functional tasks should be the extent of physical training for this population. Also, patients in NYHA class I-III that are not stable or show contraindications listed in table 3, should not perform exercises until they are stable again.

Now that the risks are known it is now important to examine the benefits of exercise on overall CHF disease progression. One study with a 3.3 year follow-up did show that cardiac mortality was reduced following exercise.(Rees et al., 2004) While this is reassuring, one study is not conclusive evidence that exercise can halt the progression of CHF or reverse its effects on the cardiovascular system. However, research has shown that the improvement in sympatho-vagal balance protects the heart from further left ventricle remodelling.(Working Group on Cardiac Rehabilitation & Exercise Physiology and Working Group on Heart Failure of the European Society of Cardiology, 2001) This, in combination with the many peripheral changes that occur with exercise, may lead to at least a delay in disease progression. Positive disease outcomes related to CHF can also be seen in improvements in NYHA class score following an exercise programme intervention. Many studies have shown improvements in NYHA class after an exercise programme.(Austin et al., 2008; Delagardelle, 2002; Kiilavuori et al., 1996; Working Group on Cardiac Rehabilitation & Exercise Physiology and Working Group on Heart Failure of the European Society of Cardiology, 2001) One example is a study by Delagardelle et al. where the average NYHA class of subjects prior to exercise initiation was 2.7 and after completion of the exercise programme, the average NYHA class was 1.5.(Delagardelle et al., 1999) A change in one class of NYHA is clinically significant, especially with the higher classes. Research has shown that the improvement of NYHA class is sustainable as long as the exercise programme continues. It is also important to remember that people with CHF who do not perform exercise not only don't improve NYHA class, but over time will decrease in NYHA class due to disease progression.

Knowing that the risks of performing exercise with CHF are low and the outcomes/benefits may be moderate to high, the risk vs. benefit analysis is in favour of the performance of exercise. This knowledge that exercise is beneficial and low risk is the first step to prescribing exercise for people with CHF. The next step is evaluating the individual person. Lastly, the actual exercise programme can be developed.

RECOMMENDATIONS FOR EXERCISE PRESCRIPTION FOR PEOPLE WITH CHF

Aerobic and resistance exercise have been evaluated in this chapter and both have been shown to have positive results in people with CHF. Prescription of either aerobic or resistance exercise will benefit the person with CHF. However, the combination of both methods of exercise will have the greatest effect.(Borg, 1982; Braith & Beck, 2008; Degache et al., 2007; Volaklis & Tokmakidis, 2005; Working Group on Cardiac Rehabilitation & Exercise Physiology and Working Group on Heart Failure of the European Society of Cardiology, 2001) The combination of both aerobic and resistance training will cause improvements in both the central and peripheral systems. This combination of exercise modes will address issues of VO_2 and EF, as well as peripheral muscle metabolism, strength, and muscle fibre type.

An assessment of the individual's present exercise tolerance, CHF status, presence of co-morbidities, medications, and physical and anthropometric measurements are necessary before the prescription of any exercise programme. Once the initial assessment is complete and none of the contraindications listed in table 3 are present, the person should be involved in selection of exercise modes. People with CHF should be referred to a comprehensive cardiac rehabilitation programme. Cardiac rehabilitation will not only be able to prescribe a safe and effective exercise programme, but most programmes also offer education on lifestyle modification and risk factors. Further discussion about cardiac rehabilitation programmes and the cardiac rehabilitation team can be found in the chapter titled: Exercise Based Cardiac Rehabilitation. When cardiac rehabilitation is not available or not appropriate, a direct referral to physiotherapy is appropriate. An individual exercise programme can be developed and monitored by the physiotherapist.

Modes of Exercise

- Circuit Training: Circuit training has been shown to be very beneficial for people with CHF.(Meyer 2006; Rees et al., 2004; Wise, 2007; Working Group on Cardiac Rehabilitation & Exercise Physiology and Working Group on Heart Failure of the European Society of Cardiology, 2001) The circuit can be comprised of both aerobic and resistance activities. Each activity can be set with an intensity and duration that is appropriate for the individual. Circuit training allows a person with CHF to get more intense peripheral exercise without putting greater stress on the cardiovascular system.(Volaklis & Tokmakidis, 2005; Working Group on Cardiac Rehabilitation & Exercise Physiology and Working Group on Heart Failure of the European Society of Cardiology, 2001) Typical circuit training for people with CHF should allow for rest in between each activity. The exercise phases are usually short (60 seconds to 120 seconds) with rest periods equal to work periods. Prescription could also be for longer duration and then a rest period that lasts until the person's HR recovers to rest + 10 bpm. The key to proper circuit training with people with CHF is to achieve a high enough intensity and duration of activity to cause changes in the periphery, yet allow long enough rest to prevent adverse stress to the cardiovascular system.

- Types of Aerobic Activities: Most general aerobic activities are acceptable for people with CHF. Bicycle ergometry, treadmill walking, general walking (indoors), stair stepping, and callisthenics, are all good modes to use for aerobic training in people with CHF.(Working Group on Cardiac Rehabilitation & Exercise Physiology and Working Group on Heart Failure of the European Society of Cardiology, 2001) Outdoor walking is safe as long as outside temperatures are in the range of $0° -27°C$. Running and outdoor biking are not safe methods of aerobic training due to the cardiovascular stress and the environmental factors that will affect work rates. Also, swimming is not advisable as mentioned in the alternative therapies section. Bicycle ergometry in the pool may be very effective however.(Meyer & Leblanc, 2008) Any aerobic activity should be examined in relation to the cardiovascular and peripheral changes it will have.

- Types of Resistance Activities: Double limb activities put a greater stress on the cardiovascular system, as do activities requiring the use of larger muscle groups.(Meyer 2006; Working Group on Cardiac Rehabilitation & Exercise Physiology and Working Group on Heart Failure of the European Society of Cardiology, 2001) Therefore, most training programmes should have the person perform the majority of the resistance exercises using a single limb and smaller muscle groups. Exercises for specific muscle groups can be utilized as long as the initial contraction intensity is low (see intensity section) and the work phase is kept short. Typical work phases are 10-20 repetitions with rest after each set. Free weights, circuit equipment, isotonic equipment and resistance bands are all appropriate means for a person with CHF to perform resistance exercise.

Frequency

Most exercise programmes for people with CHF combine aerobic and resistance exercises into one session. When prescribed this way, a frequency of 2-3 days per week is appropriate for people with CHF NYHA classes I, II and III. People with CHF in NYHA class III that are more symptomatic may still be able to perform exercise 2-3 days per week at lower intensities, or they may need to decrease frequency to 1-2 days per week.

Intensity

Intensity is a very individualized parameter of exercise, but the methods to determine intensity are universal and easily applicable. The person's NYHA class will help guide the initial intensity prescription. People in NYHA classes I and II can perform higher intensities and people in NYHA class III should perform lower intensities. In a Cochrane Review by Rees, exercise at greater intensity produced greater results, however, the confidence intervals overlapped, so the researcher stated that statistical significance of the results is questionable.(Rees et al., 2004) For this reason, it is felt that vigorous exercise intensities are not needed in order for people with CHF to improve.

For aerobic exercise, intensities that achieve a level of 40-80% VO_2 max are used.(Working Group on Cardiac Rehabilitation & Exercise Physiology and Working Group on Heart Failure of the European Society of Cardiology, 2001) Intensity should start out at the low end and then be increased slowly over several exercise sessions. HR, BP, respiratory rate, and electrocardiography should be monitored during initial exercise sessions. Rates of perceived exertion can be also be used to assess the intensity of exercise. There are many different scales utilized in the clinic. Regardless of the scale used, the person should feel like they are working at a "somewhat hard" level or less.

The person's NYHA class can guide the intensity of resistance exercise that should be used. The greater the NYHA class, the lower the initial intensity, the smaller the muscle group that should be used, and the smaller number of repetitions per set that should be performed. Research has found that an initial intensity of 40% 1 repetition max is appropriate for people with

CHF.(Delagardelle et al., 2002; Meyer 2006; Working Group on Cardiac Rehabilitation & Exercise Physiology and Working Group on Heart Failure of the European Society of Cardiology, 2001) Unilateral limbs and small muscle groups will also produce less stress on the cardiovascular system.

Duration

Duration can vary greatly among individuals. Typical cardiac rehabilitation programmes provide a total exercise time of 30-60 min including warm-up and cool down periods. This may be acceptable for many people with CHF, but not all. People with CHF that have a functional capacity of <3 METs may benefit from multiple short duration exercise sessions of 5-10 min each.(Working Group on Cardiac Rehabilitation & Exercise Physiology and Working Group on Heart Failure of the European Society of Cardiology, 2001) People with capacities of 3-5 METs may benefit from two sessions of 15 min each. Aerobic and resistance exercise durations should be looked at independently and then cumulatively. Aerobic exercise should total 30-60 min if performed alone. Aerobic activity of only 15 min may be acceptable if combined with resistance activities. Resistance exercise should be 1-2 sets of 10-20 repetitions for 2-5 muscle groups if combined with aerobic activity or 2-4 sets of 10-20 repetitions for 2-8 muscle groups if performed without aerobic exercise. The work phases for resistance exercise may last 60-120 seconds with equal rest periods.

Risk Classification

The American Heart Association, the American College of Sports Medicine, and the American Association for Cardiovascular and Pulmonary Rehabilitation have established risk categories for engaging in an exercise programme.(Fletcher et al., 2001). These risk categories may help to guide the rehabilitation professional in their initial assessment of a person's risk related to physical activity. They should help decide the individual's readiness for exercise. For example, if the individual is classified as Class A – Apparently Healthy Individual, you will have less limitations and precautions as you begin exercise with that person. If they are classified as Class D – Unstable Disease with Activity Restriction, your exercise prescription is almost exclusively functional tasks and restoring functional endurance. The risk categories should not replace the professional's initial evaluation, but enhance it.

CONCLUSION

There are many physiologic changes that occur due to the disease progression of CHF. Slowing or stopping these deleterious changes is essential in the management of CHF. Physical rehabilitation is an integral part of that disease management. There is ample evidence that aerobic and resistance training in people with CHF is safe and beneficial. Exercise will improve the person's central and peripheral symptoms of CHF, as well as QOL. In people with NYHA class I-III CHF, exercise does not cause increased risks of mortality. While it is important to provide an individual exercise programme for people with CHF, general guidelines for both aerobic and resistance exercise are given in this chapter and other resources. These guidelines should be used in conjunction with evaluation findings in order to determine each individual person's prescription of exercise. Further research should continue to examine and recommend specific parameters related to exercise prescription for people with CHF.

CASE STUDIES

Case 1

Mrs. G is a 68 year-old woman with a NYHA class II. The medical doctor asks for a phase I cardiac rehabilitation consult due to an admission to the coronary critical care unit 1 day ago. Mrs. G presented to the hospital with complaints of increased shortness of breath (SOB), bilateral lower extremity oedema, and weight gain of 2.5 kg in 6 days.

Past medical history: anterior wall myocardial infarction (MI) 3 years ago, hypercholesterolemia, osteoarthritis in bilateral knees. Current medications include: diuretic, statin, ace inhibitor and a beta-blocker.

Social history: Mrs. G lives with her husband and adult daughter in a second floor apartment with 1 flight of stairs up to the home. Until the past week, she was able to ambulate independently with a wheeled walker for at least 150 m and used a straight cane and railing for stair negotiation due to the arthritis in her knees.

Anthropometrics: She is 1.57 m tall and weighs 63.5 kg. Therefore, BMI is 25.8.

Upon your initial evaluation, Mrs. G reports a 66 on the Minnesota Living with Heart Failure Questionnaire.(Rector 1987) She is presently able to ambulate only 3-5 m. She performs all bed mobility and transfers with minimal assistance and has moderate SOB and fatigue throughout activity. You initiate a programme of transfer training, gait training, and active range of motion exercise at low intensity levels the first day. Mrs. G's vitals for this initial session are below.

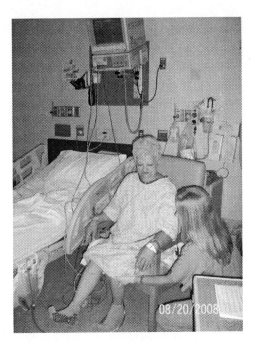

Figure 1. Mrs G. performing seated lower extremity exercise.

Vitals are as follows:

	HR bpm	BP mm/Hg	RR breaths/min	O₂ Saturations	RPE 6-20 scale	RPD 0-10 scale
At rest	86	106/85	16	97% with 2L O₂	6	6
After transfer out of bed and light single limb ex	113	126/84	24	97% with 2L O₂	10	8
After 10 min recovery	101	119/84	18	98% with 2L O₂	7	7

HR: heart rate, bpm: beats per minute, BP: blood pressure, mm/Hg: millimetres of mercury, RR: respiratory rate, RPE: rate of perceived exertion based on BORG scale(Borg, 1982), RPD: rate of perceived dyspnoea scale.

Questions to Challenge You

1 What effect will Mrs. G's medications have on her present status and as she progresses in her programme?

2 How will you modify standing and ambulation activities to accommodate Mrs. G's arthritis?

3 Do these vital sign changes represent an acceptable response to exercise for this patient at this time?

4 How will you progress her phase I rehab to encourage increased exercise tolerance and prepare for discharge from the hospital?

Case 2

Mrs. B is an 80 year-old woman with NYHA class III CHF. The MD consults in-home physiotherapy and nursing for rehabilitation after Mrs. B complained of increased shortness of breath (SOB) and decreased functional endurance at her last follow-up appointment.

Past medical history: HTN, Coronary artery bypass graft x 3 vessels CABG x3 10 years ago, hypercholesterolemia, macular degeneration. Current medications include: diuretic, statin, beta-blocker and an anti-coagulant.

Social History: Mrs. B lives alone in a 2 story house, but had a handicapped elevator installed as she is unable to ascend/descend greater than 1 step. She is able to ambulate without an assistive device and performs all ADLs independently. Her daughter takes her shopping and to all outside appointments. She owns a motorized scooter for mobility of distances greater than 50 m.

Anthropometrics: She is 1.5 m tall and weighs 72.6 kg. BMI is therefore 32.

Upon your initial evaluation, Mrs. B reports a 53 on the Minnesota Living with Heart Failure Questionnaire.(Rector, 1987) She is able to ambulate 92 m for the 6 minute walk test. She performs all bed mobility and transfers independently, but with increased time needed and some compensatory techniques. She is able to ambulate household distances independently without assistive device. You initiate a programme of aerobic and resistance training at low intensity levels the first day. You are now seeing Mrs. B for her 3rd session.

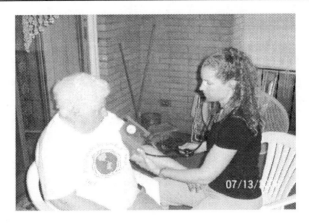

Figure 2. Assessment of Mrs. B's resting vitals.

Vitals are as follows:

	HR bpm	BP mm/Hg	RR breaths/ min	O₂ Saturations	RPE 6-20 scale	RPD 0-10 scale
At rest	75	115/78	13	99% RA	6	4
After seated single limb resistance ex	83	133/80	25	99% RA	12	7
After 10 min recovery	77	119/80	15	98% RA	6	5

HR: heart rate, bpm: beats per minute, BP: blood pressure, mm/Hg: millimetres of mercury, RR: respiratory rate, RA: room air, RPE: rate of perceived exertion based on BORG scale(Borg, 1982), RPD: rate of perceived dyspnoea scale.

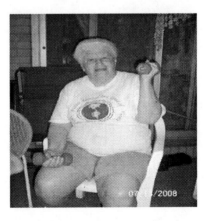

Figure 3. Mrs. B performing unilateral upper extremity resistance exercise.

Questions to Challenge You

1   Will Mrs. B's medications have any possible interactions with each other and if so, what should you look for to notify you of adverse interactions?
2   Do these vital sign changes represent an acceptable response to exercise for this patient at this time?
3   Develop an exercise programme for Mrs. B incorporating both aerobic and resistance exercise.

Case 3

Mr. N is a 74 year-old man with NYHA class II CHF. The MD consults outpatient cardiac rehab after a recent admission to the hospital for a CHF exacerbation. Mr. N has been home for 2 weeks and has no increase in his symptoms since discharge from the hospital.

Past medical history: Sub-endocardial MI 12 years ago, percutaneous transluminal coronary angioplasty (PTCA) 4 years ago, bilateral cataract surgery 2 months ago. Current medications include: diuretic and a beta-blocker.

Social History: Mr. N lives with his wife in a 2 story town house, but can stay on the first floor when his CHF symptoms are severe. He is able to ambulate without an assistive device for at least 300 m and can perform all his ADLs independently. He still works part-time as an attorney.

Anthropometrics: He is 1.8 m tall and weighs 90.0 kg. BMI is therefore 27.7.

Upon your initial evaluation, Mr. N reports a 26 on the Minnesota Living with Heart Failure Questionnaire.(Rector, 1987) He is able to ambulate 302 m for the 6 minute walk test. He performs all his daily tasks and ambulation independently, but needs increased rest as the day progresses due to shortness of breath (SOB) and occasional lower extremity oedema. You initiate a programme 3 days/week of aerobic and resistance training at low intensity levels the first day and progressing each session for the first 4 sessions. You are now seeing Mr. N for his 12th session.

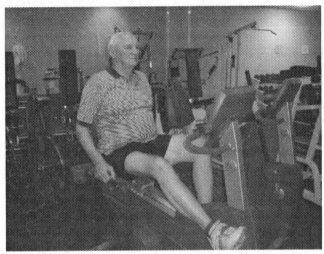

Figure 4. Mr. N performing aerobic exercise on the bicycle ergometer.

Vitals are as follows:

	HR bpm	BP mm/Hg	RR breaths/ min	O$_2$ Saturations	RPE 6-20 scale	RPD 0-10 scale
At rest	72	125/82	12	99% RA	6	1
After 40 min aerobic and resistance ex	79	144/84	25	99% RA	13	5
After 10 min recovery	73	129/81	13	100% RA	6	1

HR: heart rate, bpm: beats per minute, BP: blood pressure, mm/Hg: millimetres of mercury, RR: respiratory rate, RA: room air, RPE: rate of perceived exertion based on BORG scale(Borg, 1982), RPD: rate of perceived dyspnoea scale.

Questions to Challenge You

1 What effect will Mr. N's other medical diagnoses have on his CHF disease progression?
2 Do these vital sign changes represent an acceptable response to exercise for this patient at this time?
3 If Mr. N's BP was 159/92 after exercise, would you be concerned?
4 If the scenario in question #3 happened, what would you do at that time? How would you modify future sessions?

5   Assuming that Mr. N progresses without incident, how will you progress his cardiac rehab to encourage increased exercise tolerance and prepare for discharge from the programme?

REFERENCES

American Heart Association (2006). Heart disease and stroke statistics – 2006. Available on: http://www.americanheart.org. Accessed 16.07.08.

Austin, J, Williams, W. R., Ross, L., & Hutchinson, S. (2008). Five-year follow-up findings from a randomized controlled trial of cardiac rehabilitation for heart failure. *European Journal of Cardiovascular Prevention and Rehabilitation, 1,* 162-167.

Bartlo, P. (2007). Evidence-based application of aerobic and resistance training in patients with congestive heart failure. *Journal of Cardiopulmonary Rehabilitation and Prevention, 27,* 368-375.

Beniaminovitz, A., Lang, C. C., LaManca, J., & Mancini, D. M. (2002). Selective low-level leg muscle training alleviates dyspnea in patients with heart failure. *Journal of the American College of Cardiology, 40,* 1602-1608.

Borg, G. A. (1982). Psychophysical bases of perceived exertion. *Medicine and Science in Sports and Exercise, 14,* 377-381.

Braith, R. W. (1998). Exercise training in patients with CHF and heart transplant recipients. *Medicine and Science in Sports and Exercise, 30,* S367-S372.

Braith, R. W & Beck, D. T. (2008). Resistance exercise: training adaptations and developing a safe exercise prescription. *Heart Failure Review, 13,*:69-79.

Bjarnason-Wehrens, B., Mayer-Berger, W., Meister, E. R., Baum, K., Hambrecht, R., & Gielen, S. (2004). Recommendations for resistance exercise in cardiac rehabilitation. Recommendations of the German Federation for Cardiovascular Prevention and Rehabilitation. *European Journal of Cardiovascular Prevention and Rehabilitation, 11,* 352-361.

Coats, A. J. S., Adamopoulos, S., Radaelli, A., McCane, A., Meyer, T. E., Bernardi, L., et al., (1992). Controlled trial of physical training in chronic heart failure. Exercise performance, hemodynamics, ventilation, and autonomic function. *Circulation, 85,* 2119-2131.

Degache, F., Garet, M., Calmels, P., Costes, F., Bathelemy, J. C, & Roche, F. (2007). Enhancement of isokinetic muscle strength with a combined training programme in chronic heart failure. *Clinical Physiology and Functional Imaging, 27,* 225-230.

Delagardelle, C., & Feiereisen, P. (2005). Strength training for patients with chronic heart failure(review). *Europa Medicophysica, 41,* 57-65.

Delagardelle, C., Feiereisen, P., Autier, P., Shita, R., Krecke, R., & Beissel, J. (2002). Strength/endurance training versus endurance training in congestive heart failure. *Medicine and Science in Sports and Exercise, 34,* 1868-1872.

Delagardelle, C., Feiereisen, P., Krecke, R., Essamri, B., & Beissel, J. (1999). Objective effects of a 6 months endurance and strength training program in outpatients with congestive heart failure. *Medicine and Science in Sports and Exercise, 31,* 1102-1107.

DeTurk, W, & Cahalin, L. (2004). *Cardiovascular and Pulmonary Physical Therapy.* Ohio: McGraw-Hill.

Fletcher, G. F., Balady, G. J., Amsterdam, E. A., Chaitman, B., Eckel, R., Fleg, J., et al., (2001). Exercise standards for testing and training. A statement for healthcare professionals from the American Heart Association. *Circulation, 104,* 1694-1740.

Franciosa, J. A, Ziesche, S., & Wilen, M. (1979). Functional capacity of patients with chronic left ventricular failure. Relationship of bicycle exercise performance to clinical and hemodynamic characterization. *American Journal of Medicine, 67,* 460-466.

Franklin, B. A, Swain, D. P., & Shephard, R. J. (2003). New insights in the prescription of exercise for coronary patients. *Journal of Cardiovascular Nursing, 18,* 116-123.

Freimark, D., Schechter, M., Schwamenthal, E., Tanne, D., Elmaleh, E., Shemesh, Y., et al., (2007). Improved exercise tolerance and cardiac function in severe chronic heart failure patients undergoing a supervised exercise program. *International Journal of Cardiology, 4, 116,* 309-314.

Gademan, M. G. J., Swenne, C. A., Verwey, H. F., van de Vooren, H., Haest, J. C. W., van Exel, H. J., et al., (2008). Exercise training increases oxygen uptake efficiency slope in chronic heart failure. *European Journal of Cardiovascular Prevention and Rehabilitation. 15,* 140-144.

Giannuzzi, P., Temporelli, P. L., Corra, U., & Tavazzi, L. (2003). Antiremodeling effect of long-term exercise training in patients with stable chronic heart failure: results of the exercise in left ventricular dysfunction and chronic heart failure (ELVD-CHF) trial. *Circulation, 108,* 554-559.

Hambrecht, R., Gielen, S., Linke, A., Fiehn, E., Yu, J., Walther, C., et al.,. (2000). Effects of exercise training on left ventricular function and peripheral resistance in patients with chronic heart failure: a randomized trial. *Journal of the American Medical Association, 21,* 3095-3101.

Karlsdottir, A. E., Foster, C., Porcari, J. P., Palmer-McLean, K., White-Kube, R., & Backes, R. C. (2002). Hemodynamic response during aerobic and resistance exercise. *Journal of Cardiopulmonary Rehabilitation, 22,* 170-177.

Kelley, G. A, & Kelley, K. S. (2000). Progressive resistance exercise and resting blood pressure: a meta-analysis of randomized controlled trials. *Hypertension, 35,* 838-843.

Kiilavuori, K., Sovijarvi, A., Naveri, H., Ikonen, T., & Leinonen, H. (1996). Effect of physical training on exercise capacity and gas exchange in patients with chronic heart failure, *Chest, 110,* 985-991.

Kulcu, D. G., Kurtais, Y., Tur, B. S., Gulec, S., & Seckin, B. (2007). The effect of cardiac rehabilitation on quality of life, anxiety and depression in patients with congestive heart failure. A randomized controlled trial, short-term results. *Europa Medicophysica, 43.* 489-497.

Levinger, I., Bronks, R., Cody, D. V., Linton, I., & Davie, A. (2005). The effect of resistance training on left ventricular function and structure of patients with chronic heart failure. *International Journal of Cardiology, 2, 105,* 159-163.

Mason, D. T., Zelis, R., Longhurst, J., & Lee, G. (1977). Cardiocirculatory responses to muscular exercise in congestive heart failure. *Progress in Cardiovascular Diseases, 19,* 475-489.

McCartney, N. (1998). Role of resistance training in heart disease. *Medicine and Science in Sports and Exercise, 30,* S396-S402.

Meyer , K. (2006). Resistance exercise in chronic heart failure--landmark studies and implications for practice. *Clinical and Investigative Medicine, 29,* 166-169.

Meyer, K. (2001). Exercise training in heart failure: recommendations based on current research. *Medicine and Science in Sports and Exercise, 33,* 525-531.

Meyer, K., & Leblanc, M. C. (2008). Aquatic therapies in patients with compromised left ventricular function and heart failure. *Clinical Investigative Medicine, 31,* E90-E97.

Moffat, M., & Frowfelter, D. (2007). *Cardiovascular/Pulmonary Essentials: Applying the Preferred Physical Therapist Practice Patterns.* New Jersey: Slack Inc.

National Institute for Clinical Excellence (2003). *Management in chronic heart failure in adults in primary and secondary care. Clinical guideline 5.* London: NICE.

Pina, I. L., & Fitzpatrick, J. T. (1996). Exercise and heart failure. A review. *Chest, 110,* 1317-1327.

Pu, C. T., Johnson, M. T., Forman, D. E., Hausdorff, J. M., Roubenoff, R., Foldvari, M., et al., (2001). Randomized trial of progressive resistance training to counteract the myopathy of chronic heart failure. *Journal of Applied Physiology, 90,* 2341-2350.

Rector, T. S., Kubo, S. H., & Cohn, J. N. (1987). Patients' self assessment of their congestive heart failure. Part 2: Content, reliability and validity of a new measure, the Minnesota Living with Heart Failure questionnaire. *Heart Failure, 3,* 198-209.

Rees, K., Taylor, R. S., Singh, S., Coats, A. J. S., & Ebrahim, S. (2004). Exercise based rehabilitation for heart failure. *Cochrane Database Systematic Review, 3,* CD003331.

Rossi, P. (1992). Physical training in patients with congestive heart failure. *Chest, 101,* 350S-353S.

Selig, S. E., Carey, M. F., Menzies, D. G., Patterson, J., Geerling, R. H., Williams, A. D., et al., (2004). Moderate-intensity resistance exercise training in patients with chronic heart failure improves strength, endurance, heart rate variability, and forearm blood flow. *Journal of Cardiac Failure, 10,* 21-30.

Umpierre, D., & Stein, R. (2007). Hemodynamic and vascular effects of resistance training: implications for cardiovascular disease. *Arquivos Brasileiros de Cardiologia, 89,* 256-262.

Vatner, S. F., & Pagani, M. (1976). Cardiovascular adjustments to exercise: hemodynamics and mechanisms. *Progress in Cardiovascular Diseases, 19,* 91-108.

Volaklis, K. A., & Tokmakidis, S. P. (2005). Resistance exercise training in patients with heart failure. *Sports Medicine, 35,* 1085-1103.

Williams, A. D., Carey, M. F., Selig, S., Hayes, A., Krum, H., Patterson, J., et al., (2007). Circuit resistance training in chronic heart failure improves skeletal muscle mitochondrial ATP production rate--a randomized controlled trial. *Journal of Cardiac Failure, 13,* 79-85.

Wise, F. M. (2007). Exercise based cardiac rehabilitation in chronic heart failure. *Australian Family Physician, 36,* 1019-1024.

Working Group on Cardiac Rehabilitation & Exercise Physiology and Working Group on Heart Failure of the European Society of Cardiology (2001). Recommendations for exercise training in chronic heart failure patients. *European Heart Journal, 22,* 125-135.

World Health Organization (2008). *World Health Statistics 2008 4th ed.* Geneva: World Health Organization.

In: Physical Activity in Rehabilitation and Recovery   ISBN: 978-1-60876-400-6
Editor: Holly Blake   © 2010 Nova Science Publishers, Inc.

Chapter 7

EXERCISE BASED CARDIAC REHABILITATION

Frances Wise[*]
Cardiac Rehabilitation Unit, Caulfield Hospital, Australia.

ABSTRACT

Cardiovascular disease is the leading cause of death in developed
nations, and there is a clear link with physical inactivity. The benefits of
exercise, both aerobic and resistance training, in patients with Coronary
Heart Disease are well documented. Both modalities are important
components of cardiac rehabilitation and can contribute to secondary
prevention of heart disease with corresponding improvements in patient
survival. This chapter describes the benefits of exercise for cardiac patients,
details how exercise is prescribed in this group, and considers safety and
contra-indications.

INTRODUCTION

Cardiovascular disease, which includes coronary heart disease and stroke,
kills more people than any other disease. Coronary heart disease (CHD) itself is
the single most common cause of death in Europe, accounting for 1.92 million
deaths each year and killing over one in five men and women (WHO, 2007).
Similarly, in the USA CHD affects 16 million Americans, with over 8 million

[*] Tel: +61 3 9076 6264; Fax: +61 3 9076 6220; Email: f.wise@cgmc.org.au

myocardial infarctions occurring per year (AHA, 2008). In Australia, CHD accounts for 17% of all deaths (AIHW, 2008).

PHYSICAL INACTIVITY AND CORONARY HEART DISEASE

The link between physical inactivity and CHD is well recognised. The World Health Report 2002 estimated that over 20% of CHD in developed countries is due to lack of physical activity (less than 2.5 hours per week of moderate exercise or 1 hour per week of vigorous activity) (WHO, 2002). Data regarding physical inactivity in Europe are limited. However, in a 2005 survey, over 40% of adults in the European Union reported no moderate-level physical activity in the previous week (European Commission, 2006). In Australia, 54% of those aged 18-75 years do not undertake sufficient physical activity to obtain a health benefit, and nearly a third of these do no physical activity in their leisure time (Armstrong, Bauman, & Davies., 2000). Such findings underscore the importance of exercise in primary prevention of heart disease, and in secondary prevention measures such as cardiac rehabilitation.

OVERVIEW OF CARDIAC REHABILITATION

Since the 1960s, early mobilization following myocardial infarction has been recognised as beneficial (Goble & Worcester, 1999). Cardiac rehabilitation is now recognised as an important part of management in patients with coronary artery disease, especially after myocardial infarction, coronary artery bypass surgery or coronary angioplasty/stent (Fletcher, 1998). It is offered to individuals after cardiac events to aid recovery and prevent further cardiac illness. Cardiac rehabilitation is also of benefit for those with stable angina (Williams, et al., 2006), heart valve replacement (Gohlke-Barwolf, et al., 1992; Jairath, et al., 1995), heart transplant (Keteyian, et al., 1991), and heart failure (Belardinelli, Gergio, Ciani, & Purcaro, 1999; Ko & McKelvie, 2005; Rees, et al., 2004). Cardiac rehabilitation has been shown to improve physical health (Hevey, et al., 2003; Lavie & Milani, 1996; Yoshida, et al., 1999; Yoshida, et al., 2001), quality of life (Ades & Coello, 2000; Hevey, et al., 2003, Lavie & Milani, 1996) and decrease subsequent morbidity and mortality (Ades & Coello, 2000; Bock, 2002; Dafoe & Huston., 1997; Witt, et al., 2004). Cardiac rehabilitation programmes typically achieve this through exercise, education, behaviour change, counselling and support (Bock, 2002; Wenger et al 1995), strategies that are aimed at targeting traditional risk factors for cardiovascular disease.

The National Heart Foundation of Australia and the World Health Organisation recommend that cardiac rehabilitation be offered to everyone with cardiac disease (National Heart Foundation, 2004). Despite this, cardiac rehabilitation remains underutilised, with only 15% to 25% of eligible patients participating (Ades, 2001; Allen, Scott, Stewart, & Young, 2004).

The aims of cardiac rehabilitation are presented in table 1.

Table 1. Aims of cardiac rehabilitation

1. Broad aims of cardiac rehabilitation

i. Maximise physical, psychological and social functioning to enable people with cardiac disease to lead fulfilling lives with confidence.
ii. Introduce and encourage behaviours that may minimise the risk of further cardiac events and conditions.

2. Specific aims of cardiac rehabilitation

i. Facilitate and shorten the period of recovery after an acute cardiac event.
ii. Promote strategies for achieving mutually agreed goals of ongoing prevention.
iii. Develop and maintain skills for long-term behaviour change and self-management.
iv. Promote appropriate use of health and community services, including concordance with prescribed medications and professional advice.

From: National Heart Foundation of Australia, Australian Cardiac Rehabilitation Association. Recommended framework for Cardiac rehabilitation '04: www.heartfoundation.com.au, 2004.

PHASES AND COMPONENTS
OF CARDIAC REHABILITATION

There are three distinct phases of Cardiac rehabilitation (see figure 1):
Phase One: Inpatient rehabilitation. Shorter hospital lengths of stay (e.g. 4-6 days post-myocardial infarct) mean that Phase One cardiac rehabilitation is usually limited to early mobilization, explanation of illness or intervention, early risk factor education and appropriate referral to Phase Two rehabilitation.

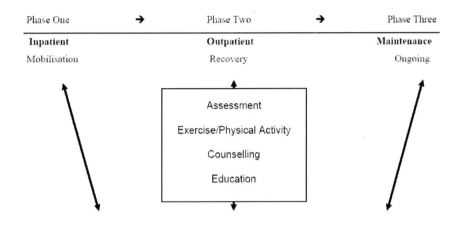

Phase One	→	Phase Two	→	Phase Three
Inpatient		**Outpatient**		**Maintenance**
Mobilisation		Recovery		Ongoing

Assessment

Exercise/Physical Activity

Counselling

Education

Medical Specialists – General Practitioner

Cardiac Rehabilitation Team Members – Allied health/Nursing

From: Outpatient cardiac rehabilitation: Best practice guidelines for health Professionals. Queensland Health 2004.

Figure 1. Phases of Cardiac Rehabilitation.

Phase Two: Ambulatory Outpatient Rehabilitation

Most cardiac rehabilitation programmes fit within this category, although they vary in content. Usually they include supervised group exercise sessions, along with education, support and counselling (See table 2). Ideally, this phase commences soon after discharge from hospital. The usual duration of Phase Two programmes is six to eight weeks, with sessions offered two or three times a week. This phase of cardiac rehabilitation is typically provided by a multi-disciplinary team of medical, nursing and allied health staff.

Table 2. Core Components of a Cardiac Rehabilitation Programme

Component	Examples of Interventions
Patient Assessment	History, examination and development of a care plan
Nutritional Counselling	Designed to reduce total caloric intake, maintain appropriate intake of nutrients and fibre, and increase energy expenditure.
Lipid Management	Provide nutritional counselling, weight management, exercise, alcohol moderation, etc; and monitor drug treatment in concert with primary healthcare provider
Hypertension Management	Monitor, and provide lifestyle modifications including exercise, weight management, moderate sodium restriction, alcohol moderation, smoking cessation, and drug therapy
Smoking Cessation	When readiness to change is confirmed, help the smoker set a quit date and select appropriate treatment strategies
Diabetes Management	Develop a regimen of dietary adherence and weight control that includes exercise, oral hypoglycaemic agents/ insulin therapy (where appropriate), and optimal control of other risk factors.
Psychosocial Management	Offer individual and/or small group education and counselling regarding adjustment to CHD, stress management, and health-related lifestyle change
Other Education/Counselling	Provide information regarding medications (e.g. indications, side effects), investigations and procedures, cardiac health beliefs and misconceptions and the importance of follow-up by specialist, GP or other primary care provider.
Physical Activity Counselling	Provide advice, support, and counselling about physical activity needs on initial evaluation and in follow-up. Assistance with return to work. Consider simulated work testing for patients with heavy labour jobs.
Exercise Training	Develop a documented individualized exercise prescription for aerobic and resistance training that is based on evaluation findings, patient and programme goals, and resources. Exercise prescription should specify frequency, intensity, duration, and modalities. Provide written guidelines for resumption of daily activities including a home walking programme

Balady et al 2007; National Heart Foundation 2004.

Phase Three: Maintenance

The long-term maintenance phase which follows the ambulatory outpatient rehabilitation supports patients in ongoing risk factor modification and physical activity. The exact format varies and is not clearly defined; for example, it may comprise review appointments with a doctor or nurse, or ongoing exercise classes. Phase Three programmes are less common compared with Phases One and Two.

The remainder of this chapter will focus upon the exercise component of Phase Two cardiac rehabilitation. This will mainly concern patients with CHD-related diagnoses such as myocardial infarction, coronary artery bypass grafts (CABG), stents, and angina. Exercise and heart failure will be dealt with in a separate chapter. Unless specified, exercise training or physical activity refers to aerobic or endurance training; strength or resistance training is discussed separately.

SPECIFIC BENEFITS OF EXERCISE IN CARDIAC REHABILITATION

Meta-analyses of the benefits of cardiac rehabilitation indicate it can reduce total mortality by 20% and cardiac mortality by 26% (Taylor, et al., 2004). While results regarding non-fatal myocardial infarction (MI) are mixed, at least one controlled trial demonstrated a significant decrease in MI recurrence following cardiac rehabilitation (Hedback, Perk, & Wodlin, 1993). Exercise-based rehabilitation also reduces hospital re-admissions in patients following myocardial infarction (Ades, Pashkow, & Nestor, 1997), CABG (Hedback, Perk, Hornblad, & Ohlsson, 2001), and percutaneous coronary interventions (PCI) including stenting (Belardinalli, et al., 2001). Many of the benefits of Cardiac Rehabilitation are mediated through the exercise component.

Exercise and Cardiovascular Pathophysiology

Exercise training results in multiple health benefits, many of which are particularly relevant to patients recovering from cardiac illness. In terms of cardiovascular dynamics, aerobic training results in improved exercise performance, which depends on an increased ability to use oxygen to derive energy for work.

Regular aerobic physical activity results in improved maximal cardiac output and peripheral oxygen extraction, which in turn increases maximal oxygen uptake (Giannuzzi, et al., 2003). Aerobic exercise also leads to decreased myocardial oxygen demands for the same level of physical work performed, thus reducing the risk of myocardial ischaemia (Fletcher, et al., 2001; US Dept of Health and Human Services, 1996).

Exercise training leads to increased fibrinolysis and decreased coagulability, thus promoting conditions that benefit patients with existing CHD (El-Sayed, El-Sayed, & Ahmadizad, 2004; Rauramaa, Li., & Vaisanen, 2001). Exercise also enhances endothelial function, thus potentially reducing the risk of coronary re-stenosis (Milani, Lavis, & Cassidy, 2004; Patti, et al., 2005). In patients with stable angina, myocardial ischaemia can be reduced by exercise training via improved endothelium-dependent vasodilatation and myocardial blood flow (Gielen & Hambrecht, 2001). This in turn may explain research findings where exercise training in angina patients resulted in less severe angina (Redwood, Rosing, & Epstein, 1972), and in fewer subsequent coronary events compared with patients treated with coronary stenting (Hambrecht, et al., 2004).

Exercise also improves autonomic function in patients with CHD (Goldsmith, et al., 2000; Malfatto, et al., 2005). Specifically, exercise increases vagal activity and reduces sympathetic hyperactivity, thereby potentially reducing the risk of sudden death and contributing to increased survival rates in cardiac rehabilitation patients (Williams, et al., 2006).

Exercise and Cardiovascular Risk Factors

Physical activity also has a beneficial effect on many of the known risk factors for cardiovascular diseases (Fletcher, et al., 2001; US Dept of Health and Human Services, 1996). Exercise training itself has been reported to:

- reduce blood pressure in those with hypertension and normal blood pressure (Rogers, et al., 1996),
- increase high-density lipoprotein cholesterol levels by approximately 8% to 10% (Brochu, et al., 2000),
- decrease elevated triglycerides by over 20% (Brochu, et al., 2000),
- contribute modestly to body weight control (Schairer, et al., 1998).

The benefits conferred by exercise upon lipid levels (including low-density and high-density lipoproteins and triglycerides), insulin resistance and weight are increased when combined with dietary modification (Haskell, et al., 1994; Pasanisi, et al., 2001; Singh, et al., 1996; Schuler, et al., 1992).

Overall, regular exercise training can improve the CHD risk profile and retard the development of atherosclerosis, thus decreasing the risk of mortality and morbidity from coronary artery disease.

Exercise and Disability

Limitation in functional independence, whether in terms of paid work or leisure activities, is frequently observed following myocardial infarction, coronary artery bypass grafts or stents, and other diagnoses including angina. Such disabilities are reduced by improved fitness, strength and exercise tolerance resulting from the exercise component (both aerobic and strength training) of cardiac rehabilitation (Brochu, et al., 2002; Pollock, et al., 2000; Wenger, et al., 1995; Witt, et al., 2004). Improved exercise capacity (as measured by peak oxygen uptake) is also a predictor of survival in CHD (Kavanagh, et al., 2002). Finally, exercise training in CHD and heart valve replacement has been reported to improve physical performance of activities of daily living and return to work (Brochu, 2002; Gohlke-Barwolf, et al., 1992).

Exercise and Psychological Wellbeing

Depression, anxiety, and decreased quality of life or psychological well-being are known sequelae of cardiac diagnoses such as myocardial infarction, CABG, PCI and angina (Shephard & Franklin, 2000). Close to one in three individuals suffering acute myocardial infarction have been found to suffer some form of depression (Lesperance, Frasure-Smith, & Talajic, 1996; Schleifer, et al., 1989). Symptoms of depression and anxiety potentially result in reaction to clinical manifestations of cardiac disease such as reduced functional capacity and potential for hospital re-admissions or further life-threatening events (Shephard & Franklin, 2000).

Meta-analyses of non-cardiac literature indicate that both aerobic and resistance exercise, whether moderate or vigorous, can reduce the symptoms of depression (Dunn, Trivedi, & O'Neil, 2001). Similar findings have emerged from cardiac rehabilitation research where improvements in measures of depression and quality of life (QOL) have been observed following exercise training. These benefits have been observed post-myocardial infarction (Oldridge, et al., 1998; Milani, Lavie, & Cassidy, 1996; Taylor, et al., 1986), following valve replacements (Ueshima, et al., 2004) in older patients (Stahle, et al., 1999) and in women (Lavie, Milani, Cassidy, & Gilliland, 1999), where improvements in exercise capacity were accompanied by reduced depression, anxiety, and/or enhanced QOL. Strength or resistance training in cardiac patients has also been reported to result in improvements in QOL scores (specifically in the emotional health domain of the SF-36), depression and fatigue. (Beniamini, Rubenstein, Zaichkowsky, & Crim, 1997; Izawa, et al., 2004).

Accordingly, clinical guidelines (Wenger, et al., 1995) now advise that exercise training in cardiac rehabilitation generally results in improvement in measures of psychological status and functioning and is recommended to enhance psychological and social functioning.

EXERCISE PRESCRIPTION

Exercise Testing

Before a patient commences exercise training in cardiac rehabilitation, an assessment should be undertaken to establish any potential risks and to prescribe an appropriate exercise regimen. Apart from documenting the patients' medical history and performing a limited physical examination (e.g. blood pressure, pulse, cardiovascular examination), it has been recommended by several authors that an exercise test be performed (Fletcher, et al., 2001; Foster, et al., 2001). Frequently this is performed using a treadmill or stationary bike, and following MI is usually either sub-maximal (a pre-determined end point e.g. peak MET[1] level of 5, or 70% of predicted maximal heart rate) or symptom limited (Fletcher, et al., 2001). There are some shortcomings with such testing; for example, the fact that a treadmill test does not necessarily predict a patient's physiological response to different types or duration of exercise he or she may encounter in cardiac rehabilitation (Williams, 2001). Nevertheless, exercise testing can be used to guide the intensity of exercise training. It must, however, be conducted by well-

---

[1] MET = Metabolic Equivalent (3.5 ml/kg/min of oxygen uptake) – One MET indicates a unit of sitting, resting oxygen uptake. Moderate household tasks are around 3.5 METS, while vigorous exercise is usually around 6 METS or more.

trained and experienced personnel, as up to 10 myocardial infarcts or deaths per 10,000 tests have been reported in those with CHD (Gordon & Kohl, 1993).

Exercise Intensity

Because exercise testing is not available to all cardiac rehabilitation units (e.g. most cardiac rehabilitation programmes in Australia do not have ready access to treadmill testing for the purposes of pre-exercise assessment) exercise intensity can be determined by a variety of methods.

- Maximal oxygen uptake (VO_2 max). This is considered the best measure of cardiovascular fitness and exercise capacity, but there are technical difficulties inherent in its measurement. Exercise training in cardiac rehabilitation initially aims for 40%-60% of VO_2 max, which equates to moderate levels of exercise (Fletcher, et al., 2001; US Department of Health and Human Services, 1996).
- Maximal heart rate. This is determined as either peak heart rate on exercise testing, or 220 minus patient's age. Exercise training in cardiac rehabilitation aims for 50-70% of this figure, which equates to moderate levels of exercise (Fletcher, et al., 2001; US Department of Health and Human Services, 1996).
- Karvonen Method of calculating Heart Rate Reserve (HRR). This calculates heart rate using peak heart rate, resting heart rate and target percentage (e.g. somewhere from 45% to 60%) as follows (Williams, 2001):
  ((Peak heart rate – resting heart rate) x target percentage) + resting heart rate = target heart rate.
- Rating of Perceived Exertion. This is achieved using the Borg Scale (Borg, 1970). This scale of 6 to 20 allows patients to rate their own exercise intensity, and it is recommended that in cardiac rehabilitation they aim for a rating of 11 to 13 (see table 3). This level corresponds to approximately 40% to 60% of VO_2 max, or moderate-intensity exercise (Fletcher, et al., 2001; US Department of Health and Human Services, 1996). This method is particularly useful if patients have difficulty checking their own heart rate, or are on beta-blockers or are post-cardiac transplant, where the heart rate response to exercise is blunted (Williams, 2001).

Table 3. Borg Scale of Perceived Exertion

6	No exertion at all
7	Very, Very Light
8	
9	Very Light
10	Fairly Light
11	
12	
13	Somewhat Hard
14	
15	Hard
16	
17	Very Hard
18	
19	Very, Very Hard
20	Maximal exertion

- Other. If the patient experiences exertional angina, exercise intensity should be set at around 10 beats/minute below the heart rate at which ischaemia is known to occur (e.g. angina or ≥ 1 mm ST segment depression during exercise testing) (Fletcher, et al., 2001). Other signs and symptoms below which exercise intensity should be set include:

  o Plateau or decrease in systolic blood pressure

  o Systolic blood pressure > 240 mmHg

  o Diastolic blood pressure > 110 mmHg

  o Increasing frequency of ventricular arrhythmias

  o Other significant ECG changes

  o Other signs of exercise intolerance (e.g. dizziness, tiredness ≥ 24 hours post-exercise)

Exercise Frequency

Ideally exercise sessions should occur 3 to 5 times per week. This is usually achieved through a combination of formal cardiac rehabilitation sessions 2 to 3 times per week, plus a home programme of walking or other aerobic exercise.

Exercise Duration

For patients who are deconditioned following their cardiac event, exercise sessions may initially be as short as 10 to 15 minutes.

Exercise Modalities

Exercises which utilise large muscle groups such as walking (on treadmill or walking track), cycling, arm ergometry and rowing. The specific choice is usually guided by comorbidities which preclude certain activities (e.g. arthritis), by patient choice, and by available resources. High impact exercises such as jogging on hard surfaces should be avoided to prevent injury.

For a patient's home programme, walking is a preferred modality. It is low-impact and safe, and usually represents an intensity of around 40% to 70% of VO_2 max (Fletcher, et al., 2001). Patients can commence with 10 to 15 minute sessions and gradually increase up to 60 minutes.

Exercise Progression

Patients' exercise can be progressed in terms of duration and intensity according to their exercise tolerance. As the patient's fitness improves, exercise sessions can be increased every 1 to 3 weeks up to 30 to 40 minutes or more, although intensity of exercise may initially need to be reduced when duration is increased. In terms of health benefit, physical effort expending 700 to 2000 kilocalories or more per week is recommended, which can be accumulated in sessions of at least 10 minutes' duration. However, programmes emphasising moderate intensity training with sessions of longer duration (e.g. 30 minutes or more) are recommended for most adults for cardiovascular fitness (Pollock, et al., 1998).

During the course of a cardiac rehabilitation programme, exercise intensity can also be increased. For example, over the course of an 8 to 12 week programme, adjustments of 5% to 10% can be made every 4 weeks in terms of target heart rate. Ultimately, a workload of 85% of maximal heart rate (high intensity exercise) may be aimed for if tolerated by the patient, but moderate intensity exercise will also afford a health benefit.

Exercise may need to be reduced if signs or symptoms of exercise intolerance are observed, e.g. angina, abnormal blood pressure response, Borg rating ≥ 14 or significant cardiac arrhythmia (Williams, 2001).

Home Exercise Programme

A home exercise programme is designed for each patient, including guidelines on heart range for exercise (patients are taught how to check their own pulse) or Borg scale, recovery heart rate (within 10 beats of resting heart rate, 2-5 minutes post-exercise), type of exercise, duration of exercise sessions, and total exercise time per day. Patients are educated to recognise signs of over-exercise (see table 4)

Table 4. Patient Guidelines

Patient Guidelines Signs of Over-Exercise
■ Angina/chest pain. Stop immediately and take Anginine as directed. ■ Shortness of breath. It is expected that you may feel a little puffed with exercise, but not gasping for breath. You should be able to talk. Normally you can recognise this before it becomes severe and therefore slow down. ■ Heart rate greater than desired maximum heart rate. Slow down or stop if necessary. ■ Taking longer than 2-5 minutes to recover. Next time do not exercise as hard or as long. ■ Cold and clammy. It is normal to be hot and sweaty, but not cold, clammy, or very heavy perspiration. Lower intensity of exercise and stop if necessary. ■ Tired and weak in the evening or next morning post-exercise. Next time do not exercise as hard or as long. ■ Dizziness, stomach upsets or other signs of being unwell. Don't exercise.

RESISTANCE EXERCISE

Resistance (or strength) training is now accepted as an important component of cardiac rehabilitation, despite previously-held fears that it increased the risk of cardiovascular complications (Bjarnason-Wehrens, et al., 2004). Some of its benefits for patients with CHD have already been discussed. Resistance training can result in improvements in muscle strength, endurance, mass, and metabolism, as well as enhanced exercise capacity, functional independence, self-efficacy, mood and quality of life (Bjarnason-Wehrens, et al., 2004; McCartney, 1998; Williams, et al., 2007). There is also evidence that resistance training can also reduce blood pressure levels (Cornelissen & Fagard 2005), visceral fat (Treuth, et al., 1994; Treuth, et al., 1995), and glucose control in diabetics (Castaneda, et al., 2002). However, aerobic or endurance training produces greater improvements in cardiovascular function and CHD risk factors (Williams, et al., 2007). Resistance training should be considered an important modality *additional* to aerobic training.

Before commencing resistance training in cardiac rehabilitation, a patient should be assessed for appropriateness. Exclusion criteria for both aerobic and strength training are discussed later in this chapter. Resistance training is contra-indicated in Phase I (inpatient) cardiac rehabilitation (Bjarnason-Wehrens, et al., 2004). Patient's post-MI should wait 2 to 3 weeks before starting strength training (Pollock, et al., 2000).

At the beginning of outpatient cardiac rehabilitation, patients should undergo at least 2 weeks of aerobic training before commencing resistance training. Patients with chest wall wounds (e.g. following CABG) should avoid exercises which cause sternal tension for up to 2 to 3 months post-surgery (Fletcher, et al., 2001).

As with aerobic exercise, resistance training should be considered in terms of frequency, intensity, duration, and modalities.

Resistance Training Intensity

Intensity relates to the actual weight lifted during training. To determine the appropriate weight, the patient's 1-repetition maximum (the maximum weight that can be lifted or moved to complete 1 repetition, 1-RM) is used. Patients then lift a certain percentage of the 1-RM during each set of each exercise. Initially, weights should be around 30% of 1-RM, to ensure correct implementation of each exercise and thus prevent the likelihood of musculoskeletal injury.

Resistance Training Frequency

Two or three sessions per week is recommended (Bjarnason-Wehrens, et al., 2004; Williams et al, 2007). Patients should have a minimum of 48 hours rest between each resistance training session.

Resistance Training Modalities

Resistance training can be performed using a variety of devices including free weights/dumbbells, ankle weights, pulleys or strength training machines. Patients should be educated in correct technique, i.e. a slow controlled movement through the full range of motion, with no breath-holding or Valsalva manoeuvre. One exercise per major muscle group is used, for example:

- Chest press
- Shoulder press
- Triceps extension
- Biceps curl
- Lower back extension
- Latissimus dorsi pull down
- Abdominal crunch
- Quadriceps extension
- Leg (hamstring) curl
- Calf raise

Each exercise is repeated 8 to 10 times per set initially. Weight loads which allow 8 to 15 repetitions usually result in improved muscular strength and endurance (Williams, et al., 2007).

Resistance Training Duration

Initially a single set (maximum 2 sets) of each exercise is recommended (Williams, et al., 2007). A rest period of 30 to 120 seconds between sets is recommended (Dunstan et al 2002; Williams, 2001).

Resistance Training Progression

Patients should increase the number of repetitions performed in each set and the number of sets (maximum 3 sets), before increasing resistance or weight. When a patient is able to perform 3 sets of 10 to 15 repetitions with ease, weight loads can be increased by approximately 5%, and repetitions reduced again. Up to 80% of 1-RM may eventually be achieved in selected patients (Graves & Franklin,, 2001; Volaklis & Tokmakidis, 2005).

As with aerobic training, the Borg scale can be used to monitor exertion during resistance training. Patients should work between 11 and 14 on the scale ("fairly light" to "somewhat hard") (Williams, et al., 2007). Blood pressure and heart rate can also be monitored, although this is not always practical, and heart rate may not rise in proportion to myocardial stress.

SAFETY AND CONTRA-INDICATIONS

Exercise-based cardiac rehabilitation has been demonstrated to be safe for patients who are appropriately assessed and selected. Mortality rates during cardiac exercise programs range from 1 per 116,400 to 1 per 784,000 hours of exercise (Haskell, 1994; Van Camp & Peterson, 1986). The risk of adverse events can be reduced by considering contraindications for participation in aerobic or resistance training as outlined in table 5.

Patients with CHD, valvular or congenital heart disease, or cardiomyopathy can be risk-stratified according to various clinical characteristics (see table 6). For the majority of patients attending outpatient cardiac rehabilitation, they will fall into Class B (low risk for cardiovascular complications with vigorous exercise) or Class C (moderate to high risk for cardiovascular complications with vigorous exercise). Class B patients can be supervised by appropriately trained non-medical cardiac rehabilitation staff, while Class C patients should be under medical supervision during exercise sessions until their safety is established (Fletcher, et al., 2001). For both groups, exercise should be individualised and prescribed by qualified individuals.

Table 5. Absolute and Relative Contraindications
to Aerobic and Resistance Training

Absolute
Unstable Coronary Heart Disease (unstable angina) Within one week of acute myocardial infarction Decompensated Heart Failure Uncontrolled arrhythmias including sinus tachycardia Severe pulmonary hypertension (mean pulmonary arterial pressure >55 mm Hg) Severe and symptomatic aortic stenosis Acute myocarditis, endocarditis, or pericarditis Acute systemic illness or fever Uncontrolled hypertension (>180/110 mm Hg) Postural hypotension ($\geq$ 20 mmHg drop in systolic blood pressure with symptoms of dizziness or light-headedness) Aortic dissection Marfan syndrome Recent embolism Thrombophlebitis High-intensity resistance training (80% to 100% of 1-RM) in patients with active proliferative retinopathy or moderate to severe non-proliferative diabetic retinopathy
Relative (should consult a physician before participation)
Major risk factors for CHD Diabetes at any age Uncontrolled hypertension (>160/>100 mm Hg) Low functional capacity (<4 METs) Musculoskeletal limitations Individuals who have implanted pacemakers or defibrillators

From: AACPR, 1999; Williams, et al., 2007.

Table 6. Risk Stratification for Exercise Training

Class B: Low risk (must include all of the following)	Class C: Moderate to high risk (any of the following)

• New York Heart Association Class 1 or 2
• Exercise capacity ≤ 6 METS
• No evidence of congestive heart failure
• No evidence of myocardial ischaemia or angina at rest or on exercise testing ≤ 6 METS
• Appropriate rise in systolic blood pressure during exercise
• No ventricular tachycardia at rest or with exercise
• Ability to satisfactorily self-monitor intensity of exercise
	• New York Heart Association Class 3 or 4
	• On exercise testing:
	  o Exercise capacity < 6 METS
	  o Myocardial ischaemia or angina at workload <s 6 METS
	  o Fall in systolic blood pressure below resting levels during exercise
	  o Non-sustained ventricular tachycardia with exercise
	• Previous episode of primary cardiac arrest (not in presence of myocardial infarction)
	• A medical problem that patient's physician believes may be life-threatening

From: Fletcher, et al., 2001.

In addition, the following guidelines (AACPR, 1999; Fletcher, et al., 2001; Thompson 2005; Williams, et al., 2007) should be considered:

- After bypass surgery, patients can commence aerobic training 1 to 2 weeks after an uncomplicated operation, but resistance training which stresses the sternal area should be avoided for 2-3 months.
- Patients with postoperative wound infections should not participate until they have been treated with antibiotics for at least a week and activities which compromise the wound should be avoided until the wound is fully healed.
- Patients with postoperative thrombophlebitis should be effectively anticoagulated for a minimum of 2 weeks before commencing exercise training.
- Angioplasty or stent patients who sustained access vessel injury during the procedure and required surgical intervention should avoid exercise

training until the surgical incisions are healed, and activities which compromise the wound should be avoided.

- Repetitive actions such as lifting weights can result in pacing lead fractures and dislodgment (Lampert et al 2006). Patients with implantable devices such as defibrillators or pacemakers should obtain physician clearance before commencing upper-body resistance training.

- For patients with implantable defibrillators, the target heart rate for exercise training should be 10 to 15 beats per minute lower than the threshold discharge rate for the defibrillator.

- Although patients with hypertrophic cardiomyopathy have traditionally been advised to avoid resistance training, a recent American Heart Association statement suggests that low-intensity weight training with machines may be permissible in selected individuals (Maron et al 2004).

- Older patients (over 65 years old) generally have a lower exercise capacity than younger patients. A lower level of energy expenditure (e.g. 40% to 50% of VO_2max), with smaller increases during the course of cardiac rehabilitation, is recommended.

- Patients with diabetic neuropathy are at greater risk of postural hypotension and joint and muscle injuries due to inadequate proprioception and pain perception, thus greater caution is required for these individuals when engaging in exercise training.

- Patients with retinopathy should not engage in high-intensity resistance training because of the risk of vitreous haemorrhage and retinal detachment.

CONCLUSION

Exercise training, both aerobic and resistance, in cardiac rehabilitation is safe for stable patients provided that they have been properly assessed and the training programme is appropriately tailored to each patient's individual needs and potentials. As a result most patients can expect to improve their exercise tolerance, functional ability, and quality of life. Additionally, risk of mortality and hospital re-admission is also reduced as exercise training enhances cardiovascular function and helps to modify cardiac risk factors.

REFERENCES

Ades, P., Pashkow, F.J., & Nestor, J.R. (1997). Cost-effectiveness of cardiac rehabilitation after myocardial infarction. *Journal of Cardiopulmonary Rehabilitation, 17,* 222-31.

Ades, P.A., & Coello, C.E. (2000). Effects of exercise and cardiac rehabilitation on cardiovascular outcomes. *Medical Clinics of North America, 84,* 251–65.

Ades, P.A. (2001). Cardiac rehabilitation and secondary prevention of coronary heart disease. *New England Journal of Medicine, 345,* 892–902.

Allen, J.K., Scott, L.B., Stewart, K.J., & Young, D.R. (2004). Disparities in women's referral to and enrollment in outpatient cardiac rehabilitation. *Journal of General Internal Medicine, 19,* 747-53.

American Association of Cardiovascular and Pulmonary Rehabilitation. (1999). *Guidelines for Cardiac Rehabilitation and Secondary Prevention Programs 3rd Edition.* Human Kinetics: Champaign.

American Heart Association. (2008). *Heart Disease and Stroke Statistics – 2008 Update.* Dallas, Texas: American Heart Association.

Armstrong, T., Bauman, A., & Davies, J. (2000). *Physical activity patterns of Australian adults. Results of the 1999 National Physical Activity Survey.* Canberra: Australian Institute of Health and Welfare.

Australian Institute of Health and Welfare. (2008). Retrieved 16 April, 2009, from www.aihw.gov.au/cvd/index.cfm.

Balady, G.J., Williams, M.A., Ades, P.A., Bittner, V., Comoss, P., Foody, J.M., Franklin, B., Sanderson, B., & Southard, D., American Heart Association Exercise., Cardiac Rehabilitation and Prevention Committee., the Council on Clinical Cardiology., American Heart Association Council on Cardiovascular Nursing., American Heart Association Council on Epidemiology and Prevention., American Heart Association Council on Nutrition., Physical Activity and Metabolism., & American Association of Cardiovascular and Pulmonary Rehabilitation. (2007). Core components of cardiac rehabilitation/secondary prevention programs: 2007 update: a scientific statement from the American Heart Association Exercise, Cardiac Rehabilitation, and Prevention Committee, the Council on Clinical Cardiology; the Councils on Cardiovascular Nursing, Epidemiology and Prevention, and Nutrition, Physical Activity, and Metabolism; and the American Association of Cardiovascular and Pulmonary Rehabilitation. *Circulation, 115,* 2675-2682.

Belardinelli, R., Georgiou, D., Cianci, G. & Purcaro, A. (1999). Randomised, Controlled Trial of Long-Term Moderate Exercise training in Chronic Heart Failure. *Circulation, 99,* 1173-1182.

Belardinelli, R., Paolini, I., Cianci, G., Piva, R., Georgiou, D., & Purcaro, A. (2001). Exercise training intervention after coronary angioplasty: the ETICA Trial. *Journal of the American College of Cardiology, 37,* 1891-1900.

Beniamini, Y., Rubenstein, J.J., Zaichkowsky, L.D. & Crim, M.C. (1997). Effects of high-intensity strength training on quality-of-life parameters in cardiac rehabilitation patients. *American Journal of Cardiology, 80,* 841–846.

Bjarnason-Wehrens, B., Mayer-Berger, W., Meister, E.R., Baum, K., Hambrecht, R., & Gielen S. (2004). Recommendations for resistance training in cardiac rehabilitation. Recommendations of the German Federation for Cardiovascular Prevention and Rehabilitation. *European Journal of Cardiovascular Prevention and Rehabilitation, 11,* 352-361.

Bock, B.C. (2002). Issues in Predicting Adherence to Cardiac Rehabilitation. *Journal of Cardiopulmonary Rehabilitation, 22,* 261-263.

Borg, G. (1970). Perceived exertion as an indicator of somatic stress. *Scandinavian Journal of Rehabilitation Medicine, 2,* 92–98.

Brochu, M., Poehlman, E.T., Savage, P., Fragnoli-Munn, K., Ross, S., & Ades, P.A. (2000). Modest effects of exercise training alone on coronary risk factors and body composition in coronary patients. *Journal of Cardiopulmonary Rehabilitation, 20,* 180–188.

Brochu, M., Savage, P., Lee, M., Dee, J., Cress, M.E., Poehlman, E.T., Tischler, M., & Ades, P.A. (2002). Effects of resistance training on physical function in older disabled women with coronary heart disease. *Journal of Applied Physiology, 92,* 672–678.

Castanedak, C., Layne, J.E., Munoz-Orians, L., Gordon, P.L., Walsmith, J., Foldvari, M., Roubenoff, R., Tucker, K.L., & Nelson, M.E. (2002). A randomized controlled trial of resistance exercise training to improve glycemic control in older adults with type 2 diabetes. *Diabetes Care, 25,* 2335–2341.

Cornelissen, V.A., & Fagard, R.H. (2005). Effect of resistance training on resting blood pressure: a meta-analysis of randomized controlled trials. *Journal of Hypertension, 23,* 251–259.

Dafoe, W., & Huston, P. (1997). Current trends in cardiac rehabilitation. *Canadian Medical Association Journal, 156,* 527-532.

Dunn, A.L., Trivedi, M.H., & O'Neal, H.A. (2001). Physical activity dose-response effects on outcomes of depression and anxiety. *Medicine and Science in Sports and Exercise, 33,* 587–S597.

Dunstan, D.W., Daly, R.M., Owen, N., Jolley, D., de Courten, M., Shaw, J., & Zimett, P. (2002). High intensity resistance training improves glycaemic control in older patients with type 2 diabetes. *Diabetes Care, 25,* 1729–1736.

El-Sayed, M.S., El-Sayed, A.Z., & Ahmadizad, A. (2004). Exercise and training effects on blood haemostasis in health and disease: an update. *Sports Medicine, 34,* 181-200.

European Commission. (2006). Health and Food Special Eurobarometer 246 / Wave 64.3 – TNS Opinion & Social. Retreived 16 April, 2009, from http://ec.europa.eu/ph_publication/eb_food_en.pdf

Fletcher, G.F., Balady, G.J., Amsterdam, E.A., Chaitman, B., Eckel, R., Fleg, J., Froelicher, V.F., Leon, A.S., Piña, I.L., Rodney, R., Simons-Morton, D.A., Williams, M.A., & Bazzarre, T. (2001). Exercise standards for testing and training: a statement for healthcare professionals from the American Heart Association. *Circulation, 104,* 1694–1740.

Fletcher, G.F. (1998). Current status of cardiac rehabilitation. *American Family Physician, 58,* 1778-82.

Foster, C., Cadwell, K., Crenshaw, B., Dehart-Beverley, M., Hatcher, S., Karlsdottir, A.E., Shafer, N.N., Theusch, C., & Porcari, J.P. (2001). Physical activity and exercise training prescriptions for patients. *Cardiology Clinics, 19,* 447-457.

Giannuzzi, A., Mezzani, A., Saner, H., Bjornstad, H., Fioretti, P., Mendes, M., Cohen-Solal, A., Dugmore, L., Hambrecht, R., Hellemans, I., McGee, H., Perk, J., Vanhees, L., & Veress, G. (2003). Physical activity for primary and secondary prevention. Position paper of the Working Group on Cardiac Rehabilitation and Exercise Physiology of the European Society of Cardiology. *European Journal of Cardiovascular Prevention and Rehabilitation, 10,* 319–327.

Gielen, S., & Hambrecht, R. (2001). Effects of exercise training on vascular function and myocardial perfusion. *Cardiology Clinics, 9,* 357-368.

Goble, A.J., & Worcester, M.U.C. (1999). *Best Practice Guidelines for Cardiac Rehabilitation and Secondary Prevention.* Melbourne: Heart Research Centre on behalf of Department of Human Services Victoria.

Gohlke-Bärwolf, C., Gohlke, H., Samek, L., Peters, K., Betz, P., Eschenbruch, E., & Roskamm, H. (1992). Exercise tolerance and working capacity after valve replacement. *Journal of Heart Valve Diseases, 1,* 189-195.

Goldsmith, R.L., Bloomfield, D.M., & Rosenwinkel, E.T. (2000). Exercise and autonomic function. *Coronary Artery Disease, 11,* 129-135.

Gordon, N.F., & Kohl, H.W. (1993). Exercise testing and sudden cardiac death. *Journal of Cardiopulmonary Rehabilitation, 13,* 381-386.

Graves, J.E., & Franklin, B.A. (Eds) (2001). *Resistance Training for Health and Rehabilitation.* Human Kinetics: Champaign.

Hambrecht, R., Walther, C., Mobius-Winkler, S., Gielen, S., Linke, A., Conradi, K., Erbs, S., Kluge, R., Kendziorra, K., Sabri, O., Sick, P., & Schuler, G. (2004). Percutaneous coronary angioplasty compared with exercise training in patients with stable coronary artery disease: a randomized trial. *Circulation, 109,* 1371–1378.

Haskell, W. (1978). Cardiovascular complications during exercise training of cardiac patients. *Circulation, 57,* 920–4.

Haskell, W. (1994). The efficacy and safety of exercise programs in cardiac rehabilitation. *Medicine and Science in Sports and Exercise, 26,* 815-823.

Haskell, W.L., Alderamn, E.L., Fair, J.M., Maron, D.J., Mackey, S.F., Superko, R., Williams, P.T., Johnstone, I.M., Champagene, A., Krauss, R.M., & Farquhar, J.W. (1994). Effects of intensive multiple risk factor reduction on coronary atherosclerosis and clinical cardiac events in men and women with coronary artery disease: The Stanford Coronary Risk Intervention Project (SCRIP). *Circulation, 89,* 975–990.

Hedback, B., Perk, J., Hornblad, M., & Ohlsson, U. (2001). Cardiac rehabilitation after coronary artery bypass surgery: 10-year results on mortality, morbidity and readmissions to hospital. *Journal of Cardiovascular Risk, 8,* 153-158.

Hedback, B., Perk, J., & Wodlin, P. (1993) Long-term reduction of cardiac mortality after myocardial infarction: 10-year results of a comprehensive rehabilitation programme. *European Heart Journal, 14,* 831–835

Hevey, D., Brown, A., Cahill, A., Newton, H., Kierns, M., & Horgan, J.H. (2003). Four-week multidisciplinary cardiac rehabilitation produces similar improvements in exercise capacity and quality of life to a 10-week program. *Journal of Cardiopulmonary Rehabilitation, 23,* 17-21.

Izawa, K., Hirano, Y., Yamada, S., Oka, K., Omiya, K., & Iijima, S. (2004). Improvements in physiological outcomes and health-related quality of life following cardiac rehabilitation in patients with acute myocardial infarction. *Circulation Journal, 68,* 315–320.

Jairath, N., Salerno, T., Chapman, J., Dornan, J., & Weisel, R (1995). The effect of moderate exercise training on oxygen uptake post-aortic/mitral valve surgery. *Journal of Cardiopulmonary Rehabilitation, 15,* 424-430.

Kavanagh, T., Mertens, D.J., Hamm, L.F., Beyene, J., Kennedy, J., Corey, P., & Shephard, R.J. (2002). Prediction of long-term prognosis in 12,169 men referred for cardiac rehabilitation. *Circulation, 106,* 666-671.

Keteyian S, Shepard R, Ehrman J, Fedel F, et al. (1991) Cardiovascular responses of heart transplant patients to exercise training. *Journal of Applied Physiology*, 70, 2627-31.

Ko, J.K., & McKelvie, R.S. (2005). The role of exercise training for patients with heart failure. *Europa Medicophysica, 41,* 35-47.

Lampert, R., Cannom, D., & Olshansky, B. (2006). Safety of sports participation in patients with implantable cardioverter defibrillators: a survey of Heart Rhythm Society members. *Journal of Cardiovascular Electrophysiology, 17,* 11–15.

Lavie, C.J., Milani, R.V., Cassidy, M.M., & Gilliland, Y.Y. (1999). Effects of cardiac rehabilitation and exercise training programs in women with depression. *American Journal of Cardiology, 83,* 1480–1483.

Lavie, C. J., & Milani, R.V. (1996). Effects of Cardiac Rehabilitation and Exercise Training Programs in Patients > 75 years of age. *The American Journal of Cardiology, 78,* 675-677.

Lesperance, F., Frasure-Smith, N., & Talajic, M. (1996). Major depression before and after myocardial infarction: its nature and consequences. *Psychosomatic Medicine, 58,* 99-110.

Malfatto, G., Blengino, S., Annoni, L., Branzi, G., Bizzi, C., & Facchini, M. (2005). Primary coronary angioplasty and subsequent cardiovascular rehabilitation are linked to a favorable sympathovagal balance after a first anterior myocardial infarction. *Italian Heart Journal, 6,* 21-27.

McCartney, N. (1998). Role of resistance training in heart disease. *Medicine and Science in Sports and Exercise 30,* S396-S402.

Maron, B.J., Chaitman, B.R., Ackerman, M.J,, Baye´s dè Luna, A., Corrado, D., Crosson, J.E., Deal, B.J., Driscoll, D.J., Estes, N.A., Arau´jo, C.G., Liang, D.H., Mitten, M.J., Myerburg, R.J., Pelliccia, A., Thompson, P.D., Towbin, J.A., & Van Camp, S.P., for the Working Groups of the American Heart Association Committee on Exercise, Cardiac Rehabilitation, and Prevention, and Councils on Clinical Cardiology and Cardiovascular Disease in the Young. (2004). Recommendations for physical activity and recreational sports participation for young patients with genetic cardiovascular diseases. *Circulation, 109,* 2807–2816.

Milani, R., Lavie, C., & Cassidy, M. (1996). Effects of cardiac rehabilitation and exercise training programs on depression in patients after major coronary events. *American Heart Journal, 132,* 926–932.

Milani, R.V., Lavie, C.J., & Mehra, M.R. (2004). Reduction in C-reactive protein through cardiac rehabilitation and exercise training. *Journal of the American College of Cardiology, 43,* 1056-1061.

National Heart Foundation of Australia & Australian Cardiac Rehabilitation Association. (2004). *Recommended Framework for Cardiac Rehabilitation '04*. National Heart Foundation of Australia. Retrieved 16 April, 2009 from, www.heartfoundation.com.au,2004.

Oldridge, N., Gottlieb, M., Guyatt, G., Jones, N., Streiner, D., & Feeny, D. (1998). Predictors of health-related quality of life with cardiac rehabilitation after acute myocardial infarction. *Journal of Cardiopulmonary Rehabilitation, 18,* 95–103.

Pasanisi, F., Contaldo, F., de Simone, G., & Mancini, M. (2001). Benefits of sustained moderate weight loss in obesity. *Nutrition and Metabolism in Cardiovascular Disease, 11,* 401–406.

Patti, G., Pasceri, V., Melfi, R., Goffredo, C., Chello, M., D'Ambrosio, A., Montesanti, R., & Di Sciascio, G. (2005). Impaired flow-mediated dilation and risk of restenosis in patients undergoing coronary stent implantation. *Circulation, 111,* 70-75.

Pollock, M.L., Gaesser, G.A., Butcher, J.D., Després, J.P., Dishman, R.K., Franklin, B., & Garber, C.E. (1998). ACSM Position Stand: The Recommended Quantity and Quality of Exercise for Developing and Maintaining Cardiorespiratory and Muscular Fitness, and Flexibility in Healthy Adults. *Medicine and Science in Sports and Exercise, 30,* 975-991.

Pollock, M.L, Franklin, B.A., Balady, G.J., Chaitman, B.L., Fleg, J.L., Fletcher, B., Limacher, M., Pina, I.L., Stein, R.A., Williams, M., & Bazzarre, T. (2000). AHA Science Advisory. Resistance exercise in individuals with and without cardiovascular disease: benefits, rationale, safety, and prescription: an advisory from the Committee on Exercise, Rehabilitation, and Prevention, Council on Clinical Cardiology, American Heart Association; Position paper endorsed by the American College of Sports Medicine. *Circulation, 101,* 828–833.

Queensland Health. (2004). *Outpatient cardiac rehabilitation: Best practice guidelines for health Professionals*. Brisbane: Queensland Health.

Rauramaa, R., Li, G., & Vaisanen, S.B. (2001). Dose-response and coagulation and hemostatic factors. *Medicine and Science in Sports and Exercise, 33,* S516-20.

Redwood, D.R., Rosing, D.R., & Epstein, S.E. (1972). Circulatory and symptomatic effects of physical training in patients with coronary-artery disease and angina pectoris. *New England Journal of Medicine, 286,* 959–965.

Rees, K., Taylor, R.S., Singh, S., Coats, A.J., & Ebrahim, S. (2004). Exercise based rehabilitation for heart failure. *Cochrane Database of Systematic Reviews, 3,* CD003331.

Rogers, M., Probbst, M., Gruber, J., Berger, R., & Boone, J.B. Jr. (1996). Differential effects of exercise training intensity on blood pressure and cardiovascular responses to stress in borderline hypertensive humans. *Journal of Hypertension, 11,* 1369–1375.

Schairer, J.R., Kostelnik, T., Proffitt, S.M., Faitel, K.I., Windeler, S., Rickman, L.B., Brawner, C.A., & Keteyian, S.J.. (1998). Caloric expenditure during cardiac rehabilitation. *Journal of Cardiopulmonary Rehabilitation, 18,* 290–294.

Schleifer, S.J., Macari-Hinson, M.M., Coyle, D.A., Slater, W.R., Kahn, M., Gorlin, R., & Zucker, H.D. (1989). The nature and course of depression following myocardial infarction. *Archives of Internal Medicine, 149,* 1785-1789.

Schuler, G., Hambrecht, R., Schlierf, G., Niebauer, J., Hauer, K., Neumann, J., Hoberg, E., Drinkmann, A., Bacher, F., Grunze, M., & Kubler, W. (1992). Regular physical exercise and low-fat diets: effects on progression of coronary artery disease. *Circulation, 86,* 1–11.

Shephard, R.J., & Franklin, B. (2000). Changes in the Quality of Life: A Major Goal of Cardiac Rehabilitation. *Journal of Cardiopulmonary Rehabilitation, 21,* 189-200.

Singh RB, Rastogi V, Rastogi SS, Niaz MA, et al. (1996) Effect of dietand moderate exercise on central obesity and associated disturbances,myocardial infarction and mortality in patients with and without coronary artery disease. *Journal of the American College of Nutrition, 15,* 592-601.

Stahle, A., Mattson, E., Ryden, L., Unden, A., & Nordlander, R. (1999). Improved physical fitness and quality of life following training of elderly patients after acute coronary events: a 1-year follow-up randomized controlled study. *European Heart Journal, 20,* 1475–1484.

Taylor, C.B., Houston-Miller, N., Ahn, D.K., Haskell, W., & DeBusk, R.F. (1986). The effects of exercise training programs on psychosocial improvement in uncomplicated post-myocardial infarction patients. *Journal of Psychosomatic Research, 30,* 581-587.

Taylor, R.S., Brown, A., Ebrahim, S., Jolliffe, J., Noorani, H., Rees, K., Skidmore, B., Stone, J.A., Thompson, D.R., & Oldridge, N. (2004). Exercise-based rehabilitation for patients with coronary heart disease: systematic review and meta-analysis of randomized controlled trials. *American Journal of Medicine, 116,* 682–692.

Thompson, P.D. (2005). Exercise prescription and proscription for patients with coronary artery disease. *Circulation, 112,* 2354-2363.

Treuth, M.S., Hunter, G.R., Kekes-Szabo, T., Weinsier, R.L., & Goran, M.I. (1995). Reduction in intra-abdominal adipose tissue after strength training in older women. *Journal of Applied Physiology, 78,* 1425–1431.

Treuth, M.S., Ryan, A.S., Pratley, R.E., Rubin, M.A., Miller, J.P., Nicklas, B.J., Sorkin, J., Harman, S.M., Goldberg, A.P., & Hurley, B.P. (1994). Effects of strength training on total and regional body composition in older men. *Journal of Applied Physiology, 78,* 614–620.

Ueshima K, Kamata J, Kobayashi N, Saito M, Sato S, Kawazoe K, & Hiramori K. (2004). Effects of exercise training after open heart surgery on quality of life and exercise tolerance in patients with mitral regurgitation or aortic regurgitation. *Japanese Heart Journal, 45,* 789- 97.

US Department of Health and Human Services. (1996). *Physical activity and health: a report of the Surgeon General.* Atlanta, GA: US Department of Health and Human Services, Centers for Disease Control and Prevention, National Center for Chronic Disease Prevention and Health Promotion.

Van Camp, S.P., & Peterson, R.A. (1986). Cardiovascular complications of outpatient cardiac rehabilitation programs. *JAMA, 256,* 1160–1163.

Volaklis, K.A., & Tokmakidis, S.P. (2005). Resistance training in patients with heart failure. *Sports Medicine, 35,* 1085–1103.

Wenger, N.K., Froelicher, E.S., & Smith, L.K. (1995). *Cardiac rehabilitation as secondary prevention. Clinical Practice Guideline No.17.* Rockville, MD: US Dept of Health and Human Services, Public Health Service, Agency for Health Care Policy and Research and the National Heart, Lung, and Blood Institute; AHCPR Publication No. 96-0672.

Williams MA. (2001) Exercise testing in cardiac rehabilitation. Exercise prescription and beyond. Cardiology Clinics, 19, 415-31.

Williams, M.A., Ades, P.A., Hamm, L.F., Keteyian, S.J., LaFontaine, T.P., Roitman, J.L., & Squires, R.W. (2006). Clinical evidence for a health benefit from cardiac rehabilitation: An update. *American Heart Journal, 152,* 835-841.

Williams, M.A., Haskell, W.L., Ades, P.A., Amsterdam, E.A., Bittner, V., Franklin, B.A., Gulanick, M., Laing, S.T., & Stewart, K.J. (2007). Resistance Exercise in Individuals With and Without Cardiovascular Disease: 2007 Update. A Scientific Statement From the American Heart Association Council on Clinical Cardiology and Council on Nutrition, Physical Activity, and Metabolism. *Circulation,* 116, 572-584.

Witt, B.J., Jacobsen, S.J., Weston, S.A., Killian, J.M., Meverden, R.A., Allison, T.G., Reeder, G.S., & Roger, V.L. (2004). Cardiac rehabilitation after myocardial infarction in the community. *Journal of the American College of Cardiology, 44,* 988-996.

World Health Organisation. (2002). *The World Health Report 2002. Reducing Risks, Promoting Healthy Life.* Geneva: World Health Organisation.

World Health Organisation. (2007). Retreived 16 April, 2009, from www.who.int/whosis/database/mort/table1.cfm

Yoshida, T., Kohzuki, M., Yoshida, K., Hiwatari, M., Kamimoto, M., Yamamoto, C., Merguro, S., Endo, N., Kato, A., Kanazawa, M., & Sato, T. (1999). Physical and psychological improvements after phase II cardiac rehabilitation in patients with myocardial infarction. *Nursing and Health Sciences, 1,* 163-170.

Yoshida, T., Yoshida, K., Yamamoto, C., Nagasaka, M., Tadaura, H., Meguro, T., Sato, T., & Kahzuki, M.M. (2001). Effects of a Two-Week, Hospitalised Phase II Cardiac Rehabilitation Program on Physical Capacity, Lipid Profiles and Psychological Variables in Patients with Acute Myocardial Infarction. *Japanese Circulation Journal, 65,* 87-93.

In: Physical Activity in Rehabilitation and Recovery   ISBN: 978-1-60876-400-6
Editor: Holly Blake   © 2010 Nova Science Publishers, Inc.

Chapter 8

"WITHIN YOU AND WITHOUT YOU": INTERNAL AND EXTERNAL FACTORS IN THE REALISATION OF EXERCISE PRINCIPLES

Alison Mckeown[*]

Department of Psychology, University of Sheffield, UK.

ABSTRACT

The main aim of this chapter is to explore internal and external motivational factors in relation to exercise and physical activity undertaken for preventative or rehabilitative reasons. A brief social context is provided and evidence for the benefits of engaging in structured exercise as part of rehabilitation and condition management programmes is discussed. Barriers to exercise are presented and the increased effect they have in the rehabilitative context. The chapter concludes with an evaluation in favour of the health benefits.

---

[*] Tel: +44 (0) 114 222 2000; Fax: +44 (0) 114 276 6515; pcp06acm@sheffield.ac.uk

INTRODUCTION

The Current Social Context for Exercise

Over the past few decades the sport and leisure industry has experienced substantial growth on an international level. The media has largely been responsible for promoting such growth. Television broadcasting has developed several shows where contestants can undergo rigorous training regimes in order to lose weight or celebrities can compete against each other to master a sport in which they have had no previous training. Daytime talk shows proclaim the benefits of exercise, in some cases encouraging viewers to participate with an instructor on screen. Also, alongside the usual reporting of competitive sporting events, there are often documentaries featuring the individual athletes with information on their training programmes and past accomplishments. Frequently, the dominant theme which emerges from these types of programme is that of the 'body beautiful' and how one needs to look good in order to feel socially acceptable. Exercise offers a means to achieve this, albeit with no quick fixes. Tabloid publications proclaim celebrity weight loss on a weekly basis and there is a wealth of exercise videos available where minor celebrities preach versions of their own personal training programmes. Furthermore, there is an abundance of mainstream magazines available to help with designing individual exercise programmes to achieve anything from weight loss and basic fitness through to muscle definition and elite performance.

Aside from the daily bombardment of healthy images showing wholesome individuals enjoying the benefits of exercise, for many people, exercise has a less positive representation. It is something which can be painful, time consuming and notoriously difficult to fit into the time available for pursuit of leisure activities. The perceived value attributed to exercise varies, with some individuals having high levels of motivation to engage in training programmes, to belong to clubs and to attend leisure facilities such as swimming pools or gyms on a regular basis. However, others find this very difficult. There are those who choose not to engage at all, believing that exercise is either too hard, they are too busy, or that it will not offer any benefit. Other people hold strong intentions or desires to pursue exercise, but struggle to maintain a programme or to overcome the initial feelings of anxiety around starting an exercise programme. Finally, there is another group of people: those attempting to return to exercise following the onset of illness, injury or disability. Prior to the incident affecting their body, it is likely that many of these people will have been engaged in a programme of regular exercise and consequently may be experiencing a strong sense of 'bereavement' in relation to previous function. For others who have not engaged in exercise before they may be confronted with the need to participate in order to improve their physical condition. However, they may be fighting an internal scepticism over the perceived benefits and at the same time having to adjust to a new lifestyle.

Furthermore, the UK government considers that exercise plays a major role in tackling perceived levels of obesity within the general population. Engaging in more physical forms of activity can also contribute to a reduced risk of developing conditions such as coronary heart disease, stroke, type 2 diabetes and certain types of cancer.

EXERCISE AND REHABILITATION

Research suggests that exercise can have a beneficial effect for people adjusting to and recovering from a variety of different health conditions. Seyler, et al., (2006) promote the need for people to maintain physical activity post joint surgery in order to preserve bone quality and because of the positive benefits of exercise for general well being. Kennedy, et al., (2006) studied a group of people who were recovering from a spinal cord injury. They observed that participation in exercise and team based activity led to a reduction in self reported anxiety and an increase in perceived ability to cope. Regular participation in exercise has also been shown to lead to improvements in functioning and ability to manage symptoms in people with a diagnosis of rheumatoid arthritis (Metsios, et al., 2008).

For some groups of people participation in exercise is more difficult than others. Fromme, et al., (2007) investigated the attitudes towards participation in exercise held by people with haemophilia. Previously, participation in exercise was denied for this group due to the high level of risk associated with the occurrence of injury. Advances in treatment have meant that participation is now possible, but risks must be carefully assessed, monitored and counterbalanced with the beneficial health effects provided by regular exercise. In relation to this group of people, exercise offers the specific benefit of muscle strengthening providing greater support to joints and decreasing the risk of damage, which leads to bleeding complications. Difficulties were noted in identifying particular exercise modalities which would be suited to this group, but exercise participation in general was viewed positively. Attitudes of respondents to the study reflected that social and enjoyment factors were the biggest sources of motivation to engage in physical activity.

PROMOTION OF EXERCISE

According to a UK Government publication (Gameplan, 2002), in comparison with other countries only forty-six percent of the UK population participate in exercise more than twelve times a year, whereas in Sweden there is a seventy percent rate of participation and in Finland participation rates are nearer to eighty percent. In the UK, roughly thirty-two percent of adults engage in the recommended thirty minutes of moderate intensity exercise five times per week, compared to Australia where fifty-seven percent of adults and Finland where seventy percent of adults engage in this level of exercise. Current recommendations (Gameplan, 2002) suggest that participating in exercise of a moderate intensity, for half an hour five times a week is beneficial for reducing the incidence of certain types of cancer, strokes, cardiovascular problems and obesity. This parallels the concept of 'Prehab' which refers to the prevention of conditions which if allowed to develop would require rehabilitation. Strategies for prevention have thus become complementary to strategies for rehabilitation.

For over fourteen years now in the UK, a number of local primary health providers have been involved in schemes with local government which have allowed General Practitioners (GPs) to prescribe exercise programmes for people with particular health needs. Evidence suggests that there are beneficial effects for the physical and mental health of individuals who participate in prescribed exercise programmes (Lord & Green, 1995). Such programmes are also a useful means of promoting active lifestyles and improving individual quality of life (Kallings, et al., 1997). King and Senn (1996) state that exercise can protect individuals from developing the symptoms of chronic disease or arrest the progress of existing disease. However, they recommend that detailed assessment should be undertaken before commencing an exercise programme so as to establish the current physical capabilities of the individual and any potential risks to their health. The mode of recruitment to an exercise programme is also important. Exercise consultation sessions have been found to be more encouraging for participation than receipt of a promotional information leaflet (Kirk, et al., 2001).

When undertaking the actual act of prescribing an exercise programme, one group of GPs reported that they had favoured providing written prescriptions for people, over solely verbal recommendations. It was believed that there were positive implications for the individual to have a formal record of the consultation and its recommendations (Swinburn, et al., 1997). GP recommendation has been found to be influential in encouraging participation in cardiac rehabilitation programmes (Fernandez, et al., 2008) but other evidence suggests that attitude and previous experiences of exercise will also have an impact upon compliance to a rehabilitation programme (Howard & Gosling, 2008).

EXERCISE PRINCIPLES

Dick (1980) identifies three main principles of exercise: specificity, overload and reversibility. Although aimed at elite athletes, these principles remain true for all individuals undertaking an exercise programme. Specificity is concerned with adaptation of the body in relation to the stress which a particular form of exercise places upon it. Overload is the gradual increase of the stress upon the body especially the muscles. Exercise should be graded in a manner which allows adaptation and increases in performance to occur. Increasing demands too rapidly may place too much pressure on the body and lead to exhaustion or injury. Reversibility refers to the effects which occur when exercise levels decrease or cease altogether. Decline in fitness will be gradual. The main effects of disengaging with exercise are muscle atrophy, reduced efficiency of the circulatory respiratory and digestive systems, potential weight gain and a possible lowering of mood. For people approaching exercise as part of the rehabilitation process, fitness is likely to have been restricted in the ways mentioned above and possibly complicated by injuries which will have an impact upon ability to perform. When commencing an exercise programme it takes time for the metabolism to adjust. Therefore, changes will not occur straightaway.

Key factors which require consideration when designing an exercise programme are deciding on an activity, arranging set times when the activity will occur, the frequency and duration of sessions and the intensity level of the activity. Appropriate rest may be taken at defined intervals but it is important that momentum is maintained or motivation and performance will begin to decline. Periodically, changing demands upon the body will produce improvements. Maintenance of exercise levels at the same level of demand will lead to a plateau in performance over time. Exercise schedules can be varied by participating in alternative exercise modalities to an equal level of intensity after an initial graded transition period. Traditionally, exercise modalities have had seasonality in the types of activity undertaken. Seasonality still exists within personal sport, but developments in technology have meant that professional sport has extended its seasons to become virtually year round.

Undertaking exercise as part of condition management or rehabilitation from injury can be a painful and slow process. However, it is important that the individual continues to engage with some form of activity. Decline in activity will lead to decline in fitness and function which will have implications for recovery (Dick, 1980). Exercise provides physical conditioning and stimulates the production of endorphins which naturally lift the mood. The satisfaction provided by progress in ability contributes to an increased sense of self-esteem.

LIFESTYLE CHANGES

The type of exercise that an individual will choose to engage in will be influenced by their lifestyle. People with structured, goal focused lifestyles will have more of a tendency towards endurance activities with repetitive training patterns, whereas people with more impulsive lifestyles are likely to prefer physical activities involving more sudden activity, like ball games (Svebak & Kerr, 1989). Unfortunately the requirements of rehabilitation preclude making motivational choices about the mode of exercise. Incorporating exercise into one's daily activities involves making adjustments. Training sessions will need to be structured and designed to allow for improvement in fitness levels and ability and hopefully to facilitate it. Schedules are usually based around the time period of a week in order to accommodate other activities, such as work. If we consider the relevance of this for rehabilitation, certainly in the early stages, the structure of work may not be an issue as chronic illness or injury may prevent attendance at work. In some cases people are not able to return to work, but for others, the maintenance of an established exercise programme becomes a consideration when return to work is imminent. However, to return to the idea of commencing an exercise programme during an early stage of rehabilitation, timetabling would have to allow for possible attendance at hospital appointments and access to facilities. Approaches to exercise may need to be adapted in order to meet successfully the diverse needs of individuals. Wallin, et al., (2008) describe how a combination of structured independent performance, guided exercise and circuit training were used with a group of older adults to increase their confidence and participation in physical exercise. For many individuals, prophylactic exercise programmes are prescribed by a physiotherapist with precise exercises to target specific deficits. The case example below demonstrates the transition from hospital based exercise to the use of public facilities and some of the considerations which required addressing.

Case Example

Mr V was a 42 year old man who had experienced a stroke and was left with severe aphasia and right sided paralysis .Three days a week he was attending a rehabilitation facility to receive Speech & Language Therapy, Physiotherapy, Occupational Therapy and Clinical Psychology support. On the days when he was at home he was managing to accomplish household maintenance tasks and would visit his parents while his wife was at work. Prior to the occurrence of the stroke, Mr V had been fit, enjoying cycling and weekly games of badminton. Mr V had developed a low mood in response to his loss of speech and physical function and the consequent loss of independence. As his recovery progressed, it was decided that on days when he was at home Mr V could go to the local gym and do his exercises there. The physiotherapist from the rehabilitation facility liaised with staff at the local leisure centre and arranged for Mr V to have an induction, which she accompanied him to. Attention was paid to Mr V's difficulties with expressed language and leisure centre staff were briefed on communication strategies. A fitness instructor also consulted with Mr V and a programme was developed which would maintain the specific progress he had made during physiotherapy whilst allowing him to continue improving his general fitness. Mr V was encouraged to use the swimming pool at the leisure centre as well as the gym facilities but he was less motivated to engage with this as his physical disability was more pronounced in the water, posing an increased safety problem. It is also likely that he struggled with having to change his clothing and disliked others observing him struggle. Although the swimming was not maintained, Mr V continued to attend the gym and expressed enjoyment at the independence this afforded him as well as the physical benefit. The extent of Mr V's residual disability meant that it was not possible for him to return to work but the exercise schedule offered him regular and meaningful activity.

BARRIERS TO COMMENCING EXERCISE AS PART OF THE REHABILITATION PROCESS

A change in lifestyle, behaviour or simply having a new experience can be anxiety provoking for many people. This is best summarised by the German term "*schwellenangst*" (Fortey, et al., 2003) which literally refers to fear of crossing the threshold, hence fear of starting something new. If we apply this concept to exercise, entering a facility can be difficult for individuals as it raises mini challenges such as which room to go to, where to change and where to leave belongings. All of this is tempered with existing anxiety concerning ability to perform and the human need to conform to the behaviour of others (Asch, 1955). If one has a visible disability then this may be heightened with anxiety about accessing facilities. Participation in exercise in a public setting leaves one open to comment and vulnerable to criticism. Many activities require wearing fewer clothes or specialist clothing and this can both impact upon a person's body image and alter the way they view themselves, or their prevailing perception of themselves may prevent them from engaging with the activity. Bain, Wilson, and Chaikind (1989) found that the perceptions and motivations of women attempting to overcome obesity were influenced by past social experiences relating to criticism of body size.

Moreover, for some people it is likely that they will not have participated in organised or structured physical activity since leaving school. Experiences of school based physical activity are often reported as being negative. A study examining young people's attitudes towards exercise revealed that school based physical activity was perceived by some respondents as boring, potentially humiliating, restricted in choice and intrusive towards personal privacy (Mulvihill, Rivers, & Aggleton, 2000). By contrast, other respondents reported that they enjoyed the social aspects of team games. For the individuals concerned, all of these perceptions will serve to influence their future beliefs about exercise participation. The beliefs of people attending rehabilitation or being encouraged to participate in exercise for health reasons will also have been subject to the early influence of school based physical activity. Consequently, this may lead to a resurgence of memories from this time, particularly if negative experiences occurred in the past. Such memories may contribute to feelings of resistance towards exercise or incite feelings of reduced confidence within the individual. Therefore, sensitivity and awareness of possible past experiences should be applied when encouraging participation.

Heavy or complicated equipment also presents a challenge for people and can often be perceived as intimidating. In the interests of Health and Safety, good public gyms offer an induction for users to learn how to use the equipment and how to make best use of the services available. Having someone introduce one to the equipment helps to allay fears about looking foolish and allows space to ask questions. This may be of particular importance for user groups with physical disabilities or health problems as particular needs can be addressed. As demonstrated in the case example of "Mr V", this may be just as much about the leisure centre staff learning how best to accommodate the needs of the user as the user learning about the service. Certain conditions such as asthma, epilepsy or diabetes should be disclosed to leisure centre staff if it is possible that an attack may occur whilst on the premises. Understandably, it may feel intrusive for individuals with these conditions to tell strangers about their medical history and one hopes that they will be met with sensitivity. However, it is often common practice now for many leisure facilities to include questions on medical history as a routine part of all induction sessions. Failure to do so leads towards the question of due diligence in law. Many fitness classes begin with the instructor enquiring about the existence of any medical conditions or injuries within the group.

THE STAGES OF CHANGE MODEL (MILLER AND ROLLNICK, 1991) AND THE REHABILITATION/EXERCISE CONTINUUM

Miller and Rollnick (1991) propose a five-stage model of change. They state that change begins with a "pre-contemplation" phase where the individual does not recognise a need to change. This progresses to the "contemplation" phase where the individual is beginning to identify the possibility of making a change and what this might involve. The next stage is the "preparation" phase when the individual makes plans to implement the change, including the removal of potential obstacles and the acquisition of potential supports. Following this is the "action" phase where the change is actively implemented and then the "maintenance" phase where the individual endeavours to preserve the change. Across time, other factors in the individual's life may evolve and this might necessitate revisiting some of the earlier stages in order to revise the change and facilitate continued maintenance.

Let us now apply this model to physical health and the idea of commencing exercise as part of rehabilitation. For an individual who did not previously recognise exercise as a need, they would have to consider which activity they would like to engage in and the influence of their own physical capabilities. The preparation phase might involve researching local exercise facilities (e.g. classes, opening times, cost etc.) and making sure that they possess any necessary equipment such as training shoes or a swimming costume. This will be followed by the action phase where the individual will begin to participate in regular exercise and the maintenance phase, which -involves ensuring continued participation. The departure from rehabilitation to 'normal' exercise may not involve a discernible transition.

MOTIVATION

A successful exercise programme requires commitment and effort over a sustained period of time. For many people this can seem a daunting prospect, especially as the benefits are not immediately forthcoming. This contrasts with behavioural theories (Skinner, 1961, 1974) of motivation which propose that there needs to be a reinforcing factor for the behaviour to be repeated. Delayed gratification means that the individual has to motivate themselves cognitively in the initial stages of an exercise programme, visualising the prospect of future feelings of strength and fitness. Sullivan, et al., (2008) showed that the perceived benefits of undertaking exercise and self-efficacy in relation to exercise were the two most important determinants of exercise intentions.

In relation to exercise, motivation has several strands. The individual must motivate themselves to undertake each isolated session as well as the programme as a whole. Individuals have different motivations for participation in exercise. These motivations will probably be subject to daily variation (Frey, 1993) and those with a chronic condition are likely to be influenced by the intensity of the symptoms being experienced (Charmaz, 1997). Starting an exercise session requires an initial burst of effort which then has to be maintained for the duration of the session. For example, it may take some resolve to get up and leave the house for a walk; but if the wind is blowing strongly, it begins to rain or tiredness simply sets in, it might take extra effort to complete the activity. Likewise, if one is feeling fatigued or in physical discomfort before the session commences, then it could be difficult to generate the desire to undertake activity, which at times will possibly contribute to an exacerbation of these sensations. Those with chronic conditions will experience what Charmaz (1997) characterises as "good days" or "bad days". The difference between the two may reflect psychological states and physiological conditions, which are either conducive to exercise or adverse to it. Furthermore, when illness becomes established as a core feature of the self identity it can be difficult to envisage an alternative future where illness experiences will play a less dominant role. The planning and conduct of exercise presupposes a future of betterment in some measure.

Aesthetic factors have been found to contribute to motivation for engaging in exercise (Pretty, et al., 2005). Running, walking or cycling through the countryside produces a sensation of having travelled to somewhere; this is different from using a treadmill or static exercise bike in the gym. One also has that connection with the seasons and the diversity in the landscape and unfortunately at times the weather! Exercising in a natural environment has been found to have a positive impact upon mood (Pretty, et al., 2005). The losses which accompany the onset of chronic illness or acquired disability frequently result in low mood (Gadalla, 2008; Gureje, 2008; Mulley, 2008). Prolonged periods spent in confinement can produce sensations of incarceration which will also impact upon the mood of the individual. Therefore, a factor which can contribute to lifting the mood is beneficial for those who are able to participate. However, individuals who are undergoing rehabilitation may experience an increased sense of vulnerability exercising in the outside environment depending on the nature of their condition and whether or not support is available.

A further source of motivation is provided by vicarious experiences. Observing others performing and achieving can provide the impetus to encourage the individual to continue attempting to reach their goals (Bandura, 1977). Once goals begin to be accomplished, this can then spur the individual into setting more advanced or difficult goals for themselves, thus continuing their own development. The achievement of goals has beneficial effects for self-efficacy and assists in the development of a positive self concept (Bandura, 1977).

Individual belief systems are instrumental in commencing and adhering to an exercise programme. Individual decisions to engage repeatedly in behaviour are influenced by perceptions of how this behaviour was previously received by others (Albarracin & Wyer, 2000). Positive beliefs about the beneficial effects of exercise can serve as a large source of motivation. These beliefs may not be near the forefront whilst engaged in the effort of physical activity, but noticed afterwards when experiencing the benefits of having undertaken exercise (Kerr, 1997). Analysis of people's beliefs about participation in exercise has identified that health benefits are the largest source of motivation for engaging people in exercise, within a non rehabilitation context (Zunft, et al., 1999). Other influential reasons were relaxation and increased fitness. Weight loss was recognised as beneficial, but endorsement of this view was relatively low. The main obstacles preventing regular participation in physical activity were work activities and individuals believing that they were not the sort of person who enjoys or is good at exercise. Similar barriers apply within a rehabilitation context with the addition of a further range including reduced mobility, fear of further injury, reduced vision, cognitive impairment, dizziness, exacerbation of persistent pain and increased fatigue.

Some individuals have been observed to display a disparity between their thoughts and beliefs and the actions that they choose to pursue. Festinger (1957) refers to this disparity as "cognitive dissonance". He postulates that being in a state of cognitive dissonance is uncomfortable for the individual concerned. Such discomfort will usually serve as a motivation to take action which will remove the disparity and lead to a more consistent interaction between thoughts, beliefs and behaviour. When this theory is applied to the decision to undertake exercise, it is frequently observed that there are individuals who talk about wanting to participate, but this is not reflected in their behaviour. Likewise, there are people who undertake massive amounts of exercise at risk of detrimental effects to their physical wellbeing yet expound the view that their efforts are minimal and they need to do more. At this point it is worth noting that like many behaviours, exercise holds the potential to be considered an addiction if taken to excess. Individuals who use exercise to reinforce their self esteem may develop a dependency on physical exercise as a means by which to continue supporting their personal sense of self (Groves, et al., 2008). However, this is a large area of concern and beyond the scope of this chapter, although it does raise concerns for the physical rehabilitation of individuals who have sustained serious injury as a result of excessive levels of exercise. Nevertheless, for the average individual undertaking rehabilitation, there is often a small amount of cognitive dissonance between goals and actual activity undertaken but this can be overcome through modification of the goals until agreement is reached on what is realistic and achievable.

LOCUS OF CONTROL: INTERNAL FACTORS VS. EXTERNAL FACTORS

Locus of control refers to the level of responsibility that an individual adopts in relation to their experience in the world (Phares, 1976). Beliefs may be global or specific and are situated along a continuum of attribution ranging from internal factors to external factors. Rotter (1966) discovered that the relationship between internal and external beliefs is curvilinear; with individuals whose beliefs are situated at either extreme of the continuum will experience mood difficulties. If one takes too much personal responsibility, the weight can be crippling to manage. Conversely, if one does not take any personal responsibility, then one loses a sense of choice or accomplishment. The key is for the individual to discover a balance between the internal and the external. Let us now consider the relevance of this concept for motivating participation in exercise.

INTERNAL FACTORS RELEVANT TO EXERCISE

Internal factors are important when engaging in exercise as they allow the individual to develop a sense of agency alongside a sense of mastery. Perceived choice and belief in one's ability contribute to a sense of self-esteem, helping to reduce feelings of low mood or low self worth. Schwarzer, et al., (2008) studied people engaged in cardiac or orthopaedic rehabilitation and found that adherence to exercise programmes was more likely to occur if the individual possessed internal responsibility for their recovery and participated in scheduling their own activity.

As outlined earlier, individual beliefs are large internal factors influencing an individual's ability to engage with participation in exercise, or indeed one could argue most forms of activity. Consequently, beliefs about potential harm might impair ability to participate. These beliefs frequently arise in rehabilitation settings and need to be identified and explored or even challenged if the individual is to participate successfully. Familiarity might also have a detrimental effect upon motivation. Many exercise programmes, whether general exercise or rehabilitative, are repetitive in nature and hold the potential to evoke sensations of boredom within the individual. Therefore, efforts should be made to ensure that the activity remains interesting and occasionally novel. Wherever possible efforts should be made to try and preserve a sense of recreation and enjoyment.

EXTERNAL FACTORS RELEVANT TO EXERCISE

Exercise in a group can be highly motivating for individuals as it carries social benefits such as forming new relationships or receiving support from others. Illness or injury usually carries a recuperation period. If this is prolonged then it may mean that the individual becomes socially isolated. The social contacts offered by group exercise and the identity provided by group membership (Carless & Douglas, 2008) may help to foster a sense of belonging and lead to increased self-esteem. Team based activities carry social pressures not to 'let the side down', emphasising the need for consistent performance. The 'Hawthorne effect' (Mayo, 1927- 1932) demonstrates that being watched generates a sense of observed performance which can lead to wanting to perform to a higher standard and may introduce an element of competition.

In a similar vein, the increasing trend of people employing a personal trainer or coach reflects the need for external motivation at times when internal motivation may flag. Essentially, one is purchasing an audience as well as technical expertise. It may be seen that personal strategies for exercise have been borrowed from rehabilitation. In rehabilitation settings, exercise is usually introduced under the guidance of a physiotherapist, who will often undertake a facilitative and motivational role in engaging the individual with an exercise programme. For example, physiotherapists may lead group based exercise sessions in the management of chronic pain conditions (Holden, et al., 2008).

CONCLUSION

Exercise can have positive health benefits for all people, including those already in full health, those engaged in rehabilitation and those who have been diagnosed with a health condition. Commencing and maintaining an exercise programme requires preparation, motivation and delayed gratification. Motivation will vary across different individuals and will depend on various other factors such as the health condition itself, the duration for which it has been experienced, the intensity and severity of symptoms, the stage of rehabilitation and the nature of any other treatments being undertaken. These varied factors need to be acknowledged and allowed for when designing an exercise programme.

REFERENCES

Albarracin, D., & Wyer, R.S. (2000). The Cognitive Impact of Past Behaviour: Influences on Beliefs, Attitudes and Future Behavioural Decisions. *Journal of Personal and Social Psychology, 79(1),* 5-22.

Asch, S.E. (1955). Opinions and Social Pressure. *Scientific American, 193(5),* 31-35.

Bain, L.L., Wilson, T., & Chaikind, E. (1989). Patient Perceptions of Exercise Programmes for Overweight Women. *Research Quarterly for Exercise and Sport, 60(2),* 134-143.

Bandura, A. (1977). Self-efficacy: Toward a Unifying Theory of Behavioural Change. *Psychological Review, 84,* 191-215.

Carless, D., & Douglas, K. (2008). Narrative, Identity and Mental Health: How Men with Serious Mental Illness Re-story their Lives through Sport and Exercise. *Psychology of Sport and Exercise, 9(5),* 576-594.

Charmaz, K. (1997). *Good Days Bad Days: The Self in chronic Illness and Time.* New Jersey: Rutgers University Press

Department of Culture, Sport and Media. *More Sport for Everyone.* Retrieved April 4, 2009, from http://www.culture.gov.uk/what_we_do/sport/3466.aspx.

Department of Culture, Sport and Media and The Strategy Unit, The Cabinet Office. (2002). *Gameplan: A strategy for delivering Government's sport and physical activity objectives.* Retrieved April 4, 2009, from http://www.sportdevelopment.org.uk/gameplan2002.

Dick, F. W. (1980). *Sports Training Principles.* London: Lepus Books.

Fernandez, R.S., Salamonson, Y., Griffiths, R., Juergens, C., & Davidson, P. (2008). Sociodemographic Predictors and Reasons for Participation in an Outpatient Cardiac Rehabilitation Programme Following Percutaneous Coronary Intervention. *International Journal of Nursing Practice, 14(3),* 237-242.

Festinger, L. (1957). *A Theory of Cognitive Dissonance.* California: Stanford University Press.

Fortey, S., Kopleck, H., Galloway, H., & Schnoor, V. (Eds) (2003). *Collins German English Dictionary* (4th Edition). Glasgow: HarperCollins Publishers.

Frey, K. (1993). Distance Running: A Reversal Theory Analysis. In, J.H. Kerr, S. Murgatroyd and M.J. Apter (Eds). Advances in Reversal Theory. Lisse: Swets and Zeitlinger. In, Kerr, J.H. (1997). *Motivation and Emotion in Sport: Reversal Theory.* Hove: Taylor and Francis.

Fromme, A., Dreeskamp, K., Pollmann, H., Thorwesten, L., Mooren, F.C., & Volker, K. (2007). Participation in Sports and Physical Activity of Haemophilia Patients. *Haemophilia, 13,*323–327.

Gadalla, T. (2008). Association of Comorbid Mood Disorders and Chronic Illness with Disability and Quality of Life in Ontario, Canada. *Chronic Disease in Canada, 28(4), 148*-154.

Groves, M., Biscomb, K., Nevill, A. and Matheson, H. (2008) Exercise Dependence, Self-esteem and Identity Reinforcement: A Comparison of Three Universities in the United Kingdom. *Sport in Society, 11(1),* 59-73.

Gureje, O. (2008). The Relation Between Multiple Pains and Mental Disorders: Results from the World Mental Health Surveys. *Pain, 135 (1-2),* 82-91.

Holden, M.A., Nicholls, E.E., Hay, E.M., & Foster, N.E. (2008). Physical Therapists' Use of Therapeutic Exercise for Patients with Clinical Knee Osteoarthritis in the United Kingdom: In Line with Current Recommendations? *Physical Therapy, 88(10),* 1109-1121.

Howard, D.B., & Gosling, C.M. (2008). A Short Questionnaire to Identify Patient Characteristics Indicating Improved Compliance to Exercise Rehabilitation

Programmes: A Pilot Investigation. *International Journal of Osteopathic Medicine, 11(1)*, 7-15.

Kallings, L.V., Leijon, M., Hellénius, M.L., & Ståhle, A. (2007). Physical activity on prescription in primary health care: a follow-up of physical activity level and quality of life. *Scandinavian Journal of Medicine & Science in Sports, 18(2)*, 154-161.

Kennedy, P., Taylor, N., & Hindson, L. (2006). A Pilot Investigation of a Psychosocial Activity Course for People with Spinal Cord Injuries. *Psychology, Health & Medicine, 11(1)*, 91–99.

Kerr, J.H. (1997). Motivation and Emotion in Sport: Reversal Theory. Hove: Taylor and Francis

King, C.N., & Senn, M.D. (1996). Exercise Testing and Prescription: Practical Recommendations for the Sedentary. *Sports Medicine, 21(5)*, 326-336.

Kirk, A. F., Higgins, L. A., Hughes, A. R., Fisher, B. M., Mutrie, N., Hillis, S., & MacIntyre, P. D. (2001). A Randomized, Controlled Trial to Study the Effect of Exercise Consultation on the Promotion of Physical Activity in People with Type 2 Diabetes: a Pilot Study. *Diabetic Medicine, 18*, 877-882.

Lord, J.C. & Green, F. (1995). Exercise on Prescription: Does it Work? *Health Education Journal, 54(4)*, 453-464.

Mayo, G.E. (1927-1932). *The Hawthorne Studies*. Retrieved 4 April, 2009, from http://www.nwlink.com-Hawthorneeffect.

Miller, W.R., & Rollnick, S. (1991). *Motivational Interviewing: Preparing People for Change*. New York: Guilford Press

Metsios, G.S., Stavropoulos-Kalinglou, A., Veldhuijzen van Zanten, J.J.C.S., Treharne, G.J., Panoulas, V.F., Douglas, K.M.J., Koutedakis, Y., & Kitas, G.D. (2008). Rheumatoid Arthritis, Cardiovascular Disease and Physical Exercise: A Systematic Review. *Rheumatology, 47(3)*, 239-248.

Mulley, G. (2008). Depression in Physically Ill Older Patients. In, S. Curran and J.P. Wattis (Eds) (2008). *Practical Management of Affective Disorders in Older People: A Multi Professional Approach*. Abingdon: Radcliffe.

Mulvihill, C., Rivers, K., & Aggleton, P. (2000). Views of young People Towards Physical Activity: Determinants and Barriers to Involvement. *Health Education, 100(5)*, 190-199.

Phares, E.J. (1976). *Locus of Control in Personality*. New Jersey: General Learning Press.

Pretty, J., Peacock, J., Sellens, M., & Griffin, M. (2005). The Mental and Physical Health Outcomes of Green Exercise. *International Journal of Environmental Health Research, 15(5)*, 319-337.

Rotter, J.B. (1966). Generalized Expectancies for Internal Versus External Control of Reinforcement. *Psychological Monographs, 80(1),* 1-28.

Skinner, B.F. (1961). Cumulative Record. London: Methuen. In, A. Slater and D. Muir, (1999). *The Blackwell Reader in Developmental Psychology.* Oxford: Blackwell Publishing.

Skinner, B.F. (1974). About Behaviourism. New York: Knopf. In, V.H. Vroom and E.L. Deci (Eds), (1992). *Management and Motivation: Selected Readings* (2nd Ed) London: Penguin.

Schwarzer, R., Luszczynska, A., Ziegelmann, J.P., Scholz, U., & Lippke, S. (2008). Social-Cognitive Predictors of Physical Exercise Adherence: Three Longitudinal Studies in Rehabilitation. *Health Psychology, 27(1 Suppl),* S54-63.

Seyler, T. M., Mont, M. A., Ragland, P.S., Kachwala, M.M., & Delanois, R.E. (2006). Sports Activity after Total Hip and Knee Arthroplasty: Specific Recommendations Concerning Tennis. *Sports Medicine, 36(7),* 571-583.

Sullivan, Karen A. and White, Katherine M. and Young, Ross M., & Scott, Clinton J. (2008). Predictors of intention to exercise to reduce stroke risk among people at risk of stroke: An application of an extended Health Belief Model. *Rehabilitation Psychology.* (In Press)

Svebak, S., & Kerr, J.H. (1989). The Role of Impulsivity in Preference for Sports. *Personality and Individual Differences, 10(1),* 51-58.

Swinburn, B.A., Walter, L.G., Arroll, B., Tilyard, M.W., & Russell, D.G. (1997). Green Prescriptions: Attitudes and Perceptions of General Practitioners Towards Prescribing Exercise. *British Journal of General Practice, 47(422),* 567-569.

Thurston, M., & Green, K. (2004). Adherence to Exercise in Late Life: How Can Exercise on Prescription Programmes be Made More Effective? *Health Promotion International, 19(3),* 379-387.

Wallin, M., Talvitie, U., Cattan, M., & Karppi, S.L. (2008). Construction of Group Exercise Sessions in Geriatric Inpatient Rehabilitation. *Health Communication, 23(3).* 245-252.

Zunft, H-J.F., Friebe, D., Seppelt, B., Widhalm, K., de Winter, A-M.R., de Almeida, M.D.V., Kearney, J.M., & Gibney, M. (1999). Perceived Benefits and Barriers to Physical Activity in a Nationally Representative Sample in the European Union. *Public Health Nutrition, 2,* 153-160.

In: Physical Activity in Rehabilitation and Recovery   ISBN: 978-1-60876-400-6
Editor: Holly Blake   © 2010 Nova Science Publishers, Inc.

Chapter 9

REPRESENTATION AND PERCEPTIONS OF INJURY IN SPORT AND EXERCISE: THE 'COMMON SENSE' MODEL

Martin S. Hagger[*]

School of Psychology, University of Nottingham, UK.

ABSTRACT

The common-sense model of illness perceptions (Leventhal, Meyer, & Nerenz, 1980) suggests that people's lay representations of illness assist them in coping with health threats by guiding their coping responses to produce adaptive illness outcomes. The present theoretical and empirical chapter reviews the literature with respect to the common-sense model and reports an empirical study that sought to examine relations among lay perceptions of sport-related musculoskeletal injuries, generalized coping strategies to deal with injury, and important functional and emotional outcomes in injured sports participants and athletes. Specifically, the cross-lagged effects between injury perception and coping procedures were tested among sport injured athletes ($N = 126$, 81 men, 45 women, mean age = 21.46, $SD = 6.42$) over a period of four weeks. Confirmatory factor analyses supported the construct validity of self-report measures of injury perception dimensions (identity, serious consequences, time, personal control, and treatment control), coping dimensions (active and planning coping and venting emotions), and the emotional (anxiety, depression) and functional (sport functioning, physical

---

[*] Tel: +44(0)115 8467929; Fax: +44(0)115 9515324; Email: martin.hagger@nottingham.ac.uk.

functioning) outcomes. Autoregressive path analyses revealed a moderate degree of stability in the illness perception constructs over a 4-week period. There was only one cross-lagged relationship with personal control (time1) predicting active coping (time 2) and vice-versa. Personal control was the most prominent predictor of both functioning and emotional outcomes. In addition, planning coping was negatively related to emotional outcomes, while injury identity was important in predicting physical functioning and both emotional outcomes. Importantly, few of the injury perceptions at time 1 predicted outcomes at time 2, indicating that immediate beliefs about the injury and coping styles are most relevant. Results are discussed with respect to the common-sense model and practical recommendations to change cognitive perceptions of injury such as personal control and emotional representations that impact upon anxiety and depression. It is proposed that practitioners adopt planning and active coping strategies to improve injury outcomes.

INTRODUCTION

Sports injuries constitute a major problem to athletes and health care providers alike. Estimates of the incidence of injuries among sports participants range from three to five million per annum in the United States (Bijur et al., 1995; Kraus & Conroy, 1984). Incidence rates in European Union countries are estimated at five per thousand (Petridou et al., 2003). In addition, there is evidence suggesting that sports-related injuries are on the increase (Renstrom, 1991; Watson, 1993). In the US, over 1.5 million hospital emergency department visits are made for sports-related injuries from the five major sporting activities: basketball, baseball, softball, football, or soccer (National Center for Injury Prevention and Control, 2002). In the United Kingdom, it is estimated that between 1 and 1.5 million episodes of exercise-related morbidity result in attendance at hospital casualty departments (Nicholl, Coleman, & Williams 1991), with participants from rugby, soccer, martial arts, hockey, and cricket making up the majority of the admitted cases (Nicholl & Coleman, 1996).

Musculoskeletal injuries make up a large proportion of sports injuries and have emerged as an important health problem with a substantial cost burden on health care providers (American Sports Data, 2003; National Center for Injury Prevention and Control, 2002; Nicholl, Coleman, & Williams, 1993). Musculoskeletal injuries sustained by recreational sports participants can result in time lost in sports participation and training, which can be acute lasting a few days to months and years (I. W. Ford, Eklund, & Gordon, 2000). In addition, sport-injured athletes, particularly with chronic injuries, experience considerable psychological trauma (Crossman, 1997), depression (Smith, Scott, & Wiese, 1990), and grief (Evans & Hardy, 1995). Studies have suggested that problem-focused coping behaviours such as attendance to rehabilitation programs will ameliorate the adverse psychological effects of the injury (e.g. Smith et al., 1990) and are positively related to clinical outcomes (B. W. Brewer, van Raalte et al., 2000).

Recent research has adopted theoretical frameworks from social psychology to explain the relationships among key psychosocial, emotional, and outcome constructs, namely, injury stress, coping responses, injury occurrence, rehabilitation adherence and clinical and emotional outcomes. Prominent among these theories are stress process and cognitive appraisal models (Wiese-Bjornstal, Smith, Shaffer, & Morrey, 1998; Williams & Andersen, 1998), loss-of-health models (Smith et al., 1990), personality models (Wittig & Schurr, 1994), causal attributions (B. W. Brewer, Cornelius et al., 2000), self-efficacy theory (Magyar & Duda, 2000), and protection-motivation theory (B. W. Brewer et al., 2003; Taylor & May, 1996). This chapter presents a study that aims to build upon this research by adopting Leventhal, Meyer and Nerenz's (1980) common-sense model of illness perceptions to explain the cognitive antecedents of coping responses and emotional and functional outcomes in sport-injured athletes. The theory has received a recent resurgence in interest in explaining adjustment and adherence to treatment regimes for chronic illnesses and conditions (Leventhal, Leventhal, & Contrada, 1998). It is attractive for use in an athletic injury context as it integrates many of the components of previously adopted social-cognitive approaches, namely beliefs, emotional responses, coping procedures, and clinical and emotional outcomes (Wiese-Bjornstal et al., 1998). The theory is useful because it provides an explicit, testable framework to understand the mechanisms by which social cognitive constructs influence the coping procedures of sport-injured people.

The common-sense model of illness perceptions was developed in the context of chronic illness and the processing of information from health threatening messages (Leventhal et al., 1980). A core hypothesis of the model is that individuals form a lay representation or perception of their illness or condition on the basis of three sources of information: the general pool of lay information available regarding the illness or condition, expert sources of information such as general practitioners and physiotherapists, and current and past experience with the illness or condition. The illness perception has both cognitive and emotional content, but these components are not considered orthogonal; it is expected that there may be some shared variance between these two sets of representations. According to the theory, if the illness or condition is represented as sufficiently threatening by an individual, they will be compelled to search for appropriate coping procedures to ameliorate the perceived threat (see figure 1). The adopted coping procedures may be active (behavioural) or passive (psychological). The theory proposes that coping procedures are adopted in response to the cognitive and emotional components of the representation simultaneously in a parallel process (figure 1). In turn coping is proposed to mediate the impact of illness representations on illness outcomes like functioning and emotional responses. In addition, the theory explicitly cites a role for the appraisal of adopted coping procedures. Appraisals are hypothesised to mediate the impact of lay representations on themselves over time. This is because appraisals of coping as effective will determine whether a person modifies their lay view of the illness (figure 1).

Research has suggested that illness perceptions have five core dimensions: identity, causes, serious consequences, timeline, and personal control. Leventhal et al. (1984) proposed that there was a logical organization among these dimensions and they form a 'schematic' representation of the illness or condition. The Illness Perception Questionnaire (IPQ, Weinman, Petrie, Moss-Morris, & Horne, 1996), and its revised form (IPQ-R; Moss-Morris et al., 2002) are the most frequently used. In this inventory, items measuring the *identity* subscale refer to a person's beliefs about the symptoms of the illness or condition. The items used are typically symptom lists, although some researchers (e.g., Moss-Morris et al., 2002) have criticized this approach because it does not capture other elements of the meaning of the illness to the person. The *cause* dimension reflects the factors that the individual believes caused their illness or condition. A number of different cause factors have been identified in research on illness perceptions and a number of underlying dimensions have been derived intuitively or from factor analysis. Examples of the dimensions that have been identified are biological cause, emotional cause, environmental cause, and psychological cause (Heijmans, 1998; Heijmans & De Ridder, 1998; Moss-Morris et al., 2002; Rutter & Rutter, 2002). The *serious consequences* dimension reflects a person's evaluation of the impact that the illness or condition will have on their life and activities. Serious consequences often reflect the threat of the illness on personal, financial, social, and occupational activities. The *timeline* dimension refers to an individual's perception of the course of the illness or condition, chronic or acute. The *control/cure* scale is the evaluation of whether there are effective measures

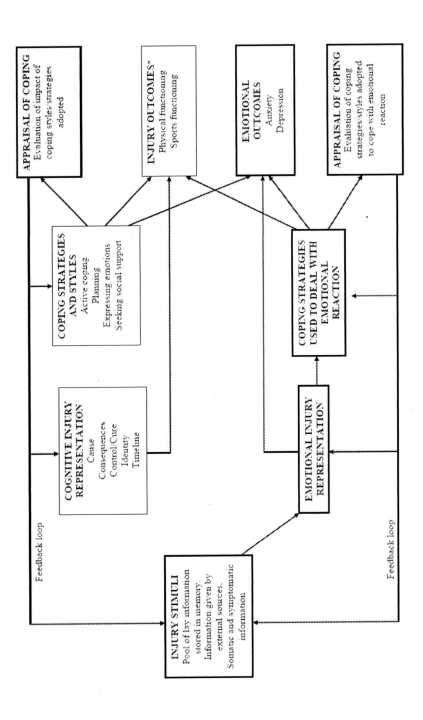

Figure 1. Schematic representation of Leventhal et al.'s (1980) common sense model adapted for injury representations.

available to the individual to control or cure the illness or condition. It has been typically measured using items relating to personal control over the illness, that is, whether the illness or injury sufferer can take action and change the course of the condition. Together these perceptions form a person's cognitive representation of illness threat.

Recent interpretations of the common-sense model have resulted in further development of the measures of illness perceptions. Moss-Morris and co-workers (2002) have presented a revised version of the illness perception questionnaire (IPQ-R). The revised version offers further differentiation of the illness perception dimensions to form a more complete map of the cognitive perceptions. For example, the cure/control dimension is divided into *personal control* and *treatment control*. Personal control beliefs reflect personal efficacy to change or alter the course of the illness, and treatment control refers to beliefs about the efficacy of medication or other treatments to control the illness. Research using this revised instrument has indicated that the revised scales retain adequate validity and reliability across a number of illnesses (Moss-Morris et al., 2002) and has been supported by confirmatory factor analysis (Hagger & Orbell, 2005). The study presented in this chapter will therefore adopt this augmented version of the IPQ-R to examine the structure of perceptions of injury in a sport context and the impact of injury perceptions on coping mechanisms and outcomes in sport-injured participants.

There has, however, only been limited support for the factor structure of the IPQ-R dimensions. Moss-Morris and coworkers (2002) supported their measure using a combination of exploratory factor analysis and concurrent validity tests with like measures. Additional support in other domains come from a study by Hagger & Orbell (2005) who used confirmatory factor analysis to support the proposed factor structure of the IPQ-R in a cervical screening context. This is the first and only confirmatory factor analytic test of the IPQ-R and supported the proposed structure of the core illness perception components but required some modifications specifically tailored for the specific causes and symptoms of the illness, as expected. The promise of this rigorous approach is that it provided a confirmatory test in which the a priori factor structure was tested against observed data from a population suffering from the conditions. However, few studies have adopted this approach because of its demand for large sample sizes. The present study aims to address this relative dearth of research by providing a confirmatory factor analysis of the IPQ-R modified for musculoskeletal injuries. It is expected that the a priori structure will hold for the core IPQ-R constructs and provide excellent goodness-of-fit with the data.

There is evidence to support the hypothesised relationships among illness perceptions and coping procedures in studies adopting the common-sense model with chronic conditions. The identity, serious consequences, and timeline cognitive illness perception dimensions have been associated with maladaptive and passive coping strategies such as avoidance and denial and venting emotions (Fortune, Richards, Main, & Griffiths, 2000; Rutter & Rutter, 2002). Positive relations have also been noted between the personal control construct and more adaptive, problem-focused coping procedures such as active coping, cognitive reappraisal and seeking social support (Heijmans, 1998, 1999). These relations have been supported by meta-analytic findings across studies (Hagger & Orbell, 2003).

Relationships between illness perceptions and illness outcomes are typically strong and adhere to a consistent pattern across studies of chronic illnesses and conditions (Heijmans, 1998; Orbell, Johnston, Rowley, Espley, & Davey, 1998). Meta-analytic findings have suggested that strong positive relationships exist between the identity, serious consequences and timeline cognitive perception dimensions and maladaptive outcomes such as anxiety and depression, although these dimensions tend to be negatively related to adaptive outcomes such as functioning and psychological well-being (Hagger & Orbell, 2003). The personal control dimension tends to be positively related to adaptive outcomes and negatively related to maladaptive outcomes (Heijmans, 1998; Heijmans & De Ridder, 1998). Recently, research has indicated that emotional perceptions are positively related to both emotional outcomes and functioning (Moss-Morris et al., 2002). The study reported in this chapter aims to extend the body of literature in the field by examining relations among injury perceptions, generalized coping styles, and key emotional and functional outcomes in sports participants and athletes with musculoskeletal injuries.

One recent avenue of research has been the translation of research findings from the common sense model into interventions to change illness perceptions that will have a concomitant effect on coping behaviours in practical contexts (Moss-Morris & Yardley, 2008). For example, Petrie et al. (2002) used a randomised controlled trial with an intervention that targeted illness perceptions among coronary heart disease patients undergoing rehabilitation from surgery. The intervention comprised structured sessions in which nurses targeted beliefs about heart disease including causes and helped patients develop plans to manage their illness post-hospitalization. The intervention reduced perceptions of cause, consequences, and timeline and increased perceptions of control among patients receiving the intervention. There were also increases in recovery time and self-management behaviours like physical activity. Similar interventions have shown or proposed to be equally efficacious in changing beliefs in medical and health settings such as asthma and diabetes (McAndrew et al., 2008), end-stage renal disease (Karamanidou, Weinman, & Horne, 2008), head and neck cancer (Humphris & Ozakind, 2008), and chronic fatigue syndrome (Deary, 2008). Wearden and Peters (2008) outline the flexibility of the model in producing wide-ranging, comprehensive interventions which target illness or injury threat like Petrie et al.'s intervention, but also the emotional components of the model such as those used by Cameron and Jago (2008) and Humphris and Ozakinci (2008). These studies demonstrate the applicability of the model in providing target constructs for intervention. The present study seeks to identify the proximal and distal targets for intervention based on this model with a view to identifying whether short and long term interventions may be effective in producing changes in functioning and emotional outcomes in sport-injured athletes.

To date, no study has examined the temporal stability of illness perceptions. This is important as it illustrates the relative changeability in such perceptions over time. This is important if the constructs have effects on key outcome variables. A lack of stability may mean that the contribution to that outcome variable may decay over time if stability is not high and there are no other extraneous variable to maintain the relationship. In such cases, the effect may be reduced to zero, in what is called an *entropic* model (Hertzog & Nesselroade, 1987). This is relevant practically as it will provide those interested in promoting rehabilitation and improving injury recovery with information as to whether changing injury perceptions will result in concomitant changes in outcomes and changes that will have lasting effects. The present study will therefore test the stability of these perceptions over time in a sport injury context using an autoregressive path analysis model in which the effect of an injury perception variable is regressed on itself over time.

The autoregressive model will also be used to test the nature of the relationships between injury perceptions and coping strategies over time. This will provide a better estimate of the directionality of relations among these key constructs from the common sense model. The model proposes that perceptions of injuries, if sufficiently threatening, will compel a person to select coping procedures to address the threat. However, another plausible effect might be that a given coping style, such as a problem-focused coping style which is usually deemed to be adaptive, will provide information that will assist in the modification of injury perceptions. For example an active coping style may result in people feeling that they have more personal control over the injury or people who adopt an emotion-venting coping style may report more symptoms (higher levels if injury identity) or perceive more serious consequences. The present study will evaluate whether these relationships are unidirectional or bidirectional (reciprocal). This is important as it will perhaps identify which perceptions should be the targets for intervention in order to change injury outcomes.

RESEARCH HYPOTHESES

The study reported in this chapter will examine the hypotheses of the common-sense model in athletes and sport participants with sport-related musculoskeletal injuries. It is expected that modelling the processes within the common-sense model will support and extend the recent theoretical investigations into sport-related injury coping and rehabilitation (e.g., B. W. Brewer et al., 2003; Taylor & May, 1996). This research is unique in that it aims to provide a test of the differential effects of injury perceptions on emotional responses and functional outcomes in sport-related injury sufferers. It will also make a unique contribution to the literature by testing the unidirectional or bidirectional (reciprocal) relationships between injury perceptions and coping procedures or styles. This may provide useful information on the mechanisms driving coping responses and outcomes as the result of an individual's cognitive processing of information about their sport-related injury.

Specifically, it is hypothesised that cognitive and emotional perceptions of injury will exhibit a theoretically predictable pattern of inter-correlations. It is anticipated that positive relations will be observed among the identity, serious consequences, and timeline injury perceptions. Negative relationships are expected between these constructs and the personal and treatment control dimensions. It is also expected that the identity, serious consequences, and timeline dimensions will be negatively related to adaptive coping procedures such as active coping and planning and positively related to a maladaptive coping strategy, namely venting emotions. In addition, it is expected that the personal and treatment control dimensions will be positively related to adaptive coping procedures active coping and planning and negatively related to venting emotions, a maladaptive coping procedure.

It is also expected that the injury perceptions and coping styles will demonstrate a reasonable degree of stability over time. We will measure injury perceptions and generalized coping styles at two points in time four weeks apart to examine the relative temporal stability of the perceptions and coping styles over time. In addition, in accordance with the common sense model, significant and positive cross-lagged relations are expected between the personal and treatment control dimensions and active and planning coping styles. However, reciprocal cross-lagged relations between active and planning coping styles and injury perceptions are not expected.

In addition, perceptions of personal and treatment control are expected to predict sport and physical functioning outcomes, measured at the second time point, in accordance with the common sense model and previous research (Hagger & Orbell, 2003). Sport and physical functioning are also expected to be negatively related to injury identity, serious consequences, and timeline at time point 2. Problem-focused forms of coping, active and planning coping are expected to be positively related to functioning outcomes. Importantly, it is expected that the immediate perceptions of injury and coping styles will be the most proximal predictors of these outcomes, mediating the impact of the time 1 constructs on the outcomes. It is also expected that problem-focused forms of coping will mediate the impact of injury perceptions measured at the previous time point, in accordance with the common sense model and previous research (e.g., Rutter & Rutter, 2002). Finally, injury perceptions, namely, identity, serious consequences, and timeline are expected to be positively related to emotional outcomes of anxiety and depression, while personal and treatment control are expected to be negatively related to these outcomes. It is also expected that adaptive coping strategies such as active and planning coping will be negatively related to these emotional outcome variables.

METHOD

Participants

Participants were recruited from undergraduate students at two University sites and from a University-based sport centre by two graduate assistants as part of a larger study on the psychological antecedents of sports injuries. Participants completed an initial consent and screening form and were required to self-report the regularity of their sports participation and their musculoskeletal injury status. Of the 525 screened, 259 reported they were currently injured and were competitive or recreational athletes (men = 168, women = 91; mean age = 23.51, SD = 8.79). Average injury duration was 7.2 months (median = 3.35). The screened participants completed baseline (Time 1) self-report measures of injury perceptions and coping styles.

Participants at Time 1 were followed-up four weeks later at Time 2 ($N = 126$, 81 men, 45 women, mean age = 21.46, $SD = 6.42$). Participants in the follow-up sample reported an average injury duration of 7.76 months (median = 4.00). These participants completed repeat measures of injury perceptions and coping styles as well as self-report measures of physical functioning, emotional outcomes (anxiety and depression), and sports functioning.

Measures

Injury Perceptions

The common-sense model constructs were measured by a modified version of the revised illness perception questionnaire (IPQ-R; Moss-Morris et al., 2002) which made reference to sport-related injuries. The core dimensions of identity, serious consequences, timeline, personal control, and treatment control were assessed. The IPQ-R has exhibited satisfactory factor structure and concurrent validity in studies of a number of chronic illnesses (e.g., Hagger & Orbell, 2005; Moss-Morris et al., 2002).

Coping Styles

We used the active coping, planning coping, and emotion venting dimensions from the COPE inventory to tap typical *problem-focused* and *emotion-focused* coping styles adopted by the present sample to deal with musculoskeletal injuries (Carver, Scheier, & Weintraub, 1989). These scales have been shown to have satisfactory factorial validity and reliability in development studies (Carver et al., 1989). The scales were adapted to make reference to sport-related injuries.

Injury Outcomes

The *anxiety* and *depression* scales from the Mental Health Inventory (MHI, Veit & Ware, 1983) were used to tap emotional responses to injury. These measures have been developed based on cognitive-emotional-relational theories of emotion and have been used extensively in research in cognition and emotion (Heubeck & Neill, 2000; Ostroff, Woolverton, Berry, & Lesko, 1996). A generic measure of physical functioning was also administered adapted from the Medical Outcomes Survey 36-item Short Form Health Survey (MOS-SF36, Ware & Sherbourne, 1992). We also developed a five-item sports functioning scale based on modal responses from an open ended questionnaire in a series of brief pilot interviews. This scale has been shown to be valid and reliable in previous research with sports injured athletes (Gladwell, Head, Hagger, & Beneke, 2006).

DATA ANALYSIS

The EQS computer program (Bentler, 2004) was used to develop confirmatory factor analytic (CFA) models to test the adequacy of the factor structure of the measures in the present study. This was a preliminary step before a path model testing the proposed associations between the study constructs could be estimated. Data from Time 1 were used to test the validity of the injury perception and coping variables and data from Time 2 were used to test the validity of the injury outcomes. A robust maximum likelihood method was used for all analyses to protect the estimation of the models from any violations of the assumption of normality (Satorra & Bentler, 1988). The adequacy of the proposed models was evaluated using the comparative fit index (CFI, Bentler, 1990), non-normed fit index (NNFI, Marsh, Balla, & McDonald, 1988), standardized root-mean square of the residuals (SRMR, Hu & Bentler, 1995), and root-mean square error of approximation (RMSEA, Hu & Bentler, 1999). Values greater than .90 for the CFI and NNFI indexes were considered acceptable for a well-fitting model (Bentler, 1990), although values greater than .95 are preferable (Hu & Bentler, 1999). Values of .05 or less for the SRMR and 0.8 or less for the RMSEA are indicative of adequate model fit (Hu & Bentler, 1999). In addition to the examination of overall goodness-of-fit indexes, we also examined the adequacy of the solution estimates of the model in each sample, such the parameter estimates that represent the relative contribution of each indicator to the hypothesised latent factor or factor loading, largest standardized residuals, and composite reliability (ρ_c) estimates as recommended by Jöreskog (1993).

The hypothesised longitudinal effects of injury perceptions and coping styles on sport injury outcomes were tested by path analysis using non-latent composite variables derived from the CFA (see figure 2). The path analysis was conducted by simultaneous process using a maximum likelihood estimation method with the EQS computer program. Goodness-of- fit of the proposed models was evaluated using the goodness-of-fit chi-square and the incremental fit indexes cited earlier.

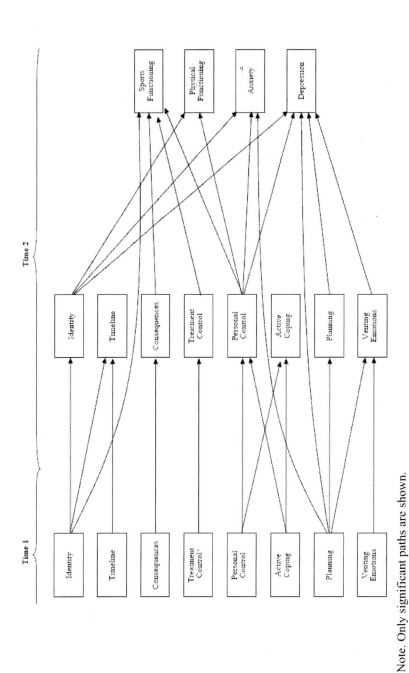

Note. Only significant paths are shown.

Figure 2. Final path model depicting relations among common sense model components, coping styles, and musculoskeletal injury emotional and functional outcomes.

RESULTS

Participants

The average age of participants who were followed up at Time 2 (mean age = 21.47, SD = 6.42) was lower than those who dropped out after Time 1 (mean age = 25.45, SD = 10.22) a difference that was statistically significant (t (1,257) = -3.73, $p < .01$), although the size of the effect was comparatively small (partial η^2 = .051). The gender ratio did not differ significantly between participants followed up relative to those who dropped out. The most frequently cited injury by the final sample was strains and sprains of muscles, ligaments, tendons and joints (N = 48), followed by muscle, ligament and tendon tears and ruptures (N = 19), bone fractures and stress fractures (N = 21), dislocation or subluxation of joints (N = 7), and tendonitis (N = 4). The remaining injuries were small incidences of other injuries such as cartilage injuries, bursitis and synovitis, and trapped nerves (van Michelen, 1997). Eighty-six participants sought treatment for their injury, with the majority attending a physiotherapist (62.79%).

Confirmatory Factor Analyses

The construct validity of the injury perception constructs, coping style constructs from the COPE, and the injury outcomes constructs was tested using confirmatory factor analyses (CFA) models. The CFA models were hypothesised to explain the variance/covariance matrices among the sets of items measuring each construct. The first model tested the factor structure of the key constructs from the IPQ-R, namely, identity, timeline, consequences, treatment control, and personal control. The second model tested the factor structure of the key constructs from the COPE inventory, namely, active coping, planning, and emotion venting. A third model tested the adequacy of the factor structure of injury outcomes, namely, anxiety and depression from the MHI, physical functioning from the MOS SF-36, and the sport functioning constructs. Each factor was set a priori to be indicated by the items hypothesised to ostensibly measure the target construct. Each hypothesised relationship between the latent factor and indicant item or factor loading was a free parameter in the model with the exception of a single item which was randomly set to unity to define the scale of the factor, as is the norm in CFA models. The initial models were modified to exclude items that were not adequately explained by the proposed latent factor or contributed substantially to any misspecification in the model. Items were scheduled for deletion were associated with large standardized residuals ($> \pm$ 2.00) or exhibited low factor loadings (J. Ford, MacCallum, & Tait, 1986; Motl & DiStefano, 2002).

Goodness-of-fit statistics for the hypothesised CFA model representing the covariances among the IPQ-R items for sports injuries items for the proposed perceived autonomy support scale were unacceptable ($\chi^2 = 928.090$, $df = 454$, $p <$ .01; CFI = .767; NNFI = .787; SRMR = .064; RMSEA = .064; 90% confidence intervals lower bound (CI$_{90}$ LB) = .058; 90% confidence intervals upper bound (CI$_{90}$ UB) = .069). However, five items was responsible for the standardized residuals greater than ± 2.00 and exhibited a low factor loadings that were below the acceptable .400 minimum (J. Ford et al., 1986). Examination of the content of these items revealed at two were personal control items ("Nothing I do will affect my injury"; "I had the power to influence the state of my injury"), two were identity items ("Sleep difficulties"; "Discomfort walking"), and one related to treatment control ("There is nothing that helped improve the course of my injury"). Research using CFA suggests that post priori modifications of unsatisfactory models should be conducted using multiple criteria including statistical (factor loadings, largest standardized residuals) and conceptual (item content) artifacts. In the present study it can be seen that two of the items responsible for large residuals referred to vague aspects "nothing" while other items referred to specific consequences or control factors. The two identity items were those that were clearly less relevant than other injury-related symptoms like "tenderness" and "soreness". The final personal control item referring to "power" may also have been less related to personal responsibility compared to other items measuring control which made reference to "my actions" and "me". Therefore these items may have reflected a high degree of ambiguity relative to other content. These items were deleted from the analysis and a model revised model exhibited much improved and acceptable fit with the data ($\chi^2 = 409.603$, $df = 351$, $p < .01$; CFI = .940; NNFI = .930; SRMR = .047; RMSEA = .037; 90% CI LB = .028; 90% CI UB = .046) with no misspecifications according to the standardized residuals and factor loadings.

Table 1. Zero-Order Correlations Among Injury Representation, Emotional Responses, Coping Procedures and Demographic Variables from the First-Wave Data

	1	2	3	4	5	6	7	8	9	10	11	12	13
1. Identity (T1)	—												
2. Consequences (T1)	.164**	—											
3. Timeline (T1)	.368**	.487**	—										
4. Treatment control (T1)	.013	.361**	.294**	—									
5. Personal Control (T1)	.015	-.077	-.137*	-.207**	—								
6. Active coping (T1)	.199**	-.013	.149*	.081	-.137*	—							
7. Planning (T1)	.176*	.081	.215**	.128*	-.161**	.775**	—						
8. Venting emotion (T1)	.265**	.185**	.419**	.140*	-.099	.162*	.289**	—					
9. Identity (T2)	.548**	.197*	.348**	-.042	-.064	.203*	.120	.314**	—				
10. Consequences (T2)	.183*	.724**	.489**	.364**	-.137	.011	.100	.264**	.266**	—			
11. Timeline (T2)	.287**	.392**	.703**	.151	-.100	.132	.117	.426**	.423**	.492**	—		
12. Treatment control (T2)	-.085	.298**	.168	.527**	-.075	-.040	.004	.064	.018	.275**	.196*	—	
13. Personal Control (T2)	.017	-.147	-.114	-.062	.396**	.335**	.227*	-.060	-.163	-.238**	-.216*	-.127	—
14. Active coping (T2)	.280**	-.094	.156	-.105	.182*	.558**	.383**	.212*	.321**	.003	.193*	-.088	.307**
15. Planning (T2)	.171	.008	.111	-.034	-.007	.450**	.454**	.254**	.293**	.061	.174	-.074	.243**
16. Venting emotion (T2)	.336**	.259**	.353**	-.055	-.057	.233*	.292**	.663**	.379**	.275**	.420**	.046	-.045
17. Anxiety (T2)	.051	.131	.151	.068	-.234**	-.190*	-.250**	.264**	.058	.182*	.188*	.263**	-.211*
18. Depression (T2)	.088	.241**	.250**	.103	-.177*	-.186*	-.193*	.259**	.105	.242**	.266**	.250**	-.140

	1	2	3	4	5	6	7	8	9	10	11	12	13
19. Physical functioning (T2)	.338**	-.064	.236**	-.167	.044	.139	.079	.271**	.389**	.088	.228*	-.174	-.029
20. Sports functioning (T2)	.428**	.064	.318**	-.128	-.044	.117	.139	.289**	.358**	.229*	.327**	-.095	.015

	14	15	16	17	18	19	20
14. Active coping (T2)	–						
15. Planning (T2)	.405**	–					
16. Venting emotion (T2)	.304**	.333**	–				
17. Anxiety (T2)	-.007	-.009	.372**	–			
18. Depression (T2)	.034	.095	.372**	.822**	–		
19. Physical functioning (T2)	.166	.107	.260**	.043	.103	–	
20. Sports functioning (T2)	.092	.084	.210*	-.057	.099	.293**	–

Note. N = 145, with the exception of correlations including sports functioning, N = 100.
* $p < .05$ ** $p < .01$.

Table 2. Standardized Regression Coefficients for Autoregressive Path Analysis of Injury Perceptions, Coping Styles, and Injury Outcomes

Paths (Hypothesised)[a]	β	Paths (Hypothesised)[a]	β	Paths (Modified)[b]	β
Identity (T1→T2)	.49**	Personal Control (T2)→Anxiety (T2)	.24**	Personal Control (T1)→Active Coping (T2)	.17**
Timeline (T1→T2)	.71**	Personal Control (T2)→Depression (T2)	.21**	Planning (T1)→Venting Emotion (T3)	.14*
Consequences (T1→T2)	.66**	Personal Control (T2)→Physical Functioning (T2)	-.21**	Active Coping (T1)→Personal Control (T2)	.35**
Treatment Control (T1→T2)	.53**	Personal Control (T2)→Sports Functioning (T2)	-.14**	Planning (T1)→Anxiety (T2)	-.41**
Personal Control (T1→T2)	.35**	Treatment Control (T2)→Anxiety (T2)	-.13	Planning (T1)→Depression (T2)	-.40**
Active Coping (T1→T2)	.51**	Treatment Control (T2)→Depression (T2)	-.05	Identity (LT)→Sports Functioning (V2)	.29**
Planning (T1→T2)	.46**	Treatment Control (T2)→Physical Functioning (T2)	.04		
Venting Emotions (T1→T2)	.59**	Treatment Control (T2)→Sports Functioning (T2)	.14*		
Identity (T2)→Anxiety (T2)	-.15**	Active Coping (T2)→Anxiety (T2)	.09		
Identity (T2)→Depression (T2)	-.13**	Active Coping (T2)→Depression (T2)	.06		
Identity (T2)→Physical Functioning (T2)	.33**	Active Coping (T2)→Physical Functioning (T2)	-.01		
Identity (T2)→Sports Functioning (T2)	.15	Active Coping (T2)→Sports Functioning (T2)	-.11		
Timeline (T2)→Anxiety (T2)	.04	Planning (T2)→Anxiety (T2)	.08		
Timeline (T2)→Depression (T2)	.10	Planning (T2)→Depression (T2)	.17**		
Timeline (T2)→Physical Functioning (T2)	-.02	Planning (T2)→Physical Functioning (T2)	-.08		
Timeline (T2)→Sports Functioning (T2)	.10	Planning (T2)→Sports Functioning (T2)	-.05		
Consequences (T2)→Anxiety (T2)	-.03	Venting Emotion (T2)→Anxiety (T2)	.47**		

Paths (Hypothesised)[a]	β	Paths (Hypothesised)[a]	β	Paths (Modified)[b]	β
Consequences (T2)→Depression (T2)	.06	Venting Emotion (T2)→Depression (T2)	.40**		
Consequences (T2)→Physical Functioning (T2)	.10	Venting Emotion (T2)→Physical Functioning (T2)	.13		
Consequences (T2)→Sports Functioning (T2)	.21**	Venting Emotion (T2)→Sports Functioning (T2)	.01		

Note. [a]Paths included as part of the hypothesised model; [b]Theoretically plausible paths included in the model as a result of the Lagrange Multiplier tests.

* p < .01, p < .05.

The same procedure was followed for the CFA models for the coping and outcome variables. Goodness-of-fit statistics for the hypothesised CFA model for the coping procedures of action coping, planning coping, and emotion venting resulted in a well-fitting model with no substantial misspecifications (χ^2 = 101.833, df = 49, p < .01; CFI = .934; NNFI = .951; SRMR = .064; RMSEA = .065; CI_{90} LB = .047; CI_{90} UB = .082). Finally, the model for the outcome variables of sports functioning, physical functioning, anxiety, and depression exhibited a model that was not satisfactory according to goodness-of-fit statistics (χ^2 = 469.124, df = 293, p < .01; CFI = .878; NNFI = .865; SRMR = .080; RMSEA = .092; CI_{90} LB = .081; CI_{90} UB = .102). Examining the standardized residuals revealed that the items were contributing to the misspecification in the CFA with standardized residuals exceeding ±2.00. Two of these were anxiety items ("How much of the time did your hands shake when you were doing things?"; "How much of the time did you feel rattles, upset or flustered?") and one was a physical functioning item ("To what extent were you affected? Eating, dressing, showering/bathing, or using the toilet"). The anxiety items were perhaps did not reflect the core aspects of anxiety such as exhibiting high arousal or nervousness, these were perhaps more akin to worry. The physical functioning item was probably not relevant to people with sports-related injuries and is more applicable with other types of injury and the effects of immobilising treatment in elderly patients. Deleting these items and re-running the analysis resulted in a CFA model that exhibited good fit with the data s (χ^2 = 298.542, df = 239, p < .01; CFI = .954; NNFI = .947; SRMR = .064; RMSEA = .045; CI_{90} LB = .025; CI_{90} UB = .060). The items that comprised the latent factors were used to develop the composite variables for the path analyses.

Composite Variables for Path Analysis

Non-latent composite variables were used in a path analysis to test the main study hypotheses. Descriptive statistics and correlations for the composite variables are given in table 1. Importantly, a theoretically-predictable pattern of results emerged from the inter-relations among the injury perception factors. At time 1, the identity, consequences, and timeline constructs were all significantly and positively related as expected. Personal control was unrelated to identity and consequences and significantly and negatively related to timeline and, contrary to expectations, treatment control. Treatment control was unrelated to identity but was significant and positively related to consequences and timeline. This supports previous research, with the exception of treatment control. It may be that personal and treatment control are negatively related because the degree of treatability of an injury by medication or therapy is perhaps viewed as taking the outcome of the injury and the power ability to treat it out of the hands of the injured person. An identical pattern was found at time 2. These finding support the pattern found in many other studies of illness perceptions in chronic illness (Hagger, Chatzisarantis, Griffin, & Thatcher, 2005).

Testing Common-Sense Model Hypotheses

Stability of Injury Perceptions
We hypothesised that people's injury perceptions and coping styles would exhibit a degree of stability over the course of their injury, yet would be imperfect indicating a degree of change over time. All the autoregressive coefficients were statistically significant and ranged from .35 to .71 for the injury perception components and from .46 to .59 for the coping style components. The personal control construct was the least stable over time, indicating that this variable had the greatest propensity for change over the course of the injury. We also hypothesised that the injury perception constructs would influence forms of active coping over time. Specifically, we expected perceptions of personal control and treatment control to influence forms of problem-focused coping, namely active coping and planning over time. Personal control at time 1 significantly predicted active coping at time 2 as predicted by the common sense model. However, active coping at the time 1 also significantly predicted personal control at time 2. This suggests that those who engaged in active coping were more likely to report higher perceptions of personal control subsequently. Therefore the link between personal control and active coping is reciprocal. This is adaptive as both personal control and active coping are implicated in predicting functioning outcome variables. There was also a significant effect of planning coping (time 1) on venting emotions (time 2) but no cross-lagged relationship. No other cross-lagged relations were found.

Predicting injury outcomes. The key functioning and emotional outcomes in the present study were predicted from injury perceptions and coping strategies at time 2. Specifically, physical and sports functioning were predicted by personal control at time 1, which is consistent with previous research that has demonstrated the efficacy of personal control in terms of predicting functioning and influencing behavioural outcomes. Most importantly, this has been a variable that has been flagged as a target of interventions to change beliefs regarding illness with a view to changing health-related behaviour (e.g., Petrie et al., 2002). Sports functioning was also a function of serious consequences at time 2 and injury identity at time 1. This indicates that current perceptions of injury are not always associated with adaptive outcomes. Physical functioning was, however, predicted by identity at time 2, indicating that people reporting more symptoms are likely to improve their functioning. This may be a consequence of identity at time2 compelling a person to engage in coping strategies to manage their injury. However, the present measures of coping perhaps did not account for these influences. In terms of emotional outcomes, anxiety and depression were positively predicted by venting emotions at time 2, as expected, but also by personal control at time 2. Depression was also predicted by planning at both time points and injury identity at time 2. The strongest effect on depression was for venting emotions at time 2, which is not surprising given that emotion-venting often serves to highlight and exacerbate moods rather than reduce levels of emotion. Finally, the time 2 injury perception and coping variables that significantly predicted the functioning and emotional outcomes also mediated the effects of the time 1 versions of these constructs. This indicates that it is current perceptions that are most relevant to outcomes and mediate the effect of previous perceptions. The only exceptions were the planning at time 1 construct on anxiety and depression, which negatively predicted these outcomes directly, and identity at time 1 which predicted sports functioning directly. Overall, these results support some hypotheses from the common-sense model, but demonstrate that immediate injury perceptions are more predictive of behaviour with strong roles for identity and personal control in predicting functioning and emotional outcomes of sport-related injury.

DISCUSSION

Overall, findings from the study presented in this chapter support hypotheses from the common-sense model regarding the stability of injury-related perceptions and emotional and functioning outcomes in sport injured athletes over time. Furthermore, there is further evidence to support the construct validity of the IPQ-R for the common sense model constructs using confirmatory factor analysis, in keeping with previous research in other fields (Hagger & Orbell, 2005). Important findings from the path analysis in the present study were that both the functioning variables and emotional outcomes were predicted by concurrently-measured personal control. This demonstrates that personal control is clearly a pivotal construct within the model. In terms of specific functioning variables, sports functioning was significantly predicted by serious consequences and identity at time 1, but not time 2. This indicates that people may engage in adaptive strategies to bring about better sport-related outcomes if they perceived the injury as more serious and symptomatic in the first place. Physical functioning was also predicted by current symptom reports (identity), as well as personal control indicating that current problems limited current mobility. The emotional outcome of depression was positively predicted by current adoption of venting emotions and personal control and negatively predicted by planning as a coping strategy as well as personal control. Anxiety, on the other hand, was a function of concurrently-measured identity and planning. Similarly, anxiety was positively predicted by venting emotions, identity and treatment control, and negatively by personal control measured at time 2 and, additionally, by planning at time 1. The suggestion here is that planning coping at time 1 led to less anxiety and depression at time 2. Interestingly active coping at time 1 also lead to increased personal control at time 2. This suggests that personal control is augmented by actively making changes to cope with injury.

A unique aspect of this study was the longitudinal nature of the data. The autoregressive path-analytic model is a powerful tool to determine whether sets of constructs have unidirectional or reciprocal prediction over time (Hertzog & Nesselroade, 1987). The model also tests the extent of inter-individual change in a variable over time and provides information on its degree of stability. In the present analysis, we tested the level of stability in injury perceptions over time. Results indicated that many of the variables exhibited a moderate degree of stability over time, but suggested that within this system of variables there were still unmeasured variables external to the system accounting for the unexplained variance in the variable over time. We also tested whether there were cross-lagged relationships among these sets of variables over time. In particular, we were interested whether injury perceptions influence the selection of coping strategy over time or whether coping styles changed injury perceptions, or whether such relations were bi-directional i.e. reciprocal. In the present analysis, one reciprocal cross-lagged relationship was found between active coping and personal control. There was also a unidirectional relationship between planning coping (time 1) and venting emotions (time 2) but no reciprocal relationship. The effect of personal control on active coping supports a hypothesis of the common sense model that injury perceptions lead to the adopting of coping procedure. However, this effect was reciprocal in that the adoption of an active coping strategy was related to reporting of personal control over the injury. This may have been a function of the ways in which the current set of constructs were operationalised. Coping was measured in a very general sense – as a dispositional tendency to adopt a coping style or procedure, rather than a specific coping behaviour targeting the particular health threat, the musculoskeletal injury in this case. As a consequence, it may be that a generalized tendency to adopt a problem-focused coping style may contribute to reporting a high degree of personal control over the outcome of the injury. This suggests that such a style may be a source of information for injury perceptions just as symptomatic, expert and lay information regarding the injury may develop injury perceptions over time. As personal control seems to be adaptive in bringing about changes in sports and physical functioning, it may be reasonable to recommend that problem-focused coping styles are advocated by coaches, physiotherapists, and other practitioners involved in assisting sports participants and athletes to recover from injury.

The sports functioning construct developed for the present study represented an important domain-relevant functioning variable. The findings from these data are in keeping with the common sense model and indicate that representing the injury as having serious consequences predicts the impairment of an injury sufferer's ability to participate in and train effectively for their sport. Importantly, the positive influence of personal control on sports functioning indicates that the control over outcomes is likely to result in the individual adopting strategies that lead to injury recovery. However, it was expected that this would be mediated by active and coping planning strategies. However, this was not the case, and active coping strategies did not have a major impact on either of the coping constructs. Although these findings support relations among injury perceptions and outcomes identified in previous studies (Hagger & Orbell, 2003), they do not support the mediation hypothesis proposed by the common-sense model (Helder et al., 2002; Rutter & Rutter, 2002). It was expected that the impact of serious consequences, identity, and personal control at time 1 on sports functioning at time 2 would be mediated by active and planning coping at time 1. The non-significant finding for this mediation effect was also found by N. T. Brewer et al. (2002). One possible explanation for this is that the measures of coping strategies reflect only generalized coping tendencies (Coyne & Racioppo, 2000) and not the specific behaviours through to bring about true change in functioning outcomes. It may be that there are specific coping strategies that were unmeasured here that explained the influence of identity, consequences, and personal control on functioning variables.

Physical functioning, a more generic measure of mobility and physical aptitude, was also predicted by personal control suggesting that the same mechanisms my have been responsible for changes in this variable as sports functioning. Specifically, it is possible that higher levels of personal control may have lead to specific coping behaviours that bring about greater physical functioning, yet these behaviours are not accounted for by active and planning coping strategies measured here, but again, that may have been due to the generic nature of the coping measures. Physical functioning was also predicted by current identity perceptions, but not serious consequences. This may be because physical functioning reflects general mobility issues rather than specific impairments related to sport. Therefore, if a person is experiencing current injury symptoms, these are likely to be related to reduced physical functioning in a general sense rather than sports-specific functioning. For example a rugby player who is currently suffering from knee tendonitis is likely to have trouble walking and will therefore report lower physical functioning, while such perceptions are more likely to affect sports functioning over time, hence the effect of identity at time 1 on sports functioning rather than current symptoms.

Importantly, in all cases where injury perceptions at time 2 predicted injury outcomes, there were indirect effects of these injury perceptions at time 1 on the outcome variables mediated by the time 2 variables. Therefore, changes in the identity, consequences, treatment control, personal control, planning, and venting emotions over time were accounted for solely by the variables themselves plus some unmeasured influence, and any effects of the variable over time were accounted for by the same variable at a subsequent point in time. This meant that there were no cross-lagged effects, with the exception of the effect of active coping at time 1 on personal control at time 2. It also meant that there were no effects of time 1 injury perceptions on time 2 outcomes with the exception of the effect of planning (time 1) on depression and anxiety (time 2) and the effect of identity (time 1) on sports functioning (time 2). This is important as it illustrates that it is current perceptions of injury that have effects on the functioning variables and previous effects. It also means that after accounting for change in the injury perceptions over time, the variables remain related to injury outcomes. In a practical sense, this means that current injury perceptions are important in determining emotional perceptions and the effects of time-lagged perceptions can be accounted for by current perceptions.

PRACTICAL IMPLICATIONS

The practical implications of this research are two fold. Firstly, given the significant relationship between personal control over the injury and sports and physical functioning it seems that injury sufferers who are empowered are likely to display better functioning. This may be because they engage in practical behaviours that result in successful injury treatment. A major challenge for practitioners such as coaches and personal trainers who are dealing with injured athletes is to ensure that athletes sufficiently self-regulate in terms of adhering to treatment. This is important for athletes who do not have support staff who are constantly available to assist recovery and rehabilitation. Therefore providing means to promote greater personal control over injury outcomes is an effective intervention technique. A second important implication can be derived from the role that active coping has on personal control and, indirectly, adapting functioning outcomes. Giving the athlete information relating to the practical personal behaviours that will assist rehabilitation and outlining to them the effectiveness that coping may have on injury outcome may compel an athlete to adopt a problem-focused strategy that will, in turn, positively improve sport and physical functioning. There has been recent research to suggest that constructs from the self-regulation model can be altered by intervention, although subsequent changes in attendance behaviour were not noted (Karamanidou et al., 2008; Petrie et al., 2002; Wearden & Peters, 2008). There is also recent evidence that the common-sense model can inform interventions to change the emotional representations and influence emotional outcomes. The use of emotion regulation strategies can assist in minimising the impact of emotional representations and other cognitive representations on anxiety and depression. For example, practitioners interested in changing the emotional representations of sport-injured clients and patients can provide interventions to modify the maladaptive emotions and developing action plans for recovery (Cameron & Jago, 2008).

CONCLUSIONS AND FUTURE RESEARCH

A strength of the study reported in the chapter is that it is the first to adopt an autoregressive approach to the common sense model of injury perceptions. It aimed to explain the autoregressive, unidirectional and reciprocal effects of injury perceptions and coping strategies over time in athletes with musculoskeletal injuries. Importantly, data demonstrated the relative degree of stability of the injury perception constructs and the relatively few cross-lagged effects among to constructs. Results partly support theoretical predictions in that personal control is pivotal variable in terms of sports functioning while planning and venting emotions are important in influencing affective outcomes (Hagger & Orbell, 2003, 2006). The adoption of a longitudinal autoregressive design to study the appraisal process in the common-sense model is unique to the present study, and provides preliminary evidence to support the inclusion of appraisals in tests of the common-sense model.

Although the findings give some indication that the theory has efficacy in explaining some of the mechanisms behind emotional responses and functional outcomes, it has not provided support for the mediation hypothesis. For example, problem-focused coping strategies did not mediate the relations between the injury cognition variables and sports functioning. Instead, it appeared that an active coping style led to increased perceptions of personal control. Methodological artefacts may have been responsible for affecting this unexpected finding. Recent research has criticized the use of generalized coping measures such as the COPE (Coyne & Racioppo, 2000). More domain-specific coping measures have been recommended as possible solutions and future research may seek to address this problem when examining sports-injuries and coping procedures. In addition, these data are correlational in nature and, as a consequence, causality cannot be unequivocally supported from these findings. Further research will need to adopt experimental or intervention designs similar to that conducted by Petrie et al. (2002) to determine the impact of changing injury perceptions through the promotion of greater personal control over the injury symptoms and outcomes. Such research would permit further inference of causality by testing whether changes in injury perceptions like personal control will be associated with key outcomes like functioning.

AUTHOR NOTE

The author would like to thank Kate Green, Joanna Phanis, and Ayesha Shivji for assistance with data collection, and Joanne Thatcher for her helpful comments on an earlier draft of this chapter.

REFERENCES

American Sports Data. (2003). *A comprehensive study of sports injuries in the U.S.* Hartsdale, NY: American Sports Data Inc.

Bentler, P. M. (1990). Comparative fit indexes in structural models. *Psychological Bulletin, 107*, 238-246.

Bentler, P. M. (2004). *EQS structural equations modeling software (Version 6.1) [Computer Software]*. Encino, CA: Multivariate Software.

Bijur, P. E., Trumble, A., Harel, Y., Overpeck, M. D., Jones, D., & Schiedt, P. C. (1995). Sports and recreation injuries in U.S. children and adolescents. *Archives of Pediatric and Adolescent Medicine, 149*, 1009-1016.

Brewer, B. W., Cornelius, A. E., van Raalte, J. L., Petitpas, A. J., Sklar, J. H., Pohlman, M. H., et al. (2000). Attributions for recovery and adherence to rehabilitation following anterior cruciate ligament reconstruction: A prospective analysis. *Psychology and Health, 15*, 283-291.

Brewer, B. W., Cornelius, A. E., van Raalte, J. L., Petitpas, A. J., Sklar, J. H., Pohlman, M. H., et al. (2003). Protection motivation theory and adherence to sport injury rehabilitation revisited. *The Sport Psychologist, 17*, 95-103.

Brewer, B. W., van Raalte, J. L., Cornelius, A. E., Petitpas, A. J., Sklar, J. H., Pohlman, M. H., et al. (2000). Psychological factors, rehabilitation adherence, and rehabilitation outcome following anterior cruciate ligament reconstruction. *Rehabilitation Psychology, 45*, 20-37.

Brewer, N. T., Chapman, G. B., Brownlee, S., & Leventhal, E. (2002). Cholesterol control, medication adherence and illness cognition. *British Journal of Health Psychology, 7*, 433-447.

Cameron, L. D., & Jago, L. (2008). Emotion regulation interventions: A common-sense model approach. *British Journal of Health Psychology, 13*, 215-221.

Carver, C. S., Scheier, M. F., & Weintraub, J. K. (1989). Assessing coping strategies: A theoretically based approach. *Journal of Personality and Social Psychology, 56*, 267-283.

Coyne, J. C., & Racioppo, M. W. (2000). Never the twain shall meet? Closing the gap between coping research and clinical intervention research. *American Psychologist, 55*, 655-664.

Crossman, J. (1997). Psychological rehabilitation from sports injuries. *Sports Medicine, 23*, 333-339.

Deary, V. (2008). A precarious balance: Using a self-regulation model to conceptualize and treat chronic fatigue syndrome. *British Journal of Health Psychology, 13*, 231-236.

Evans, L., & Hardy, L. (1995). Sport injury and grief responses: A review. *Journal of Sport and Exercise Psychology, 17*, 227-245.

Ford, I. W., Eklund, R. C., & Gordon, S. (2000). An examination of psychosocial variables moderating the relationships between life stress and injury time-loss among athletes of a high standard. *Journal of Sports Sciences, 18*, 301-312.

Ford, J., MacCallum, R., & Tait, M. (1986). The application of factor analysis in psychology: A critical review and analysis. *Personnel Psychology, 39*, 291-314.

Fortune, D. G., Richards, H. L., Main, C. J., & Griffiths, C. E. M. (2000). Pathological worrying, illness perceptions and disease severity in patients with psoriasis. *British Journal of Health Psychology, 5*, 71-82.

Gladwell, V., Head, S., Hagger, M. S., & Beneke, R. (2006). Does a program of pilates improve chronic non-specific low back pain? *Journal of Sport Rehabilitation, 15*, 338-350.

Hagger, M. S., Chatzisarantis, N., Griffin, M., & Thatcher, J. (2005). Injury representations, coping, emotions, and functional outcomes in athletes with sport-related injuries: A test of self-regulation theory. *Journal of Applied Social Psychology, 35*, 2345-2374.

Hagger, M. S., & Orbell, S. (2003). A meta-analytic review of the common-sense model of illness representations. *Psychology and Health, 18*, 141-184.

Hagger, M. S., & Orbell, S. (2005). A confirmatory factor analysis of the revised illness perception questionnaire (IPQ-R) in a cervical screening context. *Psychology and Health, 20*, 161-173.

Hagger, M. S., & Orbell, S. (2006). Illness representation and emotion in people with abnormal screening results. *Psychology and Health, 21*, 183-209.

Heijmans, M. (1998). Coping and adaptive outcome in chronic fatigue syndrome: Importance of illness cognitions. *Journal of Psychosomatic Research, 45*, 39-51.

Heijmans, M. (1999). The role of patients' illness representations in coping and functioning with Addison's disease. *British Journal of Health Psychology, 4*, 137-149.

Heijmans, M., & De Ridder, D. (1998). Assessing illness representations of chronic illness: Explorations of their disease-specific nature. *Journal of Behavioral Medicine, 21*, 485-503.

Helder, D. I., Kaptein, A. A., van Kempen, G. M. J., Weinman, J., van Houwelingen, H. C., & Roos, R. A. C. (2002). Living with Huntington's disease: Illness perceptions, coping mechanisms, and patients' well-being. *British Journal of Health Psychology, 7*, 449-462.

Hertzog, C., & Nesselroade, J. R. (1987). Beyond autoregressive models: Some implications of the trait-state distinction for the structural modeling of developmental change. *Child Development, 58*, 93-109.

Heubeck, B., & Neill, J. T. (2000). Internal validity and reliability of the 30-item Mental Health Inventory for Australian adolescents. *Psychological Reports, 87*, 431-440.

Hu, L., & Bentler, P. (1995). Evaluating model fit. In R. H. Hoyle (Ed.), *Structural Equation Modeling. Concepts, Issues, and Applications* (pp. 76-99). London: Sage.

Hu, L., & Bentler, P. M. (1999). Cutoff criteria for fit indexes in covariance structure analysis: Conventional criteria versus new alternatives. *Structural Equation Modeling, 6*, 1-55.

Humphris, G., & Ozakind, G. (2008). The AFTER intervention: A structured psychological approach to reduce fears of recurrence in patients with head and neck cancer. *British Journal of Health Psychology, 13*, 223-230.

Jöreskog, K. G. (1993). Testing structural equation models. In K. A. Bollen & J. S. Long (Eds.), *Testing structural equation models* (pp. 294-316). Newbury Park, CA: Sage.

Karamanidou, C., Weinman, J., & Horne, R. (2008). Improving haemodialysis patients' understanding of phosphate-binding medication: A pilot study of a psycho-educational intervention designed to change patients' perceptions of the problem and treatment. *British Journal of Health Psychology, 13*, 205-214.

Kraus, J. F., & Conroy, C. (1984). Mortality and morbidity from injuries in sports and recreation. *Annual Review of Public Health, 5*, 163-192.

Leventhal, H., Leventhal, E., & Contrada, R. J. (1998). Self-regulation, health, and behavior: A perceptual-cognitive approach. *Psychology and Health, 13*, 717-734.

Leventhal, H., Meyer, D., & Nerenz, D. (1980). The common sense model of illness danger. In S. Rachman (Ed.), *Medical Psychology* (Vol. II, pp. 7-30). New York: Pergamon Press.

Leventhal, H., Nerenz, D. R., & Steele, D. J. (1984). Illness representations and coping with health threats. In A. Baum, S. E. Taylor & J. E. Singer (Eds.), *Handbook of Psychology and Health: Social Psychological Aspects of Health* (Vol. 4, pp. 219-252). Hillsdale, NJ: Earlbaum.

Magyar, T. M., & Duda, J. L. (2000). Confidence restoration following athletic injury. *The Sport Psychologist, 14*, 373-390.

Marsh, H. W., Balla, J. R., & McDonald, R. P. (1988). Goodness-of-fit indexes in confirmatory factor analysis: The effect of sample size. *Psychological Bulletin, 103*, 391-410.

McAndrew, L. M., Musumeci-Szabo, T. J., Mora, P. A., Vileikyte, L., Burns, E., Halm, E. A., et al. (2008). Using the common sense model to design interventions for the prevention and management of chronic illness threats: From description to process. *British Journal of Health Psychology, 13*, 195-204.

Moss-Morris, R., Weinman, J., Petrie, K. J., Horne, R., Cameron, L. D., & Buick, L. (2002). The revised Illness Perception Questionnaire (IPQ-R). *Psychology and Health, 17*, 1-16.

Moss-Morris, R., & Yardley, L. (2008). Current issues and new directions in Psychology and Health: Contributions to translational research *Psychology and Health, 23*, 1-4.

Motl, R. W., & DiStefano, C. (2002). Longitudinal invariance of self-esteem and method effects associated with negatively worded items. *Structural Equation Modeling, 9*, 562-578.

National Center for Injury Prevention and Control. (2002). *CDC injury research agenda*. Atlanta, GA: Centers for Disease Control and Prevention.

Nicholl, J. P., & Coleman, P. (1996). Acute sports injuries. *British Medical Journal, 312*, 844.

Nicholl, J. P., Coleman, P., & Williams , B. T. (1991). Pilot study of the epidemiology of sports injuries and exercise-related morbidity. *British Journal of Sports Medicine, 25*, 61-66.

Nicholl, J. P., Coleman, P., & Williams, B. T. (1993). *Injuries in sport and exercise*. London: Sports Council.

Orbell, S., Johnston, M., Rowley, D., Espley, A., & Davey, P. (1998). Cognitive representations of illness and functional and affective adjustment following surgery for osteoarthritis. *Social Science and Medicine, 47*, 93-102.

Ostroff, J. S., Woolverton, K. S., Berry, C., & Lesko, L. M. (1996). Use of the Mental Health Inventory with adolescents: A secondary analysis of the Rand Health Insurance Study. *Psychological Assessment, 8*, 105-107.

Petridou, E., Belechri, M., Dessypris, N., Moustaki, M., Alexe, D., Marinopoulos, S., et al. (2003). *Sports injuries in the EU countries in view of the 2004 Olympics: Arresting information from existing data bases*. Athens: Center for Research and Prevention of Injuries among the Young.

Petrie, K. J., Cameron, L., Ellis, C. J., Buick, D., & Weinman, J. (2002). Changing illness perceptions after myocardial infarction: An early intervention randomized controlled trial. *Psychosomatic Medicine, 64*, 580-586.

Renstrom, P. (1991). Sports traumatology today: A review of common current sports injury problems. *Annales Chirurgiae et Gynaecologiae, 80*, 81-93.

Rutter, C. L., & Rutter, D. R. (2002). Illness representation, coping and outcome in irritable bowel syndrome (IBS). *British Journal of Health Psychology, 7*, 377-391.

Satorra, A., & Bentler, P. M. (1988). *Scaling corrections for statistics in covariance structure analysis*. Los Angeles, CA: University of California at Los Angeles, Department of Psychology.

Smith, A. M., Scott, S. G., & Wiese, D. M. (1990). The psychological effects of sports injuries coping. *Sports Medicine, 9*, 352-369.

Taylor, A. H., & May, S. (1996). Threat and coping appraisal as determinants of compliance to sports injury rehabilitation: An application of protection motivation theory. *Journal of Sport Sciences, 14*, 471-482.

van Michelen, W. (1997). The severity of sports injuries. *Sports Medicine, 24*, 176-180.

Veit, C. T., & Ware, J. E. (1983). The structure of psychological distress and well-being in general populations. *Journal of Consulting and Clinical Psychology, 51*, 730-742.

Ware, J. E., & Sherbourne, C. D. (1992). The MOS 36-item short-form health survey (SF-36): I. Conceptual framework and item selection. *Medical Care, 30*, 473-483.

Watson, A. W. S. (1993). Incidence and nature of sports injuries in Ireland. *American Journal of Sports Medicine*(21), 137-143.

Wearden, A., & Peters, S. (2008). Therapeutic techniques for interventions based on Leventhal's common sense model. *British Journal of Health Psychology, 13*, 189-193.

Weinman, J., Petrie, K. J., Moss-Morris, R., & Horne, R. (1996). The Illness Perception Questionnaire: A new method for assessing the cognitive representation of illness. *Psychology and Health, 11*, 431-445.

Wiese-Bjornstal, D. M., Smith, A. M., Shaffer, S. M., & Morrey, M. A. (1998). An integrated model of response to sport injury: Psychological and sociological dynamics. *Journal of Applied Sport Psychology, 10*, 46-49.

Williams, J. M., & Andersen, M. B. (1998). Psychosocial antecedents of sport injury: Review and critique of the stress and injury model. *Journal of Applied Sport Psychology, 10*, 5-25.

Wittig, A. F., & Schurr, K. T. (1994). Psychological characteristics of women volleyball players: Relationships with injuries, rehabilitation, and team success. *Personality and Social Psychology Bulletin, 20*, 322-330.

In: Physical Activity in Rehabilitation and Recovery   ISBN: 978-1-60876-400-6
Editor: Holly Blake   © 2010 Nova Science Publishers, Inc.

Chapter 10

THE ROLE OF PHYSICAL EXERCISE IN OCCUPATIONAL REHABILITATION

Amanda Griffiths and Alec Knight**

Institute of Work, Health and Organisations,
University of Nottingham, UK.

ABSTRACT

Given the accepted role of physical exercise in rehabilitation in healthcare settings, it is surprising that exercise has been subject to little research in occupational environments. Employers, on the other hand, are beginning to credit exercise with some potential significance. This chapter presents the scientific evidence to date, and using the UK as an example, explores the disconnect between academic considerations, policy-level and employer-led imperatives. It focuses on three areas of concern to employers: (a) common mental health issues, (b) musculoskeletal disorders, and (c) cardiovascular conditions and respiratory disorders. Reviewers of the scientific literature have frequently commented upon the lack of methodological rigour in relation to the extant evidence. However, such criticisms should be tempered by a realistic appreciation of the nigh-impossibility of conducting experimental or quasi-experimental investigations in the turbulent world of real organisations. The authors

* Tel: +44 (0)115 8466637; Fax: +44 (0)115 8466625; Email: Amanda.Griffiths@nottingham.ac.uk
* Tel: +44 (0)115 8232213; Fax: +44 (0)115 8466625; Email: Alec.Knight@nottingham.ac.uk

conclude that although evidence remains mixed at present, the role of physical exercise in occupational rehabilitation looks promising.

INTRODUCTION

In many countries there is increasing recognition of the extent of work incapacity. For example, a government-led review of the health of Britain's working age population in 2008 estimated that the annual costs to the economy of ill-health in terms of lost working days and worklessness (defined as not being in paid employment and not actively seeking work) was over £100 billion – equivalent to the annual running costs of the National Health Service (Department for Work and Pensions & Department of Health, 2008a). The Confederation of British Industry, one of the main lobbying organisations for the country's businesses, estimated that in 2007, absence from work, to the tune of 172 million days, cost employers £13 billion. On any single day between 2 and 3 per cent of the workforce is absent from work due to ill-health (Department for Work and Pensions, 2004). Evidence suggests that once out of work on a long-term basis, the risks to mental health, physical health and social exclusion increase. In principle, providing that it is 'good' work, work has a protective effect on health (Waddell & Burton, 2006). There is an increasing recognition at policy-level that with better healthcare and workplace management, many people with long-term health conditions can be assisted to remain in, or to return to, work and that work itself should be regarded as one of the best forms of 'welfare' for people of working age (Department of Work and Pensions, 2004; Department for Work and Pensions, & Department of Health, 2008b). The British Government has stated that it wishes to see "increasing recognition among employers that they should support their staff to remain in and return to work following illness" (Department for Work Pensions, & Department of Health, 2008b, p.70). Despite developments in the evidence base, and policy-level support, a widely-held view remains that people should refrain from work when they have a health condition.

In Britain, government initiatives to reduce worklessness and lost working days include a national education programme for GPs, electronic 'fit-notes' (which focus on what people can do, as opposed to medical certificates that focus on what they cannot), and the creation of employment advisers in various settings. Also proposed is better support for employers in ensuring that workplaces are healthy and safe, that employee well-being is promoted, and that return to work can be facilitated when people develop a health condition or impairment.

Many enlightened employers recognise the importance of a swift and supportive response to employee ill-health and make use of vocational rehabilitation (VR) or occupational rehabilitation (OR) programmes to assist their employees to work. The British Government's Department for Work and Pensions (2004) described VR as "a process to overcome the barriers an individual faces when accessing, remaining or returning to work following injury, illness or impairment. This process includes the procedures in place to support the individual and/or employer or others (e.g. family and carers), including help to access VR and to practically manage the delivery of VR; and, in addition, VR includes the wide range of interventions to help individuals with a health condition and/or impairment overcome barriers to work and so remain in, return to or access employment" (pp.14-15).

Such rehabilitation programmes are described as comprising two essential elements: (a) an employment goal (e.g. return to work, or to access employment for the first time), and (b) a balanced mix of appropriate interventions to help an individual overcome barriers to work. In practice, interventions can include the provision of flexible working options, support in getting back to work (such as access to psychological therapies), adjustments to working conditions on return to work, and access to occupational health services. Physical exercise (either alone, or as a single component of a more complex OR programme) has also been used to attempt to help employees with a variety of common health problems, but as yet, is rare. In Britain, rehabilitation does not normally commence until an employee has been off work for an average of nine weeks (Chartered Institute of Personnel and Development, 2008), although, as is evident from the Case Study below, some organisations increasingly believe that earlier interventions are more effective.

Traditionally in organisational practice, and in much of the research literature, OR has been concerned solely with assisting absent employees to return to work, regardless of whether their incapacity is work-related. It should be said that it is recognised that employers have a duty to prevent work-related ill-health rather than simply address it after the event (Tehrani, 2004). Nevertheless, this chapter draws a distinction between OR and the broader issue of the prevention of work-related ill-health. This chapter focuses on the former, specifically on improving the work capability of employees absent due to common health problems: usually those that are manageable and widespread in people of working age. Common mental health disorders, mild to moderate musculoskeletal disorders, and cardiovascular conditions and respiratory disorders, are typical targets for OR. Together, these conditions account for approximately two-thirds of all sickness absence from work, long-term incapacity and ill-health retirement in the UK (Waddell, Burton & Kendall, 2008)[1].

Case Study I – Centrica

Centrica is an integrated energy company that sources, generates, processes and supplies energy, and provides a range of related services. During the busy period in the build up to winter, their engineers were prone to injury and musculoskeletal disorders (MSDs). Their occupational health services instigated a programme in 2007 where managers could refer all engineers who had a history of sickness absence due to MSDs to a rehabilitation programme. The aim was to strengthen engineers by means of 'prescription gym' (at a gym near their home) and a back or knee workshop according to individual need. Participants were offered 4 one-to-one coaching sessions over 5 weeks and as much access to the gym/swimming pool as required. Programmes were administered by a coach and devised according to individual need by a team comprising a physiologist, physician, sports scientist and physiotherapist.

Significant improvements in strength, mobility and motivation were achieved. Absence levels in this group were significantly less than in previous years; only 4 per cent of the rehabilitation group took any MSD related absence, compared to 41 per cent of engineers who did not participate. On the basis of this success, the programme was later made available to all engineers.

The company had previously maintained a policy of referral to the occupational health team on Day 20 of an employee's sick leave. The occupational health team provided advice and support (including recommendations about exercise) to help employees get back to work. In mid-2008, the company changed this such that Day 8 for any period of sickness absence that involved MSDs (or mental health issues) became the trigger for managers to ask for advice.

Centrica report that in addition to the clear benefits on employee return to work, such rehabilitation programmes are perceived as a real benefit ("carrot") by employees, not as punitive system designed to reduce company costs ("stick"). Thus, the company believes OR is also associated with an increase in employee engagement and ultimately with a better service for customers.

---

[1] The other major causes of sickness absence are minor illness and acute medical conditions. These are not usual targets for OR since the former are typically mild and self-limiting, while the latter require specialised treatment.

The benefits of effective OR could, in principle, be considerable for individuals and organisations alike. Individuals may benefit financially (by remaining in paid employment and maximising their career trajectory), in terms of health (which may improve as a secondary consequence of OR), and in ways that are difficult to quantify such as avoiding secondary effects of worklessness on family and dependents, social exclusion and poverty. Similarly, organisations may benefit financially (by minimising both the direct and indirect costs associated with employee absence and its management), by retaining trained and experienced personnel, and by avoiding litigation where incapacity be caused by work. Despite these clear potential benefits, OR is far from common in British organisations. It is estimated that about 60 per cent of the country's employers provide some form of rehabilitation service for their employees, although this figure disguises variation by sector and size. Public service employers are more likely to provide OR than private sector organisations, and very few small businesses offer any formal provision at all (Chartered Institute of Personnel and Development, 2008).

It is established that risk factors for numerous common mental and physical conditions decrease with regular physical activity (Pate, et al., 1995; Scully, Kremer, Meade, Graham, & Dudgeon, 1998) and that such activity can improve the overall health of employees (Kerr, Griffiths, & Cox, 1996). But, can physical activity help employees make a sustainable return to work where their ill-health has been significant enough to prevent them from attending work? This chapter explores the relevant evidence for exercise's role in OR from two standpoints. The first perspective is academic, and examines published research evidence largely from the international scientific literature. The second perspective is applied, which highlights the policy need for action in one country (Britain), and provides two case studies (in figures 1 and 2) of major British organisations that have implemented exercise interventions as part of their rehabilitation strategies, and who believe them to have been effective.

RESEARCH ON EXERCISE AND OCCUPATIONAL REHABILITATION

A large amount of descriptive research exists on exercise and work, reporting beneficial effects such as reduced absenteeism and employee turnover (e.g. Cox, Sherhard, & Corey, 1981; Kerr & Vos, 1993; Lechner & de Vries, 1997). However, much research is cross-sectional and correlational in nature, and does not help to determine whether exercise inhibits absenteeism (i.e. has a preventative effect), or assists employees to recover from illnesses and return to work more quickly (i.e. has a rehabilitative effect), or if there is a more complex relationship. It is unclear whether exercise affects the different causes of sickness absence in different ways. Exercise is often included and evaluated in the context of a wider workplace health promotion programme (Griffiths, 1996) and, therefore, its precise role made difficult to ascertain. The following sections of this chapter discuss focused research that explores the effectiveness of OR with specific reference to exercise in three areas of concern to employers: (i) common mental health issues, (ii) musculoskeletal disorders, and (iii) cardiovascular conditions and respiratory disorders.

COMMON MENTAL HEALTH ISSUES

Increasingly, employers are recognising a broad view of mental health as a continuum from poor health to good health. In addition to those with clinically-diagnosed mental illnesses such as schizophrenia or bipolar disorder, there are a large number of individuals who suffer low mental well-being that manifests itself variously as emotional distress, low self-esteem, a sense of hopelessness, chronic stress, anxiety, depression or other 'negative' psychological states. Taken together, common mental illnesses and low psychological well-being (here referred to collectively as *common mental health issues*) are currently viewed by employers as the leading cause of sickness absence in Britain (Chartered Institute of Personnel and Development, 2008). Occupational health specialists have identified common mental health issues as the leading priority for specialist support and action in the workplace (Leka, Khan, & Griffiths, 2008). Common mental health problems accounted for approximately 13.8 million lost working days in the UK in 2006/7 (Health and Safety Executive, 2008) and statistics suggest that they are the largest and fastest growing reason for incapacity benefits. Figures from other developed countries indicate that this scenario is common. In addition to keeping employees away from work, psychological ill-health can have a significant negative effect on the productivity of employees when they are at work (commonly referred to as 'presenteeism'). Research has suggested that the financial impact of presenteeism may be even larger than the impact of absenteeism, and was estimated to cost the UK economy £15.1 billion in 2006 (The Sainsbury Centre for Mental Health, 2007).

Exercise may have an important role to play in reducing the costs of absenteeism and presenteeism, by rehabilitating absent employees and improving the work capability of present employees. There is increasing evidence from the scientific literature that exercise can aid recovery from depression and enhance psychological well-being in the general population (Craft & Landers, 1998; Department of Health, 2004). In addition, exercise has been positively associated with self-esteem, self-efficacy, subjective well-being, mood, cognitive functioning and health-related quality of life, and negatively associated with depression, anxiety and reports of stress (Altchiler & Motta, 1994; McAuley, 1994). However, it is difficult to interpret work with regard to 'stress' since much research is based on responsivity to acute stressors and is conducted in laboratories. This kind of research has little ecological validity with regard to stress experienced at work, which tends to be chronic in nature. Nonetheless, there are several plausible mechanisms by which exercise might provide some protection from the experience of chronic stress (Griffiths, 1996a). Some authors have pointed to the likelihood that it is moderate activity and participation rather than fitness itself that is associated with improved mental health and mood (Thirlaway & Benton, 1996). One implication for employers is that better gains may be achieved by encouraging the majority of employees to exercise moderately, rather than providing 'high end' facilities for the already fit.

Traditionally, researchers have paid a large amount of attention to the effect of exercise on common mental health issues among elderly and clinical populations. Relatively little attention has been paid to the working population. Even less research exists on the effect of exercise on employment-related outcomes such as absence and performance (Griffiths, 1996b), and the research that has been published often has low external validity. Sjogren, Nissinen, Jarvenpaa, Ojanen, Vanharanta, & Malkia (2006) conducted a randomised-controlled trial (RCT) with office workers to examine the effect of light exercise training on a number of mental health variables. The authors concluded that their exercise intervention resulted in a very slight improvement in subjective physical well-being, but had no effect on anxiety, self-confidence, mood or stress. However, participants were all healthy volunteers, whose psychosocial functioning and general subjective well-being were high at the outset of the trial. The authors conceded that the physical activity intervention may not have been sufficiently demanding or prolonged to have any effect on the participants. Importantly, however, there was no measure relating to employment outcomes. Proper, Staal, Hildebrandt, van der Beek, and van Mechelen (2002) conducted a systematic review of the literature on the relationship between exercise and mental health at work, and surmised that the evidence was inconclusive. The evidence base for this conclusion was very narrow, with only four studies meeting all of the review inclusion criteria. The review also failed to consider the impact of exercise on employment outcomes. Conversely, Bruning, and Frew (1987) reported that an aerobic exercise intervention resulted in reduced stress among members of staff at a hospitality equipment facility. Long (1988) concluded that an intervention combining stress-inoculation training and exercise was effective at reducing anxiety and stress among school workers. However, in both of these studies the researchers did not include employment outcomes as measures, so it is not clear whether the exercise interventions may have had a beneficial effect on employment variables above and beyond the beneficial effect on mental health.

The studies cited above highlight important limitations in the research literature on exercise, work and mental health. The literature typically refers to organisational interventions with individuals who are at work and in good health whereas OR concerns processes that assist individuals to make a sustainable return to work. Despite the potential importance of the field, and the large amount of evidence in related research areas, direct evidence on exercise in OR for common mental health issues is rare. While the possible effect of exercise on people's psychological states is increasingly recognised, and is important in preventative and therapeutic contexts, the role of exercise in affecting occupational outcomes is not well established in the scientific literature. As Long and Flood (1993) noted, research in this field may have been inhibited by a lack of understanding of how exercise can enhance employees' mental health, or the inconsistency of previous research in finding statistically significant positive effects on mental health. In addition, while psychiatric conditions have clear diagnostic criteria, other common mental health issues such as stress and anxiety are notoriously difficult to diagnose and measure. Clearly, more research is required to establish whether (and if so, how) exercise is beneficial in rehabilitating employees with common mental health issues.

MUSCULOSKELETAL DISORDERS

Musculoskeletal disorders (MSDs) is a term used to describe over 200 conditions affecting the muscles, joints, tendons, ligaments, nerves and the localised blood circulation system. MSDs are a leading cause of short-term and long-term absence among both manual and non-manual workers in many countries throughout Europe and the rest the world (European Agency for Safety and Health at Work, 2007). In the UK, as many as 10.7 million working days were lost in 2006 as a result of MSDs. Moreover, it is forecast that the incidence and impact of these conditions will intensify with the ageing of the workforce, growing obesity and reductions in exercise, physical activity and fitness in the general population (Bevan, Passmore, & Mahdon, 2007). MSDs may be specific (e.g. rheumatoid arthritis, ankylosing spondylitis) or non-specific (e.g. back pain, upper limb disorders). However, the majority are non-specific, may occur only periodically, and are difficult to diagnose (Bevan et al., 2007). Disorders may be broadly categorised according to their body region, and are often referred to as: (a) Upper Limb Disorders (e.g. neck pain); (b) Back Pain (e.g. lower-back pain); and (c) Lower Limb Disorders (e.g. knee pain). While there is a large body of research relating to exercise interventions for the rehabilitation of MSDs (especially for lower-back pain), most studies are clinical in nature and relatively few include employment outcome measures.

Exercise is reported to have consistently beneficial effects on MSDs both for employees at work (Linton & van Tulder, 2001; Maher, 2000) and for those who are absent from work (Elders, van der Beek & Burdorf, 2000; Hlobil, Staal, Uegako, Smid & van Mechelen, 2005). Maher (2000) reviewed 13 RCTs and concluded that exercise was effective in preventing low back pain. However, Maher criticised many studies for having low methodological rigour, and for lacking consistency in terms of the type and intensity of the exercise intervention. Linton and van Tulder (2001) also noted a lack of high quality exercise studies in the OR literature for MSDs. However, these researchers' analysis supported a moderate positive effect of exercise on prevention of back and neck pain. In relation to research focusing on restoration of occupational function, a number of OR studies have reported successful outcomes for exercise interventions. Lindstrom, Ohlund, Eek, Wallin, Peterson, Fordyce et al. (1992) reported that industrial workers absent from work with low-back pain returned to work more quickly and had lower levels of long-term absenteeism when they took part in an OR programme involving exercise. However, the positive effect of the OR could not be attributed exclusively to physical exercise, as it was not the sole element of the programme. Torstensen, Ljunggren, Meen, Odland, Mowinckel and Geijerstam (1998) concluded that a medical exercise programme resulted in reduced sick leave-related costs compared to an unguided exercise programme in a sample of Norwegian office workers. There was, however, no difference in the time taken to return to work between intervention groups. Similarly, Hlobil et al (2005) reported that a graded exercise intervention resulted in reduced rates of sick leave and hastened return to work among a group of airline workers who were absent from work with lower-back pain.

Case Study II: Royal Mail

Over its 300 year history, the Royal Mail has provided British postal communications, and has offered occupational health services for its employees for 150 years. In 2003 the company began a holistic (biopsychosocial) rehabilitation programme for employees who had been on sick leave with musculoskeletal disorders.

The programme, undertaken in a central London Mail Centre, lasted for 1 day per week for 6-12 weeks. The programme which included an educational and CBT (cognitive behavioural therapy) approach focused both on restoring function and confidence to work via self management, goal setting, and intensive exercise sessions in groups. Clinical outcomes included lifting capability and confidence, pain, mood and beliefs regarding pain, fear of movement and work activities; all demonstrated significant gains. From 250 cases off work, 84 per cent returned to work: 75 per cent returned to full duties within 12 weeks and a further 9 per cent returned to modified duties within 12 weeks. At six month review, recurrent absence in this group was reduced by approximately 89 per cent. Royal Mail estimated that this provided a return on investment of 320 per cent.

Employees who had a major history of back and neck pain reported the programme as a 'lifeline', giving them back their confidence, and enabling them to resume normal activities both in and outside of work. A 49-year old, for example, with a 2 year history of significant lower-back pain who had been off work for 6 months returned to work in 4 weeks and remained well afterwards.

The programme is being rolled-out nationally.

Such studies demonstrate that it is possible to conduct OR research on exercise for absent workers, and that exercise interventions may assist some of these employees to make a sustained return to work. These studies also demonstrate some of the problems of conducting OR research, which frequently suffer from a number of limitations. Studies have largely failed to determine the unique contribution of exercise in OR, have lacked meaningful comparison groups, and have employed a large range of different interventions and outcome measures. These limitations affect the external validity of research, thus making generalisations between contexts problematic. Moreover, the literature has tended to focus on a few specific conditions (e.g. back and neck pain), despite a very large range of MSDs. Large gaps remain in the research literature, while existing research requires replication and verification. Nonetheless, some employers are convinced of the role of exercise in rehabilitation, and as is demonstrated in Case Study II, have evaluated its effects and cost benefits very positively.

CARDIOVASCULAR CONDITIONS AND RESPIRATORY DISORDERS

Mental health issues and MSDs account for the vast majority of sickness absence caused by common health problems. Accordingly, research on the role exercise is most extensive in those areas. Nevertheless, there has been some OR research on exercise for other groups of common health problems. Two such groups are cardiovascular conditions and respiratory disorders.

Cardiovascular conditions include myocardial infarction, heart failure and angina, as well as hypertension and arrhythmia. Exercise has been shown to be highly beneficial to the health of those with serious cardiovascular conditions, such as myocardial infarction (Thomson, 1999). Rønnevik (1988) noted that individuals with a high exercise capacity were more likely to return to work following myocardial infarction than those with lower exercise capacity. Moreover, there is recognition that return-to-work should be a goal of cardiac rehabilitation (Waddell & Burton, 2006). Nevertheless, provision of support and research on rehabilitation of cardiovascular conditions has tended to focus on severe cases, and not on employment-related outcomes. For example, in the UK, less than 1 per cent of patients receiving cardiac rehabilitation are given vocational assessment, and occupational outcomes are rarely reported in the scientific literature (Waddell et al., 2008). However, a few researchers have directly examined the effect of exercise on return to work behaviour of those with cardiovascular conditions. Dugmore et al (1999) reported that post-myocardial infarction patients returned to work significantly earlier and resumed full-time employment more quickly following an exercise training intervention. Moreover, participants had a significant improvement in vocational status over a five year follow-up period. There is minimal evidence on the effectiveness of exercise in OR for cardiovascular conditions other than myocardial infarction.

There are three common categories of respiratory disorders, which affect working people in developed countries. These three categories together affect up to 3 million people in the UK's workforce. First, minor upper respiratory tract infections are a common reason for sickness absence from work in the UK, although not generally considered a target for OR as they tend to have a limited impact on health. Second, work-related asthma and breathing problems affect up to 142,000 people in the UK, and up to one quarter of all adult asthma sufferers may find their condition is aggravated by their work (Health and Safety Executive, 2007). Third, chronic obstructive pulmonary disease (chronic bronchitis and emphysema) and respiratory disorders are a major cause of sickness absence in the UK. Respiratory conditions are often undiagnosed, and research tends to focus on the more severe cases (commonly in workers close to retirement age) where the medical condition is often severe and progressive. Similarly, cardiovascular conditions have been under-researched as a whole in the OR literature, and more specifically with respect to the effectiveness of exercise in improving work capability. Despite the fact that these conditions are a significant cause of sickness absence, research has, again, largely focused on clinical rather than occupational outcomes. Exercise has been shown to have a beneficial effect on clinical outcomes in chronic obstructive pulmonary disease (Berry, Rejeski, Adair, & Zaccaro, 1999; Casaburi, Porszasz, Burns, Carithers, Chang & Cooper, 1997) and so it may also have a role to play in OR. However, the lack of direct empirical evidence prohibits firm conclusions. However, evidence suggests that rehabilitation in later stages of occupational asthma has little effect on work outcomes (Monninkhof, van der Valk, van der Palen, van Herwaarden, Partridge, & Zielhuis, 2003). Therefore, rather than OR, the most appropriate aims initially may be to improve occupational risk assessment, workplace management, and early detection and treatment of respiratory conditions (Waddell et al., 2008).

RESEARCH SYNTHESIS

Overall, there is little consensus or consistency among OR researchers on the most appropriate research methods, intervention strategies and outcome measures in research on common health problems. Moreover, research has provided little consistent evidence to support a beneficial effect of exercise on improving the work capability of absent employees; for those research papers that suggest exercise is beneficial in improving employees' capability to work, there are often as many research papers reporting no significant beneficial effect. Reviewers of the research literature have also often commented on the lack of methodological quality among the research that has been published (e.g. Proper et al., 2002). While there is tentative support for the effectiveness of exercise in improving work capability of employees absent due to more common MSDs and cardiovascular conditions, very little research exists on assisting individuals to access employment for the first time, or to return to work after long-term disability. Instead, research focuses on assisting employees to return to work with their present employer. Aside from these criticisms, OR research on exercise and common health problems has other significant limitations. It has rarely acknowledged comorbidity – several health problems presenting in one individual. Research has demonstrated that physical and mental conditions often co-occur (Buist-Bouwman, de Graaf, Vollebergh, & Ormel, 2005) and physical and psychological work-related illnesses may have a shared set of causal factors (e.g. MSDs and depression; Lloyd, Waghorn, & McHugh, 2008). However, individuals with multiple conditions are routinely excluded from OR intervention research and systematic literature reviews. By excluding individuals with multiple conditions, researchers have reduced the extent to which their results can be generalised and thus limited the value of their research. Organisational research is inherently complex, and control of 'extraneous' variables is not always possible or even desirable.

Researchers have often criticised the OR research literature on exercise and common health problems, on the grounds that it is largely composed of papers employing low-quality research methods. The current dominant approach in judging research on many forms of organisational interventions in relation to health matters is driven by an experimental, natural science paradigm (Griffiths, 1999), associated with the movement for evidence-based policy and practice espoused by healthcare professions. Distinct quality standards exist within this field, with a focus on a limited range of research methods (in particular RCTs) that are designed to assess evidence of the effectiveness of clinical interventions. However, as Waddell et al (2008) make clear, the aims, research population and environment of OR are clearly distinct from the aims of clinical treatments. Clinical treatment aims to treat pathology and/or reduce symptoms in patients, while OR aims to improve capability to work of absent employees such that they can return to work. Accordingly, healthcare-type research on OR has been criticised by organisational researchers for its oversights (notably the lack of systems-level variables and a failure to adopt qualitative methods where appropriate). There is a supposition that certain research methods should be held in higher regard than others (Boaz & Ashby, 2003; Cox, Karanika, Griffiths & Houdmont, 2007). In particular, some have failed to appreciate the potential value of research that does not employ an experimental or RCT method or is not large scale (epidemiological) in nature. In reality, experiments are probably impossible to conduct in real working organisations, particularly where they are addressing the sort of complex questions that are important for employers, but perhaps less interesting or feasible for researchers (Griffiths, 1999). It must be recognised that absence of evidence means many things: that the issue has not been studied enough, that the issue has not been published, or that the issue presents methodological challenges that are hard to overcome given dominant research paradigms. A less blinkered approach to the strengths and weaknesses of various research methods should be adopted in future, both by researchers and by those who judge them.

CONCLUSION

Returning to the policy imperatives, given that the scientific literature on exercise in OR is neither firm nor consistent in one direction, some may be surprised that OR is used at all by organisations in the 'real world'. This is an example of a not infrequent disconnect between research and business practice. While academics argue the minutiae of research methods, employers have real problems to solve, and are happy to continue to explore possible solutions where harm seems unlikely. But in the case of OR, such a disconnect also exists between academic research and policy positions. For example, the UK's Department for Work and Pensions' publication on VR states (2004, p.11), "The Government does not see the current inconclusive evidence base as a reason not to start considering how to move forward on VR and in particular consider how to address stakeholders' VR needs. Indeed, the implementation of VR processes, based on the evidence we do have, and the subsequent evaluation of such projects to show whether they work and are cost effective, can only help to improve this evidence base and inform the development of future VR approaches."

Researchers have focused on the evaluation of OR, but there has been a lack of evaluation of rehabilitation practice by employers themselves. In the UK, it is estimated that just over one third of the organisations providing rehabilitation services evaluate the business impact of providing such support (Chartered Institute of Personnel and Development, 2008). Similarly, only about 40 per cent of organisations monitor the cost of absence, even though 8 out of 10 employers rate sickness absence as a significant or very significant cost to the business. Nonetheless, some forward looking employers recognise the value of OR, the value of moving in with such support far more swiftly than has been traditional, and have begun to credit some significance to the role of physical exercise in rehabilitation. Future research should clarify the remaining questions. If exercise has a role in occupational rehabilitation, and the current authors suspect it has, more convincing evidence is required, accompanied by clear exposition of the business case, before organisations implement such initiatives more widely.

REFERENCES

Altchiler, M., & Motta, R. (1994). Effects of aerobic and nonaerobic exercise on anxiety, absenteeism, and job satisfaction. *Journal of Clinical Psychology, 50*(6), 829-840.

Berry, M. J., Rejeski, W. J., Adair, N. E., & Zaccaro, D. (1999). Exercise Rehabilitation and Chronic Obstructive Pulmonary Disease Stage. *American Journal of Respiratory and Critical Care Medicine, 160*(4), 1248-1253.

Bevan, S., Passmore, E., & Mahdon, M. (2007). *Fit for work?* London: The Work Foundation.

Boaz, A., & Ashby, D. (2003). *Fit for purpose? Assessing research quality for evidence based policy and practice.* London: Economic and Social Research Council.

Bruning, N. S., & Frew, D. R. (1987). Effects of Exercise, Relaxation, and Management Skills Training on Physiological Stress Indicators: A Field Experiment. *Journal of Applied Psychology, 72*(4), 515-521.

Buist-Bouwman, M. A., de Graaf, R., Vollebergh, W. A. M., & Ormel, J. (2005). Comorbidity of physical and mental disorders and the effect on work-loss days. *Acta Psychiatrica Scandinavica, 111*, 436-443.

Casaburi, R., Porszasz, J., Burns, M. R., Carithers, E. R., Chang, R. S., & Cooper, C. B. (1997). Physiologic benefits of exercise training in rehabilitation of patients with severe chronic obstructive pulmonary disease. *American Journal of Respiratory and Critical Care Medicine, 155*(5), 1541-1551.

Chartered Institute of Personnel and Development. (2008). *Absence Management.* London: Chartered Institute of Personnel and Development.

Cox, M., Sherhard, R. J., & Corey, P. (1981). Influence of an employee fitness programme upon fitness, productivity and absenteeism. *Ergonomics, 24*(10), 795-806.

Cox, T., Karanika, M., Griffiths. A., & Houdmont, J. (2007). Evaluating organisational-level work stress interventions: Beyond traditional methods. *Work & Stress, 21(4),* 348-362.

Craft, L. L., & Landers, D. M. (1998). The effect of exercise on clinical depression: A meta-analysis. *Medicine & Science In Sports & Exercise, 30*(5), 339-357.

Department for Work and Pensions. (2004). *Building Capacity for Work: A UK Framework for Vocational Rehabilitation.* London: Stationery Office.

Department for Work and Pensions, and Department of Health. (2008a). *Dame Carol Black's review of the health of Britain's working age population: Working for a Healthier tomorrow.* London: The Stationary Office.

Department for Work and Pensions, and Department of Health. (2008b). *Improving health and work: Changing lives. The Government's Response to Dame Carol Black's review of the health of Britain's working age population.* London: The Stationary Office.

Department of Health. (2004). *At Least Five a Week.* London: The Stationary Office.

Dugmore, L. D., Tipson, R. J., Phillips, M. H., Flint, E. J., Stentiford, N. H., Bone, M. F., et al. (1999). Changes in cardiorespiratory fitness, psychological wellbeing, quality of life, and vocational status following a 12 month cardiac exercise rehabilitation programme. *Heart, 81*, 359-366.

Elders, L. A. M., van der Beek, A. J., & Burdorf, A. (2000). Return to work after sickness absence due to back disorders - a systematic review on intervention strategies. *International Archives of Occupational and Environmental Health, 73*(5), 339-348.

European Agency for Safety and Health at Work. (2007). *Work-related musculoskeletal disorders: Back to work report.* Luxembourg: Office for Official Publications of the European Communities.

Griffiths, A. (1996a). Employee exercise programmes: Organisational and individual perspectives. In J. Kerr, A. Griffiths & T. Cox (Eds.) *Workplace Health, Employee Fitness and Exercise.* London: Taylor & Francis.

Griffiths, A. (1996b). The benefits of employee exercise programmes: A review. *Work & Stress, 10*, 5-23.

Griffiths, A. (1999). Organizational interventions: Facing the limits of the natural science paradigm. *Scandinavian Journal of Work, Environment & Health, 25*(6), 589-596.

Health and Safety Executive. (2007). *Occupational Asthma.* London: HSE Books.

Health and Safety Executive. (2008). *Self-reported work-related illness and workplace injuries in 2006/07: Results from the Labour Force Survey.* London: HSE Books.

Hlobil, H., Staal, B., Uegako, K., Smid, T., & van Mechelen, W. (2005). Graded exercise: A Cognitive Behavioural Approach to Return-to-Work for Workers with Non-Specific Low Back Pain. *Medicine & Science In Sports & Exercise, 37*(5(S)), 414-415.

Kerr, J. H., & Vos, M. C. H. (1993). Employee fitness programmes, absenteeism and general well-being. *Work & Stress, 7*(2), 179-190.

Kerr, J., Griffiths, A., & Cox, T. (1996). *Workplace health: Employee fitness and exercise*. London: Taylor & Francis.

Leka, S., Khan, S., & Griffiths, A (2008). *Exploring health and safety practitioners' training needs in workplace health issues*. Wigston: Institution for Occupational Safety and Health.

Lechner, L., & de Vries, H. (1997). Effects of an Employee Fitness Program on Reduced Absenteeism. *Journal of Occupational & Environmental Medicine, 39*(9), 827-831.

Lindstrom, I., Ohlund, C., Eek, C., Wallin, L., Peterson, L. E., Fordyce, W. E., et al. (1992). The Effect of Graded Activity on Patients with Subacute Low Back Pain: A Randomized Prospective Clinical Study with an Operant-Conditioning Behavioral Approach. *Physical Therapy, 72*(4), 279-290.

Linton, S. J., & van Tulder, M. W. (2001). Preventive Interventions for Back and Neck Pain Problems: What is the Evidence? *Spine, 26*(7), 778-787.

Lloyd, C., Waghorn, G., & McHugh, C. (2008). Musculoskeletal disorders and comorbid depression: Implications for practice. *Australian Occupational Therapy Journal, 55*, 23-29.

Long, B. C. (1988). Stress Management for School Personnel: Stress-Inoculation Training and Exercise. *Psychology in the Schools, 25*(3), 314-324.

Long, B. C., & Flood, K. R. (1993). Coping with work stress: Psychological benefits of exercise. *Work & Stress, 7*(2), 109-119.

Maher, C. G. (2000). A systematic review of workplace interventions to prevent low back pain. *Australian Journal of Physiotherapy, 46*, 259-269.

McAuley, E. (1994). Physical activity and psychosocial outcomes. In C. Bouchard, R. J. Shephard & T. Stephens (Eds.), *Physical activity, fitness, and health* (pp. 551-568). Leeds: Human Kinetics Europe.

Monninkhof, E., van der Valk, P., van der Palen, J., van Herwaarden, C., Partridge, M. R., & Zielhuis, G. (2003). Self-management education for patients with chronic obstructive pulmonary disease: a systematic review. *Thorax, 58*, 394-398.

Pate, R. R., Pratt, M., Blair, S. N., Haskell, W. L., Macera, C. A., Bouchard, C., et al. (1995). Physical activity and public health: A recommendation from the Centers for Disease Control and Prevention and the American College of Sports Medicine. *Journal of the American Medical Association, 273*(5), 402-407.

Proper, K. I., Staal, B. J., Hildebrandt, V. H., van der Beek, A. J., & van Mechelen, W. (2002). Effectiveness of physical activity programs at worksites with respect to work-related outcomes. *Scandinavian Journal of Work, Environment & Health, 28*(2), 75-84.

Rønnevik, P. K. (1988). Predicting return to work after acute myocardial infarction. Significance of clinical data, exercise test variables and beta-blocker therapy. *Cardiology, 75*(3), 230-236.

Scully, D., Kremer, J., Meade, M. M., Graham, R., & Dudgeon, K. (1998). Physical exercise and psychological well-being: a critical review. *British Journal of Sports Medicine, 32*, 111-120.

Sjogren, T., Nissinen, K. J., Jarvenpaa, S. K., Ojanen, M. T., Vanharanta, H., & Malkia, E. A. (2006). Effects of a physical exercise intervention on subjective physical well-being, psychosocial functioning and general well-being among office workers: A cluster randomized-controlled cross-over design. *Scandinavian Journal of Medicine & Science in Sports, 16*(6), 381-390.

Tehrani, N. (2004). *Recovery, Rehabilitation and Retention: Maintaining a Productive Workforce.* London: Chartered Institute of Personnel and Development.

The Sainsbury Centre for Mental Health. (2007). *Mental Health at Work: Developing the business case.* London: The Sainsbury Centre for Mental Health.

Thomson, P. (1999). A review of behavioural change theories in patient compliance to exercise-based rehabilitation following acute myocardial infarction. *Coronary Health Care, 3*(1), 18-24.

Thirlaway, K., & Benton, D. (1996). Exercise and mental health: The role of activity and fitness. In Kerr, J., Griffiths, A., & Cox, T. (Eds.) *Workplace health: Employee fitness and exercise.* London: Taylor & Francis.

Torstensen, T. A., Ljunggren, A. E., Meen, H. D., Odland, E. R. N., Mowinckel, P., & Geijerstam, S. P. T. (1998). Efficiency and Costs of Medical Exercise Therapy, Conventional Physiotherapy, and Self-Exercise in Patients With Chronic Low Back Pain: A Pragmatic, Randomized, Single-Blinded, Controlled Trial With 1-Year Follow-Up. *Spine, 23*(23), 2616-2624.

Waddell, G., & Burton, A. K. (2006). *Is work good for your health and well-being?* London: The Stationery Office.

Waddell, G., Burton, A. K., & Kendall, N. A. S. (2008). *Vocational Rehabilitation: What works, for whom, and when?* London: The Stationery Office.

In: Physical Activity in Rehabilitation and Recovery   ISBN: 978-1-60876-400-6
Editor: Holly Blake   © 2010 Nova Science Publishers, Inc.

Chapter 11

EXERCISE INTERVENTIONS IN THE TREATMENT OF DEPRESSION

*Sumaira Malik[1], Phoenix Kit Han Mo[1] and Holly Blake[2]**

[1] Institute of Work, Health & Organisations,
University of Nottingham, UK.
[2] Faculty of Medicine and Health Sciences, University of Nottingham, UK.

ABSTRACT

Depression is a common psychiatric problem affecting millions of people worldwide. Whilst conventional treatments for depression have involved the use of antidepressant medications or 'talking' therapies, in recent years the concept of exercise therapy has received increasing attention as a potential alternative or supplementary treatment for depression. Research suggests that exercise interventions can be beneficial for alleviating depressive symptoms in individuals with a diagnosis of depression. Furthermore, it appears that exercise may be equally as effective as the use of antidepressant medications or psychotherapy. However, there are methodological shortcomings in much of the published literature, which may limit the generalisability of findings. There is a need for further well-designed research to clarify the role of exercise in the treatment of depression. Recommendations for future research and practice are outlined in this chapter.

---

* Tel: +44 (0)115 8231049; Fax: +44 (0)115 8230999; Email: Holly.Blake@nottingham.ac.uk

INTRODUCTION

It is well established that exercise can have positive effects on mental health and well-being, and there is a general consensus that exercise offers many advantages to both the individual and health care resources as a supplement to traditional forms of treatment for depressed patients. Internationally, depression is one of the most common psychiatric problems in the general population. Estimates suggest that around 121 million people worldwide are affected by some form of depression (World Health Organisation, 2008). The common symptoms of depression typically include feelings of sadness, irritability, hopelessness, anxiety, reduced energy, loss of interest in enjoyable activities and diminished activity, and changes in eating and sleeping habits (Hale, 1997; Gelder, Harrison & Cowen, 2006; Semple, Smyth, Burns, Darjee, & McIntosh, 2005). Patients are generally diagnosed with major depression when a persistent and pervasive low mood is accompanied by a range of disabling symptoms that interfere with the normal functioning of the individual (National Institute of Clinical Excellence, 2004). According to the National Institute of Health and Clinical Excellence (2004), the prevalence of major depression among 16-65 year olds in the UK is 17 per 1,000 for men and 25 per 1,000 for women. However, when focusing on prevalence figures for mixed depression and anxiety, this figure rises significantly to 98 per 1,000 (71/1000 males and 124/1000 females). Depression can be a recurrent illness, with statistics suggesting that approximately half of those with major depression will have at least one further episode (Eaton, Shao, Hestadt 2008; Kupfer, 1991). As a result depression is often described as the 'common cold of psychiatry' (Garland, 1996).

As such depression presents an important and increasingly pervasive concern for public health. The impact of this condition on the individual, society and health care resources is substantial, with research evidence showing that depression is a significant cause of physical illness, disability and mortality internationally (Greden, 2001; Lawlor & Hopker, 2001). Results from World Health Surveys reveal that depression produces the greatest decrement in health and world-wide disease impact than any other chronic health condition including ischaemic heart disease, cerebrovascular disease, and tuberculosis (Moussavi et al., 2007; Paluska & Schwenk, 2000). Furthermore, a recent report published by the World Health Organisation (2008) states that depression is projected to become the second most common cause of disability adjusted life years in the world by 2020. One of the disturbing consequences of depression is the increase in suicide risk in sufferers, with approximately two thirds of all deaths by suicide occurring among depressed patients (American Psychiatric Association, 2000;

Sartorius, 2001; World Health Organization, 2008). Without effective treatment, depression can therefore become a chronic and recurrent condition that is associated with increasing functional disability overtime (Andrews, 2001; Solomon et al., 2000; World Health Organisation, 2008). Consequently, treatment and relapse prevention of depressive symptoms has become a key issue in the development of public health initiatives worldwide.

CURRENT TREATMENTS FOR DEPRESSION

Conventional treatments for depression have primarily involved the prescription of anti-depressant medications. Whilst drug treatments have largely proven to be effective in reducing depressive symptoms among individuals suffering from both 'severe' and 'mild to moderate' depression (de Maat, Dekker, Schoevers, & de Jonghe, 2006; Hale, 1997), it has been suggested that a significant proportion of depression within the general population remains inadequately treated (Greenberg et al, 2004; Gwynn et al, 2008; Lawlor & Hopker, 2001;). In fact, it has been estimated that only 25% of adults experiencing depression actually seek treatment from health care professionals (Dunn et al, 2002). Compliance with medication regimens is a significant problem, since of those who do seek help, 20-59% of patients prescribed with antidepressant medications are estimated to discontinue treatment within three weeks of prescription (Lawlor & Hopker, 2001), and only 20% of patients who are given referrals to psychotherapy ever enter treatment (Brody, Khaliq, & Thompson, 1997). Such delays in seeking and adhering to professional treatment can further lead to increased morbidity and mortality, and a higher relapse risk.

This pattern of findings may be attributed to a number of factors. Firstly, seeking help for mental health problems can be difficult for many individuals due to the societal stigma commonly associated with the diagnosis of a mental health condition, and also feelings of 'abnormality' which individuals may experience during discussions relating to depressive symptomatology (Barney, Griffiths, Jorm & Christenson, 2005; Sirey et al., 2001). Secondly, there are practical barriers to accessing mental health treatments like psychotherapy, such as high costs and lengthy waiting times, which may also deter people from seeking professional mental health treatment (Kung, 2004; Mohr et al., 2006). Thirdly, drug treatments may have other negative effects on the individual, since the use of anti-depressant medication has been associated with significant impairments in patient quality of life (Blumenthal et al, 1999; Cassano & Favo, 2004; van Geffen et al., 2007). For example, antidepressant medications are known to have several unpleasant side effects that may affect an individual's ability to carry out certain daily activities. These may include drowsiness or tiredness, insomnia, sexual problems, dizziness, indigestion problems and sickness or vomiting (Beaumont, Kasper, O'Hanlon, & Mendlewicz, 2008; Rothschild, 2000). The difficulty of fitting medication into personal routines, and forgetfulness, are other crucial reasons for nonadherence to antidepressant medications (Ayalon, Arean, & Alvidrez, 2005; Burra et al., 2007).

Attention is therefore shifting towards exploring the efficacy of alternative treatments and prevention strategies for depression in the general population. In line with international strategies to promote healthy lifestyle behaviours amongst those with chronic conditions, the concept of lifestyle exercise intervention or 'exercise therapy' is becoming increasingly popular. When compared with antidepressant medication and psychotherapy interventions, exercise therapy is relatively low cost and in the long-term, can be performed at the convenience of the individual outside of traditional medical settings, thus supporting the concept of 'self-care' in people with long-term chronic conditions (e.g. National Institute of Clinical Excellence, 2004). Furthermore, exercise is free from the stigma and side effects associated with the more conventional forms of anti-depressant treatments, and can therefore offer what may be perceived as a safer and more acceptable alternative to the individual.

DEFINING EXERCISE

Although many studies have examined the effects of exercise in the treatment of depression, a consistent definition of exercise is lacking and the terms 'exercise' and 'physical activity' are often used interchangeably in the research literature. In its broadest sense, physical activity encompasses any form of muscle movement, which results in energy expenditure (Powell, Thompson, Caspersen, & Kendrick, 1987). Exercise on the other hand is a planned physical activity that involves a repetitive structured movement of the body. Exercise therefore constitutes only one form of physical activity and the two terms are not equivalent to one another.

There are three main types of exercise: aerobic, anaerobic, and flexibility exercise (Brosse, Sheets, Lett, & Blumenthal, 2002). Aerobic exercise involves the metabolisation of oxygen to produce energy; it is typically less intense but of a longer duration (e.g. walking or jogging). In comparison anaerobic exercise does not require the use of inspired oxygen for energy and is normally higher in intensity but of a very short duration (e.g. weightlifting). Flexibility exercise lies between the two and is designed to improve range of motion (e.g. yoga, stretching). The bulk of the literature in this area examines the role of a structured programme of exercise (mainly aerobic exercise) in the treatment of depression, rather than the effects of physical activity in its broader sense.

THE ROLE OF EXERCISE IN DEPRESSION

It has long been known that exercise can have positive effects on mental health and well-being, and can exert an antidepressant effect. Cross-sectional and epidemiological studies have consistently shown an inverse association between regular lifetime exercise and depressive symptoms in both clinical and non-clinical samples (Bhui & Fletcher, 2000; de Moor et al, 2008; de Moor et al, 2006; Harris, Cronkite, & Morrs, 2006; Hassmen, Koivula & Uutela, 2000). It has also been shown in an experimental setting that exercise may be an effective alternative and adjunct treatment for depression (Craft, Freund, Culpepper, & Perna, 2007; Daley, 2008; Lawlor & Hopker, 2001; Stathopoulou et al, 2006). Although the antidepressant effects of exercise have now been recognised, the exact mechanism through which exercise influences depressive symptoms remains poorly understood.

A number of possible mechanisms and hypotheses have been outlined. These hypotheses can be divided into physiological and psychological explanations. Physiological explanations tend to revolve around three key hypotheses; firstly the endorphin hypothesis which proposes that the relationship between exercise and improved mental health status is caused by an increase in the secretion of endorphins during exercise, which are thought to promote a sense of well-being through reducing perceptions of pain and evoking a state of euphoria (Callaghan, 2004; Ernst, Olson, Pinel, Lam, & Christie, 2006; Morgan, 1985; North et al, 1990; Thoren et al, 1990). Secondly, the monoamine hypothesis that argues that, the association between exercise and depression is linked to the fact that exercise promotes the secretion of neurotransmitters like serotonin, dopamine and noradrenalin (Tsang & Fung, 2008; Ransford, 1982). This is likely to have beneficial consequences for mood as deficits in the levels of these chemicals have been widely associated with the aetiology of depression (Paluska & Schwenk, 2000). Thirdly, some authors argue that exercise can reduce stress reactivity through regulating hyperactivity of the HPA axis functioning (a nueroendocrine reaction to stress), which may in turn reduce depression (Brosse et al., 2002).

Psychological theories on the other hand argue that psychosocial mechanisms including social interaction, distraction, self-efficacy and mastery may all play an equally significant role in the antidepressant effect of exercise. For example, the distraction hypothesis proposes that exercise serves as a powerful distraction from unpleasant and negative thoughts and can thus lead to significant improvements in mood (Guszkowska, 2004; Morgan, 1985). This explanation is based on the premise of the response style theory of depression (Nolen-Hoeksema, 1991), which postulates that vulnerability to prolonged depression is associated with a ruminative style response (i.e. the tendency to focus repeatedly on one's negative thoughts and consequences). Whereas adopting a distracting response style (i.e. cognitions and behaviours that divert attention from depressed mood) is thought to contribute to the alleviation of depression. Craft (2005) outlines the numerous opportunities for individuals to distract themselves from their unpleasant thoughts, for example an exerciser's attention is often diverted to focus on bodily changes such as increased heart rate, breathing, tiredness and sore muscles, or on their exercise training goals, thus providing a temporary diversion from their depressed mood state.

Some authors suggest that through successfully completing a challenging activity such as a session of exercise, individuals experience feelings of achievement, mastery and success, which themselves contribute to an improvement in psychological well-being (Guszkowska, 2004; Johnsgard, 2004; Paluska & Schwenk, 2000). In depressed populations, this sense of achievement may lead individuals to feel an increased sense of control and confidence which transfers to other aspects of their life, and encourages them to engage in further activities that distract them from pondering on negative thoughts (Craft, 2005). Related to this, self-efficacy is also a key concept that helps to explain the link between exercise and depression (Johnsgard, 2004; North et al., 1990; Spence, Poon, & Dyck, 1997). This hypothesis suggests that as individuals gain a sense of mastery over a challenging activity like regularly exercising, their sense of self-efficacy (i.e. the individual's level of confidence in their capabilities to a meet a particular challenge) also increases. Changes in coping self-efficacy resulting from exercise may be associated with a reduction in symptoms of depression (Craft, 2005).

Other authors emphasise that social interaction may also account for the some of the positive effects of exercise (Brosse et al, 2002; Paluska & Schwenk, 2000; Ransford, 1982). Since exercise can provide new opportunities for depressed patients to meet and socialise with others, taking part in exercise may reduce the feelings of isolation experienced by many depressed people and provide them with a valuable source of support and encouragement (Tsang et al, 2006; Tsang et al, 2003; North et al, 1990; Thoren et al, 1990).

THE EVIDENCE BASE FOR EXERCISE INTERVENTIONS

On an international scale, the benefits of exercise interventions for mental health and well-being have received increasing recognition over recent years. In fact, the UK government now advises that health care professionals should offer depressed patients exercise therapy *before* considering the prescription of antidepressants or psychological therapies (National Institute of Clinical Excellence, 2004). However, despite this, whereas the effects of exercise on *physical* health are widely reported, the benefits of exercise programmes for *mental* health are still less widely reported and accepted among the general population (Mental Health Foundation, 2005). The following section provides an overview of the evidence base for the efficacy of exercise interventions in the treatment of depression among different depressed populations in order to identify directions for future research and practice.

Adolescent Populations

Although this chapter predominantly focuses on depression in adulthood, it is suggested that depression can re-occur across a lifetime and indeed research indicates that a large proportion of people have their first episode of major depression in childhood or adolescence (Fava & Kendler, 2000). It has also been suggested that the early onset of depression may be associated with a significantly higher risk of relapse in later life (Giles, Jarrett, Biggs, Guzick, & Rush, 1989). Consequently, developing safe and effective strategies for the early prevention and treatment of depression among adolescents is important. Despite this, the effect of exercise on depressive symptoms in adolescents experiencing depression has received comparatively less attention in the published literature. Whilst a number of cross-sectional studies suggest that young people with greater levels of exercise report lower levels of depression (de Moor et al, 2006; Steptoe & Butler, 1996), there is a notable paucity of experimental research to support the effectiveness of exercise interventions per se as a treatment for depression among adolescent populations. Indeed, readers are referred to a Cochrane review of exercise in the treatment of anxiety and depression among adolescents by Larun, Nordheim, Ekeland, Hagen, and Heian (2006), which identified that hard conclusions relating to the effectiveness of exercise interventions for young people were difficult to draw due to limited number of studies conducted in this population.

One randomised controlled trial of 49 female adolescents aged 18-20 years with mild to moderate depressive symptoms found that participants assigned to an 8-week exercise condition showed a significant decline in depressive symptoms as measured by the Centre for Epidemiologic Studies Depression (CES-D) scale, following the intervention compared to individuals in the usual care control group (Nabkasorn et al., 2006). These results are promising and suggest that exercise may be effective in improving depressive states among some young people, and this may be important for their mental health into adulthood. However, since this study was based on a relatively small sample of female participants only, with mild to moderate depressive symptoms, investigations with larger and more diverse samples are required to determine the effectiveness of exercise for male and female adolescents with both major and minor depression.

Adult Populations

The majority of interventional research examining the role of exercise in the treatment of depressive symptoms to date has focused predominantly on young to middle-aged adult populations (Daley, 2002; 2008). Though limited in size, this evidence base, particularly the most recent evidence, generally supports the assertion that exercise can yield positive effects on depression. There are several meta-analyses of studies in this field.

For example, two early meta-analyses (McDonald & Hodgdon, 1991; North et al., 1990) focusing on intervention studies with various modes of exercise (i.e. weight training, aerobics, walking and/or jogging) conclude that exercise is related to statistically significant reductions in depression. These effects were found to be moderate in magnitude, and to occur in participants classified as both non-depressed and clinically depressed. However, since these meta-analyses included non-randomized controlled trials and studies in which participants were not depressed at baseline, the extent to which conclusions can be drawn from these meta-analyses regarding the value of exercise specifically as a *treatment* for depression is limited. Further meta-analyses conducted in the 1990s synthesized evidence for the efficacy of exercise as a treatment for depression among depressed populations. Craft and Landers (1998) reviewed the effects of exercise on depression in studies in which participants had been diagnosed with clinical depression or co-morbid depression with another mental illness (e.g. schizophrenia, anxiety and paranoia) at baseline. Their review of 30 studies revealed that exercise was associated with sizeable reductions in depressive symptoms with an overall mean effect of -.72. Whilst from this we can certainly conclude that exercise is helpful in the reduction of depressive symptoms in those who are already depressed, again the inclusion of observational studies and non-randomised trials limits our ability to firmly conclude from this meta-analysis that exercise is effective as a treatment for depression.

However, more recent work has substantiated earlier claims that exercise is an effective treatment for depression. Lawlor and Hopker (2001) conducted a meta-analysis of exercise as an intervention in the treatment of depression. This included only randomised controlled trials in which participants were diagnosed with depression at baseline. Results from 14 studies showed an overall effect size of -1.1 for exercise interventions compared with control groups. Furthermore, the results also revealed that there was no association between the type of exercise or variations in results between studies, thus suggesting that both aerobic and non-aerobic exercise had a similar effect. These positive findings from the early 1990s have been substantiated by a more recent meta-analysis of 11 randomised control trials which also reported a large treatment effect for exercise interventions compared with control groups (Effect Size = 1.42) (Stathopoulou et al., 2006). Recently, Daley (2008) conducted a synthesis of meta-analyses and systematic reviews of randomised controlled trials in the field. Results of the review strongly suggest that exercise interventions are more effective than no treatment in the reduction of depression, and seem to be as effective as conventional treatment, notably psychotherapy and antidepressants. Taken together these results appear to provide firmer evidence for the anti-depressant effects of exercise.

Other studies published after the aforementioned reviews and meta-analyses also provide some support for the notion that exercise can be helpful in the treatment of depression. For example, Craft et al. (2007) compared the effects of a clinic versus home-based walking intervention among 32 women with depressive symptoms. Results demonstrated that upon completion of the 3-month intervention, both intervention groups experienced significant reduction in depression score as measured by the Beck Depression Inventory, suggesting that home-based and clinic-based exercise programmes can equally benefit women with depressive symptoms. This would seem to have practice implications, however, as the sample size of the study was small and there was no 'no-treatment' control group for comparison, it is difficult to conclude that the improvements in depression were directly a result of the exercise intervention.

It must be recognized that much of the published work in this field to date has been subject to methodological limitations; notably the use of small sample sizes resulting in the possible overestimation of treatment effects, and a lack of adequate long term follow-up, making it difficult to asses the long-term effectiveness of the interventions (Daley, 2008; Lawlor & Hopker, 2001).

EXERCISE VERSUS OTHER THERAPEUTIC MODALITIES

It has been suggested that exercise might be equally as effective as psychotherapy and antidepressant medication in the treatment of mild to moderate depression (North et al., 1990; Shephard, 1995) and a number of studies have compared the level of self-reported depressive symptoms in groups receiving different exercise and non-exercise treatments. In a randomized control trial, Klein et al. (1985) compared the effectiveness of an individual running programme versus group psychotherapy, and meditation-relaxation therapy among 74 individuals meeting the Research Diagnostic Criteria for major or minor depression. All treatment groups reported a significant reduction in depressive symptoms after 12 weeks of treatment, with no significant differences observed between the three groups. In addition, participants from all groups continued to report symptom reductions at 3 and 9-month follow-ups. These results suggest that all of the interventions indicated improvement, but more importantly suggests that aerobic exercise might be equally as effective as group psychotherapy and meditation-relaxation therapy when treating depression.

In another randomized control trial Blumenthal et al. (2007) compared the efficacy of a home-based versus supervised aerobic exercise intervention in reducing depression compared with an antidepressant medication condition and a placebo control group. All participants improved over time since results revealed that all treatment groups had lower Hamilton Depression Rating Scale scores after the 4-month intervention. The authors concluded however that the efficacy of exercise as a treatment for depression appeared to be comparable to the efficacy of antidepressant medications. These findings support the conclusions of earlier work suggesting that exercise can have similar effects to other forms of psychotherapy and behavioural and pharmacological interventions (Craft & Landers, 1998; Lawlor & Hopker, 2001).

Whilst these studies have reported outcomes of exercise interventions when compared with therapeutic 'talking' treatments or antidepressant medications, other studies have focused on the impact of combining exercise with other treatment modalities. However this research base is limited to a small number of studies published in the 1980s and 1990s, and findings have been inconsistent. For example, some authors suggest that the addition of exercise to psychotherapy is not more effective than either exercise or counseling alone (Harris, 1987), whilst others propose that combining psychotherapy and exercise may be more effective (Martinsen & Martinsen, 1990). In a small-scale randomised control trial, (n= 43 inpatients meeting DSM-III criteria for Major Depressive Disorder) Martinsen et al. (1985) found that compared to a group of participants who only received psychotherapy (n=19), participants who received a combination of aerobic training and psychotherapy (n=24) showed a significantly larger reduction in depression as measured by the Beck Depression Inventory and the Visual Analogue Scale.

On the other hand, Fremont and Craighead (1987) compared the effects of aerobic exercise with cognitive therapy, and a combination of cognitive therapy and aerobic exercise among 61 individuals experiencing mild to moderate depressive symptomatology. Participants were randomly assigned to one of the three conditions: running only, cognitive therapy only, or combined running and therapy. Cognitive therapy was provided in 10 weekly individual sessions, while supervised running was conducted in small groups three times a week for 10 weeks. They found that all three intervention groups showed a significant but not differential improvement in mood as measured by the Beck Depression Inventory both at completion of the intervention and at 4-month follow-up. The authors therefore concluded that exercise was as effective as psychotherapy for the treatment of depressed mood. However, when examining the effectiveness of a combination of cognitive therapy and exercise the study failed to show an additive benefit. Consequently, it appears that combination therapies based on exercise and 'talking treatments' warrants further investigation before firm conclusions about effectiveness can be drawn.

In a more recent study, Trivedi et al (2006) examined the effect of exercise as an augmentation for antidepressant medication in patients with major depression. Seventeen patients with incomplete remission of depressive symptoms participated in a 12-week exercise programme consisting of both supervised and home-based sessions while continuing their antidepressant medication. Results showed that patients (n=8) who completed the exercise program had a significant decrease in depressive symptoms as measured by the Hamilton Rating Scale for Depression and the Inventory of Depressive Symptomatology (IDS-SR). However, results of the study were limited by the very small sample size, high dropout rate, and the absence of a no-treatment control group.

AEROBIC VERSUS STRENGTH AND FLEXIBILITY TRAINING

Exercise has therefore been shown to have positive effects on depression and may be equally as effective as other, more traditional treatments. In the light of this growing body of evidence, attention has also been given to the different forms of exercise that may be beneficial in the treatment of depression, since the 1980s. Doyne (1987) randomly assigned 40 young women who met the Research Diagnostic Criteria for depression to one of three conditions: running, weight lifting, or a no-treatment control group. In this study, both forms of exercise intervention appeared to produce positive outcomes since participants in both the running and weight lifting groups showed significant reductions in depression as measured by the Beck Depression Inventory and the Hamilton Rating Scale for Depression when compared with the control group after 8 weeks of intervention. Such improvements were also maintained at the 1-year follow up, suggesting that there may be a long-term mental health benefit. Furthermore, there were no significant differences between the two exercise groups, thus indicating that it may be participation in exercise that exerts an influence on depression outcomes and that the nature of exercise modality may be less of an influential factor, although these findings are based on a small sample.

Again, the effects of aerobic exercise have been compared with strength and flexibility training on depressive symptoms among 99 hospitalised patients who met the DSM-III-R criteria for clinical depression (Martinsen, Hoffart, & Solberg, 1989). In this randomized controlled trial, participants in the aerobic exercise group only showed a significant increase in maximum oxygen uptake after the intervention, although similar reductions in depression were reported in both groups as measured by the Montgomery-Åsberg Depression Rating Scale, again suggesting that either form of exercise intervention can result in improvement in depression. However, as all the participants in the study received the intervention, there was no true control group for comparison, thus whether the improvements were a result of the intervention alone is unclear.

Similarly, Veale et al (1992) examined the effects of aerobic exercise in the adjunctive treatment of depression using two clinical trials. In the first trial, 220 patients who were depressed at baseline were randomized to an aerobic exercise group or a no treatment control group. Results of this trial showed that patients in the exercise group had better depression outcomes as measured by a standard psychiatric interview than the control group. In the second trial, the effect of an aerobic exercise programme was compared with low intensity exercise consisting of yoga, stretching, and relaxation exercise among 89 depressed patients. After 12 weeks of intervention, both groups showed a significant improvement in depression as measured by the Beck Depression Inventory. However, whilst both exercise groups improved in depression outcomes, there were no significant differences between the two groups in terms of depression reduction or maximum oxygen uptake.

Overall, these studies seem to suggest that aerobic exercise may be as effective as anaerobic exercise for the treatment of depression. However, our ability to draw robust conclusions from the current research base is limited due to a number of methodological factors including the small sample sizes, the differences in outcome measures, and the different doses and intensities of exercise across studies. Furthermore the lack of recent studies in this field point to a clear need for more well-designed studies comparing different exercise modalities.

DOSE AND INTENSITY OF EXERCISE

How frequently exercise is undertaken, at what intensity and for how long may have some influence on the impact of exercise in the treatment of depression. Recently, Dunn et al. (2002; 2005) examined the 'dose-response' relationship of exercise for the treatment of depression among 80 adults diagnosed with mild to moderate depression. Participants were randomized to one of four aerobic exercise groups that varied in total energy expenditure and frequency. Results showed that after 12 weeks of interventions, participants who exercised at a dose consistent to public health recommendations at that time (i.e. a total weekly energy expenditure of 175 kal/kg/week), showed a significantly higher reduction in depression scores on the Hamilton *Depression* Rating Scale compared with participants who exercised at a lower dose or were assigned to the no treatment control group. Therefore it would seem that exercising more frequently exerts a greater effect. However, the generalisability of these results may be limited due to the small numbers of participants in each condition and the relatively high dropout rate experienced in the control condition of the study.

Legrand and Heuze (2007) investigated both the frequency of exercise and the social impact of exercise interventions by comparing high frequency exercising in groups or alone, with low frequency exercise. In this study, the authors examined the influence of an 8-week aerobic exercise intervention among 23 individuals with moderate depression as measured by the Beck Depression Inventory. Results showed that participants assigned to either a high-frequency individual exercise condition or a group-based high-frequency exercise condition reported significantly lower depression scores than those in the low-frequency exercise group at both 4 weeks and 8 weeks after the intervention. In addition, there was no greater alleviation in depression with group high-frequency exercise condition. Therefore it would seem that exercising more frequently has greater effects, but these are unlikely to be a result of social interactions alone. As with earlier studies, however, these findings must be treated with caution due to the small sample size.

With regards to exercise duration, Dimeo et al. (2001) examined the short-term effects of an aerobic exercise intervention in 12 patients with Major Depressive Disorder (MDD) diagnosed according to the DSM IV criteria. Participants walked on a treadmill following an interval training pattern for 30 minutes a day over 10 days. Over this 10 day period, this study showed a clinically relevant and significant reduction in depression as measured by the Hamilton Depression Rating Scale, and also a reduction in self-assessed intensity of depressive symptoms at the end of programme. Although these findings suggest that aerobic exercise may produce improvements in mood over a relatively short time period, no firm conclusions can be drawn since again this study was based on a small sample size and there was a lack of no-treatment control group for comparison.

Older Adults

Depressive disorders are common in old age; estimates suggest that between 10-15% of adults over the age of 65 years are affected (Iliffe & Baldwin, 2003). Depression among this population is often chronic and recurrent with research showing a 70% risk of relapse within two years of remission (Blazer, 2002; Zis et al, 1980). In addition, there is evidence of an increased risk of morbidity and mortality and decreased physical functioning and health-related quality of life among depressed older adults (Blazer, 2003; Smallbrugge et al, 2006). Increasing levels of exercise among older adults is now universally recognised as an important element of health promotion and 'active ageing' interventions for this population. Exercise can have a range of positive effects on health and well-being amongst older people, with studies showing improvements in balance, strength and gait endurance and overall quality of life associated with physical exercise (Hill, Smith, Fearn, Rydberg, & Oliphant, 2007; Motl et al., 2005; Sjösten, & Kivelä, 2006). Importantly, cross-sectional studies have also shown higher levels of physical exercise to be linked with lower levels of depressive symptoms in older people in the general population (Cassidy et al, 2004; Kritz-Silverstein, Barrett-Connor, & Corbeau, 2001; Ruuskanen & Ruoppila, 1995). Exercise interventions might therefore help to alleviate depressive symptomatology among depressed older adults.

Although a large proportion of published research examining the effects of exercise on individuals with depression has focussed on middle-aged adult populations, the concept of exercise as a treatment for depressed older adults is increasingly being recognised. In the early 1990s, McNeil et al (1991) assigned 30 moderately depressed elderly individuals to one of three conditions i) experimenter-accompanied exercise in the form of walking ii) a social contact control condition involving weekly home visits by an undergraduate psychology student or iii) a wait-list control group. After a 6-week intervention period, significant reductions in the total and psychological subscale of the Beck Depression Inventory were observed in both the exercise and social contact group. However, only participants in the exercise condition showed significant reductions in somatic symptoms of the Beck Depression Inventory. This small study suggests that exercise might be effective in reducing a broader range of depressive symptoms when compared with social contact interventions alone. However, since the exercise intervention also involved an element of weekly contact with a research assistant, it is difficult to draw firm conclusions regarding the beneficial effects of exercise versus social interaction from this study. Furthermore, as the authors do not report any follow-up data, the extent to which an exercise intervention versus a social contact intervention is effective in producing long-term effects on depression also remains unclear.

In the late 1990s, a randomised controlled trial examined the efficacy of high-intensity progressive resistance training as a treatment for depression in the older population (Singh et al., 1997). A total of 32 elderly patients who satisfied the Diagnostic and Statistical Manual of Mental Disorders IV (DSM-IV) criteria for clinical depression were randomly assigned to a 10-week supervised progressive resistance training programme or a health education control group. The study revealed that depression scores on both the Beck Depression Inventory and the Hamilton Rating Scale of Depression were significantly reduced within the exercise group compared with the control group. While these results appear to provide support for the antidepressant effects of progressive resistance training, these study findings are also plagued by a number of methodological limitations including a small sample size and lack of follow-up assessment. Moreover, the study does not reveal the extent to which the efficacy of exercise in depression is influenced by the supervised, group-based nature of the intervention.

Singh et al. (2001) conducted a further randomised controlled trial of the efficacy of supervised and unsupervised progressive resistance training exercise in the long-term treatment of clinical depression among older adults. A total of 32 older adults who fulfilled the DSM-IV diagnostic criteria for major or minor depression or dysthymia were randomised to either a 20-week weight-lifting exercise intervention or a health education control group. Individuals assigned to the exercise intervention took part in 10-weeks of supervised high-intensity progressive resistance training sessions 3 times a week, followed by 10 weeks of unsupervised exercise at home, the laboratory or a health club setting with a weekly phone call from the research team. Results revealed that older adults randomised to the exercise condition showed significant reductions in depression on the Beck Depression Inventory when compared to older adults randomised to the health education control group. The authors further noted that reductions in depression were maintained over the 20-week intervention when the supervised exercise programme was changed to unsupervised patient-directed exercise. In addition, a follow-up assessment conducted 26-months after enrolment in the study found that reductions in Beck Depression Inventory scores were still significantly greater in exercisers compared with controls. Although this was a small sample study, this work suggests that both supervised and unsupervised independent exercise programmes may be effective in producing long-term reductions in depressive symptomatology for depressed older adults.

However, the research evidence in this area is not conclusive; Sims et al (2006) conducted a randomised controlled trial in which 32 older adults with a Geriatric Depression Scale score ≥11 were assigned to attend either a 10-week progressive resistance training programme or a control group providing information about exercise and local exercise options. The study found no statistically significant differences in Geriatric Depression Scale scores between the two groups upon completion of the programme or at a 6-month follow-up, although it was observed that more of the exercise intervention group had a reduction in depression symptoms at follow-up compared to the control group. One potential factor that might account for the non-significant results obtained in this study could be levels of adherence to the programme of exercise; the authors report that only 58% of the sample attended 60% or more of the exercise sessions. Compliance may therefore be an important factor influencing outcome results. In addition, the absence of a true attention control group within the study limits the extent to which comparisons can be made between the two conditions.

In 2006, Tsang et al. (2006) examined the effects of a qigong exercise programme on 82 elderly patients with a diagnosis of depression as assessed by the Geriatric Depression Scale. Participants assigned to the exercise programme showed significant improvements in depression scores immediately after 8 weeks of qigong practice compared to participants placed in a newspaper reading control group. However, the antidepressant effects of the intervention were not maintained at 4 and 8-week follow-up assessments. Whilst a short term positive effect of this mindful exercise intervention was demonstrated, the extent to which exercise interventions are able to produce long-term changes in depression among older adults therefore remains unclear. Overall, there remains a need for further well-designed experimental studies based on larger sample sizes in order to determine the types of exercise programmes that are most effective in reducing depression for this population in the medium to long-term.

EXERCISE VERSUS OTHER THERAPEUTIC MODALITIES

A small number of studies have directly compared the effectiveness of exercise interventions with antidepressant medications in older populations. On the whole, these studies suggest that exercise may be equally as effective as standard medications in alleviating depression amongst older people. For example, in a randomised controlled study of 37 older persons with symptoms of minor depression diagnosed using the Patient Health Questionnaire-9, participants receiving a facility-based aerobic and resistance training exercise intervention or a sertraline medication intervention, demonstrated a trend towards a decline in depression severity on both the Geriatric Depression Scale and the Hamilton Depression Rating Scale. On the other hand, participants assigned to a usual care control group showed a slight increase in depression severity (Brenes et al., 2007), thus suggesting that exercise may offer a promising alternative treatment to antidepressants for older people. However, it is important to note that the positive trend observed in this study did not reach statistical significance and the study is limited due to the small sample size and self-selected nature of the sample.

However, in a larger randomised controlled trial comparing an aerobic exercise intervention with standard medication (i.e. antidepressants) and a combined exercise and medication intervention (n=156), Blumenthal et al. (1999) found that older adults diagnosed with Major Depressive Disorder using a Diagnostic Interview Schedule and randomly assigned to all three conditions showed both statistically and clinically significant reductions in depression scores after 16 weeks of treatment. It was observed, however, that patients in the medication condition showed the most rapid initial therapeutic response, yet the authors concluded that, over time, exercise interventions can be equally effective.

A follow-up of participants enrolled in Blumenthal's study was conducted by Babyak et al. (2000) to examine what impact exercise would have on depression following completion of the intervention programme. Interestingly, the study found that 6 months after completion of the intervention, participants in the exercise condition had significantly lower relapse rates than participants randomised to the medication condition. Furthermore, engagement in independent exercise following termination of the treatment period was also associated with a reduced probability of depression at follow-up. These results further suggest that over time exercise can not only be equally as effective as drug remedies in the treatment of depression and prevention of relapse in older people but in fact may have more lasting benefits, although this requires further investigation with a true no-treatment control group for comparison. Future studies should seek to compare the effectiveness of group based supervised exercise programmes and unsupervised home-based exercise programmes with antidepressant medication in order to determine the influence of group social interaction on the results obtained in the reported studies.

There is also some evidence that exercise interventions might be an effective treatment for those elderly patients who are not responsive to anti-depressant medications. Mather (2002) examined the effects of a 10-week programme of weight-bearing exercise classes in reducing depressive symptoms among a group of 86 patients with a diagnosis of affective mood disorder who had failed to respond to antidepressant medication. In this study, participants were randomly assigned to the exercise condition or a health education (non-exercise) control group; results reveal that a significantly larger number of the exercise group experienced a greater than 30% decline in depressive symptoms as measured by the Hamilton Rating Scale for Depression. These results imply that exercise can produce modest improvements in depressive symptoms among elderly patients who have failed to respond to antidepressant medication; however, as in many studies in this area, these results are based on a relatively small self-selected sample of older adults. Further randomised controlled trials with a larger sample of individuals with unresponsive depression are required to verify these findings.

TYPE, DOSE AND INTENSITY OF EXERCISE

There has been very little research to date comparing the effects of different forms and intensities/durations of exercise in treating depression among older adults. This has been investigated through a comparison of the effects of high intensity progressive resistance training with low intensity resistance training in a randomised trial (Singh et al., 2005). In this study, 60 community dwelling older adults with major or minor depression were randomly assigned to one of three conditions for 8 weeks: i) High intensity progressive resistance training (resistance was set at 80% of the one repetition maximum on each machine) ii) Low intensity resistance training (resistance was set at 20% of the one repetition maximum for each machine) or iii) a control group receiving standard care from their general practitioner. The duration of exercise for participants in the high and low intensity groups was matched. Results revealed that improvements in depression scores were significantly greater among those participants who were assigned to the high intensity exercise condition compared with both the low intensity exercise and control group. Effects over time require further investigation.

Regarding the effectiveness of different types of exercise intervention for older people, research has shown that both aerobic and strength and flexibility exercise can be effective in treating depression in older samples (Palmer, 2005). However, few studies have conducted direct comparisons between different modes of exercise per se specifically in this population group. Penninx et al. (2002) compared the effects of aerobic and resistance exercise on depressive symptoms in a sample of 439 older adults with either low or high depressive symptomatology as assessed by the Center for Epidemiological Studies Depression Scale. When compared with a health education control group, participants in the aerobic exercise group demonstrated significantly reduced depression scores on the Center for Epidemiological Studies Depression Scale during an 18-month follow-up. In contrast, there were no significant associations identified between resistance exercise and depression scores. Further analyses revealed that reductions in depression scores were apparent among both the participants with high depressive symptomatology at baseline (n=98) and participants with low initial depressive symptomatology. The results from this study thus provide evidence for improved antidepressant effects of aerobic exercise over resistance exercise in older people.

SUMMARY AND LIMITATIONS OF THE EVIDENCE BASE

Overall, the existing literature suggests that exercise interventions may be beneficial for the treatment of depressive symptoms among depressed adults and elderly populations. Furthermore, it is suggested that exercise may be equally as effective as psychotherapy interventions and antidepressant medication. However, when drawing conclusions from the published evidence, it is important to acknowledge the various methodological limitations of the studies. For example, much of the research is based on relatively small sample sizes and short study durations, thus limiting our knowledge of the impact of exercise on depression in the medium and long-term. Variations in intensities, duration and types of exercise reported, as well as the different definitions of, and measurements for depression also means that studies are difficult to compare. Much of the research relies mainly on self-reported symptoms for the assessment of depression, rather than a full clinical psychiatric interview. Additionally, there is a great deal of heterogeneity in the depressive diagnostic categories examined both within and between studies, for example while some researchers focus solely on major depressive disorder others include both minor and major depression. To determine the efficacy of exercise in treating depression among various subgroups of depressed patients it is important for future researchers to differentiate between effects on different depressive diagnostic categories, although sample sizes in many of the studies do not permit this. Consequently, to support earlier conclusions by Lawlor and Hopker (2001), it seems that despite the evidence that various forms of exercise may be efficacious in reducing symptoms of depression in the short term and potentially longer, exercise should not yet replace standard treatment, particularly for those with severe depression.

DIRECTIONS FOR FUTURE RESEARCH

The evidence in general is supportive of a relationship between exercise and reductions in depression among individuals with depressive symptoms. However, drawing robust conclusions is difficult due to the limitations of the published studies in this field, and there remains a need for further research with larger sample sizes to clarify the role of exercise in the treatment of depression. This chapter is by no means an exhaustive review of the literature although it does present the key studies in this field and more specifically, from the overview presented here a number of key areas for future research have been highlighted.

First, there remains a lack of concrete guidance concerning the optimal intensity and type of exercise needed for the treatment of depression. Further randomised control trials are required to examine and compare the different types, intensities and doses of exercise that are most effective in reducing depression. This will allow for more accurate guidelines to be produced and disseminated to health care professionals as well as the general public.

Second, there is evidence that individuals with depression are at a high risk of relapse when treatment is discontinued. Attention should therefore focus on examining the extent to which exercise interventions can produce long-term, enduring effects on depression symptoms in order to clarify whether or not continuous exercise is required for the maintenance of positive effects and lowering relapse rates.

Third, more research is required to systematically examine the different biological and psychological mechanisms that have been implicated in the association between exercise and reductions in depression. Identifying the most significant mechanisms will aid practitioners in the design and development of exercise programmes that maximise the chances of producing positive effects on patient mental health and well-being.

Fourth, further intervention studies are required with adolescent populations in order to explore the effectiveness of exercise as a treatment of depression among young people and as prevention for further episodes in later life.

Finally, although the dose-response relationship between exercise and depression remains unclear, it is widely agreed that in order for exercise to be effective a continued adherence to the programme of exercise is required. However many studies report high dropout rates for exercise interventions, suggesting that depressed individuals may experience difficulties adhering to exercise programmes. There are many factors that might influence the extent to which patients adhere to exercise regimes including: attitudes to the importance of exercise, self-efficacy, physical health, early exercise experiences, perceived social support to exercise and knowledge about physical health and fitness (Brosse et al., 2002). Exercise adherence might be particularly difficult for individuals suffering from depression as they may lack the motivation to adopt a regular routine of exercise. Consequently, in order for exercise to be successful as a treatment for depression a related area of importance for researchers is the qualitative examination of attitudes and perceived barriers towards exercise adherence among depressed patients.

IMPLICATIONS FOR PRACTICE

Despite methodological flaws in the current body of experimental research, it seems evident that exercise interventions can be effective in reducing depressive symptoms, certainly in the short-term and possibly longer, with associated physical health benefits. Health care professionals can therefore advocate exercise therapy as a viable supplementary treatment for individuals suffering from depression. The addition of exercise into the routine care of depressed patients will not only increase the treatment options available to the patient but will also be of potential benefit to national health care resources. For example, exercise offers a low-cost alternative to the conventional prescription of expensive antidepressant drugs and there may be potential to reduce the financial burden of depression. In addition, since regular exercise is known for its numerous positive effects on physical health and well-being, the promotion of exercise among individuals suffering from depression may indirectly reduce strains on health care resources through improving the health of the general population and reducing the likelihood of secondary health conditions resulting from inactive lifestyles.

Motivation to exercise, positive outlooks towards regular exercise and increased self-efficacy are known to exert an influence on exercise participation. Having a positive attitude towards regular exercise has been identified as one of the most important antecedents of exercise (Hagger et al., 2007). Several meta-analyses examining socio-cognitive determinants of behaviour have identified attitude as the most significant predictor of behavioural performance (Armitage & Conner, 2001; Bozionelos & Bennett, 1999). Since depression is typically characterised by feelings such as low self-esteem, helplessness, hopelessness and a lack of energy, people with depression may experience particular difficulty in motivating themselves to take part in exercise (Seime & Vickers, 2006). In the first instance, health care professionals should therefore seek to promote the benefits of engaging in regular exercise, and foster the belief that exercise will bring about numerous benefits, which outweigh any potential costs to the patient.

Self-efficacy for exercise has also been identified as an important predictor of exercising behaviour, yet many people with depression suffer from reduced self-efficacy. Courneya and McAuley (1995) suggest that minimizing the perception of barriers to exercise, and helping individuals to develop strategies to overcome barriers may be useful for increasing self-efficacy in relation to exercise. Bandura (1986) argues that social modelling, mastery experience, and social persuasion can also enhance sense of control over exercise. In practice, this may be achieved by encouraging patients who have successfully engaged in regular exercise to share their positive experiences with their peers. Health care professionals can also seek to empower patients by encouraging patients to begin exercising and then offering feedback on their performance, which may assist in strengthening an individuals' sense of self-efficacy towards exercise performance (Sherwood & Jeffery, 2000).

In addition, adherence to exercise is a crucial factor for therapeutic success. People with depression might have less motivation and commitment to participate in a regular programme of physical exercise than non-depressed individuals. Indeed, high drop-out rates from exercise treatment conditions have been identified as a concern in many published intervention studies in this area. There is a need for health care professionals to help remove some of the barriers that may prevent ongoing engagement in exercise among individuals with depression. For example, depressed individuals are likely to suffer from low motivation and exercise self-efficacy, which may prevent them from engaging in exercise programmes in the first place or dropping out when they experience difficulties (Seime & Vickers, 2006). Furthermore, research suggests that depressed patients appear to be less physically active and have lower levels of fitness when compared to the general population (Goodwin, 2003; Martinsen & Martinsen,

1990). Consequently, individuals with depression may experience particular difficulties adhering to and maintaining a regular exercise routine. There are various methods that could be used to promote adherence to exercise; for instance the lifestyle approach, which involves encouraging patients to incorporate multiple low-intensity physical activities into their daily routine, is considered one of the most promising and least intimidating strategies for individuals who have no prior experiences in exercising (Heesch et al, 2003). Although the effects of lifestyle exercise have not yet been adequately examined, the approach is likely to be a useful start to help individuals to become more physically active and consequently, more likely to engage in and maintain exercise regimes.

Callaghan (2004) further suggests that nursing and mental health practitioners could incorporate exercise interventions into their day-to-day work with clients. This could involve developing lifestyle assessments (that include an exercise component) into their regular mental health assessments of patients, for instances nurses could accompany patients whilst they exercise e.g. going for a swim or a brisk walk. Within the UK, many General Practitioners (GPs) already have access to exercise referral schemes that could be utilised as a mechanism for promoting exercise therapy among depressed patients. Such schemes have been referred to in other chapters in this book, since they can be appropriate in the rehabilitation of a range of long-term conditions and in recovery from illness or injury. Exercise referral schemes typically operate in partnership with Primary Care Trusts and local leisure services and allow general practitioners to refer any patient whom they feel might benefit from a supervised programme of exercise. Once referred the patient is initially seen by a qualified exercise professional for a detailed assessment of their needs and the development of a supervised individual activity plan. The patient is then offered free or discounted access to relevant leisure services within the local community. Follow-up assessments are then conducted at regular intervals during the programme.

While initially developed for the benefit of patients suffering from physical health problems such as diabetes, high blood pressure, obesity or asthma for example, many schemes now accept referrals for depression (Mental Health Foundation, 2005). These schemes are likely to be beneficial to individuals suffering from low mood (Callaghan, 2004), as there will always be professionals on hand to offer continuous support and motivation to individuals who may otherwise have difficulty adhering to an exercise programme. In addition, the social element associated with exercising with a group of fellow patients may provide additional motivation and satisfaction to the patient.

Despite the increasing availability and potential value of exercise referral schemes, research suggests that they remain an under utilised resource for the treatment of depression. A recent British survey conducted by the Mental Health Foundation (2005) revealed that only 42% of GP's surveyed had access to an exercise referral scheme for their patients. Moreover, of those GP's with access only 5% cited that they used the schemes as one of their 3 most common responses to depression, whereas antidepressants were cited by far to be the most common response to depression. However it was also found that over half of the GP's felt that antidepressants were prescribed too often and agreed that they would prescribe less medication if alternative options were available. From the survey results exercise did not appear to be perceived as a useful alternative treatment by many GP's, as they were either unconvinced of its effectiveness or felt that most of their patients would not be able to participate in an exercise programme.

In the light of this data, it is apparent that before exercise therapy can be successfully incorporated into current practice, and offered as an alternative to traditional treatments for depression, it is necessary to first convince health care professionals of its value. In addition to recommending further research in this area, there is a further need for the development of marketing initiatives to promote the opportunities offered by exercise and the evidence of its efficacy to both practitioners as well as the general population. For example, the UK Mental Health Foundation has recently launched a campaign for more people with depression to be offered exercise on prescription through exercise referral schemes. A related aim of the campaign is to promote public understanding of the effectiveness of exercise in the management of mental health problems.

CONCLUSION

Exercise is known to have positive benefits for mental well-being. Despite a lack of understanding of exactly which *modes* of exercise intervention are most effective for people with depression, and how *intense* participation needs to be to exert positive effect, it seems apparent that exercise is associated with improvements in the mood and depressive symptoms of individuals suffering from depression, particularly in the short-term. The long-term effects of exercise intervention in depressed individuals are yet to be fully determined in the research literature, although the positive effects of active lifestyles on both physical and mental health are well-established for all age ranges. Exercise therapy thus demonstrates great promise as a potential supplementary or even alternative therapy for the treatment of depression. However, there remain major gaps in our understanding of the exact relationship between exercise and depression. In particular, it is unclear exactly what types, intensities and durations of exercise are most beneficial for those with depression, and for depressed people of different age ranges and we therefore need to know more about this before we can appropriately advocate specific exercise modalities to patients. Frequently observed reductions in depressive symptomology with exercise interventions suggest that we can certainly promote' exercise as a treatment intervention, although the heterogeneity and methodological limitations published research evidence means it is not yet possible to conclude firmly that exercise should be presented as the *preferred* treatment for depression. There may also be significant barriers to the uptake of exercise for the routine care of depressed patients, including individual difficulties with motivation and adherence to exercise programmes, and health care practitioner attitudes and perceptions towards the efficacy of exercise compared with more traditional treatments. It can thus be argued that the development of further well-designed programmes of research assessing measured outcomes of exercise interventions, and the promotion of exercise therapy to professionals goes hand in hand.

REFERENCES

American Psychiatric Association. (2000). *Diagnostic and statistical manual of mental disorders (4th ed.) text revision*. Washington, DC: American Psychiatric Association.

Andrews, G. (2001). Should depression be managed as a chronic disease? *BMJ, 322,* 419-421.

Armitage, C. J., & Conner, M. (2001). Efficacy of the theory of planned behaviour: A meta-analytic review. *British Journal of Social Psychology, 40,* 471-499.

Ayalon, L., Arean, P. A., & Alvidrez, J. (2005). Adherence to antidepressant medications in black and Latino elderly patients. *American Journal of Geriatric Psychiatry, 13,* 572-580.

Babyak, M., Blumenthal, J. A., Herman, S., Khatri, P., Doraiswamy, M., Moore, K., et al. (2000). Exercise treatment for major depression: Maintenance of therapeutic benefit at 10 months. *Psychosomatic Medicine, 62,* 633-638.

Bandura, A. (1986). *Social foundations of thought and action: A social cognitive theory*. Upper Saddle River, NJ: Prentice-Hall, Inc.

Barney, L. J., Griffiths, K. M., Jorm, A. F., & Christensen, H. (2005). Stigma about depression and its impact on help-seeking intentions. *Australian and New Zealand Journal of Psychiatry, 40,* 51-54.

Beaumont, G., Kaspar, S., O'Hanlon, J., & Mendlewicz, J. (2008). Antidepressants side effects and adverse reactions. *Depression, 2,* 138-144.

Bhui, K., & Fletcher, A. (2000). Common mood and anxiety states: gender differences in the protective effect of physical activity. *Social Psychiatry and Psychiatric Epidemiology, 35,* 28-35.

Blazer, D.G. (2002). *Depression in Later Life.* New York: Springer.

Blumenthal, J. A., Babyak, M. A., Moore, K. A., Craighead, E., Herman, S., Khatri, P., et al. (1999). Effects of exercise training on older patients with major depression. *Archives of Internal Medicine, 159,* 2349-2356.

Blumenthal, J. A., Babyak, M. A., Doraiswamy, P. M. Watkins, L., Hoffman, B. M., Barbour, K. A., et al. (2007). Exercise and pharmacotherapy in the treatment of Major Depressive Disorder. *Psychosomatic Medicine, 69,* 587-596.

Bozionelos, G., & Bennett, P. (1999). The theory of planned behaviour as predictor of exercise: The moderating influence of beliefs and personality variables. *Journal of Health Psychology, 4,* 517-529.

Brenes, G. A., Williamson, J. D., Messier, S. P., Rejeski, W. J., Pahor, M., Ip, E., et al. (2007). Treatment of minor depression in older adults: a pilot study comparing sertraline and exercise. *Aging & Mental Health, 11,* 61-68.

Brody, D. S., Khaliq, A. A., & Thompson, T. L. (1997). Patients' perspectives on the management of emotional distress in primary care settings. *Journal of General Internal Medicine, 12,* 403-406.

Brosse, A. L., Sheets, E. S., Lett, H. S., & Blumenthal, J. A. (2002). Exercise and the treatment of clinical depression in adults: recent findings and future directions. *Sports Medicine, 32,* 741-760.

Burra, T. A., Chen, E., McIntyre, R. S., Grace, S. L., Blackmore, E. R., & Stewart, D. E. (2007). Predictors of self-reported antidepressant adherence. *Behavioral Medicine, 32,* 127-134.

Callaghan, P. (2004). Exercise: a neglected intervention in mental health care? *Journal of Psychiatric and Mental Health Nursing, 11,* 476-483.

Cassano, E, & Favo, M. (2004).Tolerability issues during long-term treatment with antidepressants. *Annals of Clinical Psychiatry, 16,* 15-25.

Cassidy, K., Kotynia-English, R., Acres, J., Flicker, L., Lautenschlager, N. T., & Almeida, O. P. (2004). Association between lifestyle factors and mental health measures among community-dwelling older women. *Australian and New Zealand Journal of Psychiatry, 38,* 940-947.

Courneya, K. S., & McAuley, E. (1995). Cognitive mediators of the social influence-exercise adherence relationship: a test of the theory of planned behavior. *Journal of Behavioral Medicine, 18,* 499-515.

Craft, L.L. (2005). Exercise and clinical depression: examining two psychological mechanisms. *Psychology of Sport and Exercise, 6,* 151-171.

Craft, L. L., & Landers, D. M. (1998). The effect of exercise on clinical depression and depression resulting from mental illness: a meta-analysis. *Journal of Sport & Exercise Psychology 20,* 339-357.

Craft, L. L., Freund, K. M., Culpepper, L., & Perna, F. M. (2007). Intervention study of exercise for depressive symptoms in women. *Journal of Women's Health, 16,* 1499-1509.

Daley, A. J. (2002). Exercise therapy and mental health in clinical populations: is exercise therapy a worthwhile intervention? *Advances in Psychiatric Treatment, 8,* 262-270.

Daley, A. (2008). Exercise and depression: A review of reviews. *Journal of Clinical Psychology in Medical Settings, 15,* 140-147.

de Maat, S. M., Dekker, J., Schoevers, R. A., & de Jonghe, F. (2006). Relative efficacy of psychotherapy and pharmacotherapy in the treatment of depression: A meta-analysis. *Psychotherapy Research, 16,* 566 - 578.

de Moor, M. H. M., Beem, A.L., Stubbe, J. H., Boomsma, D. I., De Geus, E. J. C. (2006). Regular exercise, anxiety, depression and personality: A population-based study. *Preventive Medicine, 42,* 273-279.

de Moor, M. H. M., Boomsma, D. I., Stubbe, J. H., Willemsen, G., de Geus, E. J. (2008). Testing causality in the association between regular exercise and symptoms of anxiety and depression. *Archives of General Psychiatry, 65,* 897-905.

Dimeo, F., Bauer, M., Varahram, I., Proest, G., Halter, U., Dimeo, F., et al. (2001). Benefits from aerobic exercise in patients with major depression: a pilot study. *British Journal of Sports Medicine, 35,* 114-117.

Doyne, E. J., Ossip-Klein, D. J., Bowman, E. D., Osborn, K. M., McDougall-Wilson, I. B., & Neimeyer, R. A. (1987). Running versus weight lifting in the treatment of depression. *Journal of Consulting and Clinical Psychology, 55,* 748-754.

Dunn, A. L, Trivedi, M. H., Kampert, J. B., Clark, C. G., & Chambliss, H. O. (2002). The DOSE study: a clinical trial to examine efficacy and dose response of exercise as treatment for depression. *Controlled Clinical Trials, 23,* 584-603.

Dunn, A. L, Trivedi, M. H., Kampert, J. B., Clark, C. G., & Chambliss, H. O. (2005). Exercise treatment for depression efficacy and dose response. *American Journal of Preventive Medicine, 28,* 1-8.

Eaton, W. W., Shao, H., Nestadt, G., Lee, B. H., Bienvenu, J., & Zandi, P. (2008). Population-based study of first onset and chronicity in major depressive disorder. *Archives of General Psychiatry, 65,* 513-520.

Ernst, C., Olson, A. K., Pinel, J. P. J., Lam, R. W., & Christie, B. R. (2006). Antidepressant effects of exercise: Evidence for an adult-neurogenesis hypothesis? *Journal of Psychiatry & Neuroscience, 31,* 84-92.

Fava, M. & Kendler, K. (2000). Major depressive disorder. *Neuron, 28,* 335-341.

Fremont, J., & Craighead, L. W. (1987). Aerobic exercise and cognitive therapy in the treatment of dysphoric moods. *Cognitive Therapy and Research, 11,* 241-251.

Garland, A. (1996). Cognitive therapy in the treatment of depression. *Mental Health Nursing, 16,* 28-31.

Gelder, M., Harrison, P., & Cowen, P. (2006). *Shorter Oxford Textbook of Psychiatry.* Oxford: Oxford University Press.

Giles, D. E., Jarrett, R. B., Biggs, M. M., Guzick, D. S., Rush, A. J. (1989). Clinical Predictors of recurrence in depression. *American Journal of Psychiatry, 146,* 764-767.

Goodwin, R. D. (2003). Association between physical activity and mental disorders among adults in the United States. *Preventative Medicine, 36,* 698-703.

Greden, J. F. (2001). The burden of recurrent depression: Causes, consequences and future prospects. *Journal of Clinical Psychiatry, 62,* 5-9.

Greenberg, L., Lantz, M. S., Likourezos, A., Burrack, O. R., Chichin, E., & Carter, J. (2004). Screening for depression in nursing home palliative care patients. *Journal of Geriatric Psychiatry and Neurology, 17,* 212-218.

Guszkowska, M. (2004). The effects of exercise on anxiety, depression and mood. *Psychiatric Polska, 38,* 611-620.

Gwynn, C., McQuistion, H. L., McVeigh, K. H., Garg, R. K., Frieden, T. R., & Thorpe, L. E. (2008). Prevalence, diagnosis, and treatment of depression and generalized anxiety disorder in a diverse urban community. *Psychiatric Services, 59,* 641-647.

Hagger, M. S., Chatzisarantis, N. L., Barkoukis, V., Wang, J. C., Hein, V., Pihu, M., et al. (2007). Cross-Cultural Generalizability of the Theory of Planned Behavior Among Young People in a Physical Activity Context. *Journal of Sport & Exercise Psychology, 29,* 1-20.

Hale, A. S. (1997). ABC of mental health: Depression. *BMJ, 315,* 43-46.

Harris, D. V. (1987). Comparative effectiveness of running therapy and psychotherapy. . In W. P. Morgan & S. E. Goldston (Eds.), *Exercise and mental health.* (pp. 123-130). Washington, DC: Hemisphere.

Harris, A. H. S., Cronkite, R., & Moos, R. (2006). Physical activity, exercise coping, and depression in a 10-year cohort study of depressed patients. *Journal of Affective Disorders, 93,* 79-85.

Hassmen, P., Koivula, N., & Uutela, A. (2000). Physical exercise and psychological well-being: a population study in Finland. *Preventive Medicine, 30,* 17-25. _

Heesch, K. C., Masse, L. C., Dunn, A. L., Frankowski, R. F., & Mullen, P. D. (2003). Does adherance to a lifestyle physical activity intervention predict changes in physical activity? *Journal of Behavioral Medicine. 26,* 333-348.

Hill, K., Smith, R., Fearn, M., Rydberg, M., & Oliphant, R. (2007). Physical and psychological outcomes of a supported physical activity program for older carers. *Journal of Ageing and Physical Activity, 15,* 257-271.

Iliffe, S. & Baldwin, R. (2003) Guidelines for managing late-life depression. *Geriatric Medicine, 33,* 49-55.

Johnsgard, K. W. (2004). *Conquering depression and anxiety through exercise.* Amherst: Prometheus Books.

Klein, M. H., Greist, J. H., Gurman, A. S., Neimeyer, R. A., Lesser, D. P., Bushnell, N. J., et al. (1985). A comparative outcome study of group psychotherapy vs. exercise treatments for depression. *International Journal of Mental Health, 13,* 148-177.

Kritz-Silverstein, D., Barrett-Connor, & Corbeau, C. (2001). Cross-sectional and prospective study of exercise and depressed mood in the elderly - The Rancho Bernado Study. *Americal Journal of Epidemiology, 153,* 596-603.

Kung, W. V. (2004) Cultural and Practical Barriers to Seeking Mental Health Treatment for Chinese Americans. *Journal of Community Psychology, 32,* 27-43

Kupfer, D.J. (1991). Long-term treatment of depression. *Journal of Clinical Psychiatry, 52,* 28-34.

Larun, L., Nordheim, L.V., Ekeland, E., Hagen, K.B., & Heian, F. (2006). Exercise in prevention and treatment of anxiety and depression among children and young people. *Cochrane Database of Systematic Reviews, 3.*

Lawlor, D. A., & Hopker, S. W. (2001). The effectiveness of exercise as an intervention in the management of depression: systematic review and meta-regression analysis of randomised controlled trials. *BMJ, 322,* 763-770.

Legrand, F., & Heuze, J. P. (2007). Antidepressant effects associated with different exercise conditions in participants with depression: A pilot study. *Journal of Sport & Exercise Psychology, 29,* 348-364.

Martinsen, E. W., Hoffart, A., & Solberg, O. (1989). Comparing aerobic with nonaerobic forms of exercise in the treatment of clinical depression: A randomized trial. *Comprehensive Psychiatry, 30*, 324-331.

Martinsen, E. W., & Martinsen, E. W. (1990). Benefits of exercise for the treatment of depression. *Sports Medicine, 9*, 380-389.

Martinsen, E. W., Medhus, A., Sandvik, L., Martinsen, E. W., Medhus, A., & Sandvik, L. (1985). Effects of aerobic exercise on depression: a controlled study. *British Medical Journal Clinical Research Ed, 291*, 109.

Mather, A. S., Rodriguez, C., Guthrie, M. F., McHarg, A. M., Reid, I. C., & McMurdo, M. E. T. (2002). Effects of exercise on depressive symptoms in older adults with poorly responsive depressive disorder - Randomised controlled trial *British Journal of psychiatry, 180*, 411-415.

McDonald, D. G., & Hodgdon, J. A. (1991). *Psychological effects of aerobic fitness training: Research and theory.* New York: Springer-Verlag.

McNeil, J. E. A. (1991). The effects of exercise on depressive symptoms in the moderately depressed elderly. *Psychology and Aging, 6*, 487-488.

Mental Health Foundation (2005). *Up And Running? Exercise Therapy and the Treatment of Mild or Moderate Depression in Primary Care.* London: Mental Health Foundation.

Mohr, D., Hart, S. L., Howard, I., Julian, L., Vella, L., Catledge, C., & Feldman, M. D. (2006). Barriers to psychotherapy among depressed and nondepressed primary care patients. *Annals of Behavioral Medicine, 32*, 254-258.

Morgan, W.P. (1985). Affective beneficence of vigorous physical activity. *Medicine and Science in Sports and Exercise, 17*, 94-100.

Motl, R.W., Konopack, J.F., McAuley, E., Elavsky, S., Jerome, G.I., & Marquez, D.X. (2005). Depressive symptoms among older adults: long-term reduction after a physical activity interventions. *Journal of Behavioral Medicine, 28*, 385-394.

Moussavi, S., Chatterji, S., Verdes, E., Tandon, A., Patel, V., & Ustun, B. (2007). Depression, chronic diseases, and decrements in health: results from the World Health Surveys. *The Lancet, 370*, 851-858.

Nabkasorn, C., Miyai, N., Sootmongkol, A., Junprasert, S., Yamamoto, H., Arita, M., Miyashita, K. (2006). Effects of physical exercise on depression, neuroemdocrine stress hormones and physiological fitness in adolescent females with depressive symptoms. *European Journal of Public Health, 16*, 179-184.

National Institute for Clinical Excellence. (2004). *Depression: management of depression in primary and secondary care.* Clinical Guideline 23. London.

Retreived 2 August, 2008 from www.nice.org.uk/pdf/ CG023quickrefguide.pdf.

Nolen-Hoeksema, S. (1991). Responses to depression and their effects on the duration of depressive episodes. *Journal of Abnormal Psychology, 100,* 569-582.

North, T. C., McCullagh, P., & Tran, Z. V. (1990). Effects of exercise on depression. *Exercise and Sports Science Reviews, 18,* 379-415.

Palmer, C. (2005). Exercise as a treatment for depression in elders. *Clinical Practice, 17,* 60-67.

Paluska, S. A., & Schwenk, T. L. (2000). Physical activity and mental health: Current concepts. *Sports Medicine, 29,* 167-180.

Penninx, B. W. J. H., Rejeski, W. J., Pandya, J., Miller, M. E., Di Bari, M., Applegate, W. B., et al. (2002). Exercise and depressive symptoms: A comparison of aerobic and resistance exercise effects on emotional and physical function in older persons with high and low depressive symptomatology. *Journals of Gerontology - Series B Psychological Sciences and Social Sciences, 57,* P124-P132.

Powell, K. E., Thompson, P. D., Caspersen, C. J., & Kendrick, J. S. (1987). Physical Activity and the Incidence of Coronary Heart Disease. *Annual Review of Public Health, 8,* 253-287.

Ransford, C.P. (1982). A role for amines in the antidepressant effect of exercise: a review. *Medicine and Science in Sports and Exercise, 4,* 1-10.

Rothschild, A.J. (2000). Sexual side effects of antidepressants. *Journal of Clinical Psychiatry, 61,* 28-36.

Ruuskanen, J.M., & Ruoppilla, I. (1995). Physical-activity and psychological well-being among people aged 65-84 years. *Age and Ageing, 24,* 292-296.

Sartorius, N. (2001). The economic and social burden of depression. *Journal of Clinical Psychiatry, 62,* 8-11.

Seime, R.J. & Vickers, K.S. (2006). The challenges of treating depression with exercise: From evidence to practice. *Clinical Psychology, Science, & Practice, 13,* 194-197.

Semple, D, Smyth, R, Burns, J, Darjee, R, & McIntosh A. (2005). *Oxford Handbook of Psychiatry.* UK: Oxford University Press.

Shephard, R. J. (1995). Physical activity, health, and well-being at different life stages. *Research Quarterly for Exercise & Sport, 66,* 298-302.

Sherwood, N. E., & Jeffery, R. W. (2000). The behavioral determinants of exercise: implications for physical activity interventions. *Annual Review of Nutrition, 20,* 21-44.

Sirey, J.A., Bruce, M.L., Alexopoulos, G.S., Perlick, D.A., Friedman, M.S., & Meyers, B.S. (2001). Stigma as a barrier to recovery: Perceived stigma and patient-rated severity of illness as predictors of antidepressant drug adherence. *Psychiatric Services, 52,* 1615-1620.

Sims, J., Hill, K., Davidson, S., Gunn, J., Huang, N., Sims, J., et al. (2006). Exploring the feasibility of a community-based strength training program for older people with depressive symptoms and its impact on depressive symptoms. *BMC Geriatrics, 6,* 18.

Singh, N. A., Clements, K. M., Fiatarone, M. A., Singh, N. A., Clements, K. M., & Fiatarone, M. A. (1997). A randomized controlled trial of progressive resistance training in depressed elders. *Journals of Gerontology Series A-Biological Sciences & Medical Sciences, 52,* M27-35.

Singh, N. A., Clements, K. M., & Singh, M. A. F. (2001). The efficacy of exercise as a long-term antidepressant in elderly subjects: A randomized, controlled trial. *Journals of Gerontology - Series A Biological Sciences and Medical Sciences, 56,* M497-M504.

Singh, N. A., Stavrinos, T. M., Scarbek, Y., Galambos, G., Liber, C., Fiatarone Singh, M. A., et al. (2005). A randomized controlled trial of high versus low intensity weight training versus general practitioner care for clinical depression in older adults. *Journals of Gerontology Series A-Biological Sciences & Medical Sciences, 60,* 768-776.

Sjösten, N., & Kivelä, S.L. (2006). The effects of physical exercise on depressive symptoms among the aged: a systematic review. *International Journal of Geriatric Psychiatry, 21,* 410-418.

Smallbrugge, M., Pot, A.M., Jongenelis, L., Gundy, C.M., Beekman, A.T., & Eefsting, J.A. (2006) The impact of depression and anxiety on well-being, disability and use of health care services in nursing home patients. *International journal of geriatric psychiatry. 21,* 325-332.

Solomon, D. A., Keller, M. B., Leon, A. C., Mueller, T. I., Lavori, P. W., Shea, M. T., et al. (2000). Multiple recurrences of Major Depressive Disorder. *American Journal of Psychiatry, 157,* 229-233.

Spence, J. C., Poon, P., & Dyck, P. (1997). The effect of physical-activity participation on self-concept: A meta-analysis. *Journal of Sport and Exercise Psychology, 19,* S109.

Stathopoulou, G., Powers, M. B., Berry, A. C., Smits, J. A., & Otto, M. W. (2006). Exercise Interventions for Mental Health: A Quantitative and Qualitative Review. *Clinical Psychology: Science and Practice, 13,* 179-193.

Steptoe, A., & Butler, N. (1996). Sports participation and emotional well-being in adolescents. *Lancet, 347,* 1789-1792.

Thoren, P., Floras, J.S., Hoffman, P., & Seals, D.R. (1990). Endorphins and exercise: physiological mechanisms and clinical implications. *Medicine and Science in Sports and Exercise, 22, 417-428.*

Trivedi, M. H., Greer, T., Grannemann, B., Chambliss, H., & Jordan, A. N. (2006). Exercise as an augmentation strategy for treatment of major depression. *Journal of Psychiatric Practice, 12,* 205-213.

Tsang, H. W. H., & Fung, K. M. T. (2008). A review on neurobiological and psychological mechanisms underlying the anti-depressive effect of qigong exercise. *Journal of Health Psychology, 13,* 857-863.

Tsang, H. W. H., Mok, C. K., Au Yeunh, Y. T. & Chan, S. Y. C. (2003). The effect of Qigong on general and psychosocial health of elderly with chronic physical illnesses: A randomized clinical trial. *International Journal of Geriatric Psychiatry, 18,* 441-449.

Tsang, H. W. H, Fung, K. M. T, Chan, A. S., Lee, G., Chan, F., Tsang, H. W. H., et al. (2006). Effect of a qigong exercise programme on elderly with depression. *International Journal of Geriatric Psychiatry, 21,* 890-897.

van Geffen, E. C. G., Gardarsdottir, H., van Hulten, R., van Dijk, L., Egberts, A. C. & Heerdink, E. R. (2009). Initiation of antidepressant therapy: do patients follow the GP's prescription? *British Journal of General Practice, 59,* 81-87

Veale, D., Le Fevre, K., Pantelis, C., de Souza, V., Mann, A., Sargeant, A., et al. (1992). Aerobic exercise in the adjunctive treatment of depression: a randomized controlled trial. *Journal of the Royal Society of Medicine, 85,* 541-544.

World Health Organisation. (2008). *Depression.* Retrieved 5 May, 2008, from http://www.who.int/mental_health/management/depression/definition/en/

Zis, A., Grof, P., Webster, M., & Goodwin, F.K. (1980). Prediction of relapse in recurrent affective disorder. *Psychopharmacological Bulletin, 16,* 47-49.

In: Physical Activity in Rehabilitation and Recovery   ISBN: 978-1-60876-400-6
Editor: Holly Blake   © 2010 Nova Science Publishers, Inc.

Chapter 12

PSYCHOLOGICAL OUTCOME MEASURES TO EVALUATE EXERCISE INTERVENTIONS

Shirley A. Thomas* and Roshan das Nair*

Institute of Work, Health & Organisations,
University of Nottingham, UK.

ABSTRACT

Psychological outcome measures are becoming more commonplace in the evaluation of exercise interventions. This chapter provides guidance on what factors should be considered when selecting an outcome measure. It is important to evaluate the psychometric properties of the measure, how the measure is going to be completed and who you are completing it with, in order to select the appropriate measure and increase the validity of the findings. In addition, it is necessary to pre-define the primary end-point and to agree what magnitude of different on the outcome measure is clinically meaningful. This chapter includes an overview of outcome measures that have been commonly used to assess quality of life and mood in the evaluation of exercise interventions.

* Tel: +44 (0) 115 8467484; Fax: +44 (0) 115 8466625; Email: Shirley.Thomas@nottingham.ac.uk
* Tel: 0115 8468314; Fax: 0115 8466625; Email: Roshan.Nair@nottingham.ac.uk

INTRODUCTION

There is an emerging trend for the use of psychological measures, either as primary or secondary outcomes, for assessing the effectiveness of exercise interventions. Attention is also being given to the role of exercise as a therapy for the treatment or prevention of mental health problems, as a means of coping with mental illness, and improving quality of life for those with mental illness (Fox, Boutcher, Faulkner, & Biddle, 2000). The mutuality of these two aspects highlights the importance of psychological measures in planning and evaluating exercise interventions.

Three terms need to be considered at the very outset of this chapter: the notion of "psychological" phenomena, the concept of an "outcome", and the extent to and the precision with which this outcome can be "measured". This chapter only focuses on the psychological aspects of an intervention that are measured at outcome, as a discrete, yet significant, aspect of outcome measurements in exercise interventions in general. Exercise interventions often include outcome measures for a range of facets of psychological outcomes, including quality of life, mood, self-esteem and self-efficacy. This chapter focuses on quality of life and mood. It would, of course, be beyond the scope of this single chapter to outline all the available psychological outcome measures, so only the most frequently used in clinical practice and research will be addressed.

THE NOTION OF "PSYCHOLOGICAL" PHENOMENA

The notion of there being a discrete set of psychological phenomena is a contentious one, and perhaps is a hangover from Cartesian dualism, which attempted to split the body and the mind. While attempts have been made to define what is psychological, this is always as an adjectival half of a phenomenon, such as "psychological disorder", "psychological testing", "psychological coaching", etc. However, most of these terms suggest that psychological refers to phenomena directed towards the "will" or the "mind" and its relation to cognitive, affective, and conative functions (Huitt, 2001).

THE CONCEPT OF AN "OUTCOME"

The course of any intervention traverses various stages, with outcome being one of the final points (if not *the* final point) in the trajectory of patient care. Connecting this with our previous discussion on what is psychological, psychological outcomes can therefore be related to simple, discrete, outcomes related to cognition, affect, or conation, or a more holistic, complex interplay between these various aspects. Outcomes can be viewed from various perspectives, although it is reasonable to believe that there is likely to be some degree of overlap between various outcomes. For instance, the psychological outcome of interest can be from the perspective of the patients, their carers, the healthcare provider, the economy, etc. Psychological outcomes also vary in terms of the nature of the phenomenon assessed. For instance, the outcome can be dichotomous (e.g., the presence or absence of phenomena) or polytomous/scaled (e.g., the severity of phenomena). These factors, are in turn, related to the manner in which these outcomes are measured.

THE "MEASUREMENT" OF OUTCOME

Psychological outcome measures evaluate the extent to which the desired outcome (or in some cases, an undesired outcome) is manifest, following the intervention. Measures estimate the extent to which an attribute relates to a predefined standard. This standard can be based on the patient's own premorbid or baseline performance on that attribute, or could be a normative standard, based on the performance of a healthy comparison group. Although outcomes are assessed at the end of an intervention, sometimes a series of time-points can be identified for this. Frequently, outcomes are assessed immediately post-intervention, and sometimes after a specified period has lapsed since the intervention (long-term). Timing of measurement of outcomes is vital in exercise interventions to determine the extent to which the intervention has been maintained (its durability) or to assess generalisability of intervention effects. However, the primary endpoint(s) are not always pre-defined or clearly stated in papers evaluating exercise interventions. Assessments for psychological outcomes have often been included as secondary outcome measures or as part of a battery of multiple outcomes. The use of the latter can increase the error rate of findings due to the increased number of statistical comparisons performed.

Measures can also be differentiated based on whether they are "subjective" (personal accounts) or "objective" (usually performance-based, professionally-administered assessments). Subjective measures closely approximate the data obtained on interviews. These can vary on the basis of the "subject" who provides the account (e.g. patient, care-giver, healthcare professional, etc.) or the form of assessment (e.g. questionnaire, observation, rating scale, etc.).

As psychological outcome measures in exercise interventions have mainly employed questionnaires/rating scales, it is important to consider the levels of measurement associated with these formats. Typically, four levels are defined: Nominal (where attributes are named, e.g. gender), Ordinal (where attributes are hierarchically ordered, e.g. ranking ability levels on an Activities of Daily Living Scale), Interval (where the attributes are ordered and the distance between them is meaningful, e.g. temperature on the Celsius scale), and Ratio (where a meaningful absolute zero is present, e.g. length measured in centimetres) (Stevens, 1946; Trochim, 2006). These levels are hierarchically ordered, with the lowest one (nominal) being least restrictive in terms of assumptions, but also with the least sophisticated mathematical properties. Therefore, it is desirable to use interval or ratio level scales when parametric statistics are to be conducted on the data, or when change scores are to be calculated. However, given that most psychological scales are at an ordinal level, it is important to convert these to interval scales by use of techniques such as Rasch analysis.

SELECTING A MEASURE

In addition to the aspects of measures discussed previously, when selecting a psychological outcome measure to evaluate exercise interventions, special attention needs to be paid to the psychometric properties, administration, and interpretation of these measures (see figure 1).

- What is my primary psychological outcome?
- Do I want to assess severity of symptoms or obtain a diagnosis?
- How will the outcome be assessed?
- How will the measure be completed and who by?
- If it is a self-report measure, can the patient complete it him/herself?
- How long does the measure take to complete?
- Who was the measure developed for use with?

- Is the measure suitable for this patient/patient group (think demographics such as: age, educational level, language, cultural factors, physical and mental ability levels)
- Are there any somatic items on the measure which may be confounded by physical symptoms of the patient's condition?
- Has reliability of the measure been established in the patient group with which I am planning to use it?
- Has validity of the measure been established in the patient group with which I am planning to use it?
- What cut-off value is appropriate to use with this patient group (where a cut-off is relevant)?
- Can this measure be used more than once on the same patient/patient group without performance being affected by practice effect?
- Are there parallel versions of the test that can be used for repeated testing (if relevant)?
- What is a reasonable time gap between testing that will minimize practice effect for repeated testing (if relevant)?
- Has the measure been shown to be sensitive to detecting change following intervention?
- What size of difference on a measure is clinically meaningful?
- How easy is it to interpret the results from the measure used?

Figure 1. Questions to ask when choosing a psychological outcome measure.

Psychometric Properties

A measure that is reliable "consistently produces the same results, particularly when applied to the same subjects at different time periods when there is no evidence of change" (Bowling, 1997, p. 11). There are multiple components of reliability which include:

- Internal consistency – the homogeneity of the scale which is tested by assessing the correlations between scale items. The average inter-correlation between items and the number of items is reported as Cronbach's alpha (range 0-1) which should be greater than 0.7 (Nunnally, 1978).
- Inter-rater reliability – the concordance between two raters assessing the same individual on the same occasion.

- Test-retest reliability – the consistency between scores when the test is completed with the same individual on two (or more) occasions.
- Sensitivity to change – whether the measure is able to detect change. This is particularly pertinent for outcome measures and can be evaluated by correlating the scores with other measures that have detected anticipated changes (Bowling, 1997).

The validity of a measure "…is concerned with whether the indicator does actually measure the underlying attribute or not" (Bowling, 1997, p.10). The components of validity include:

- Content validity – whether the scale items include all aspects of the construct that is measured (e.g. do the items encompass all symptoms of depression?).
- Criterion validity – the correlation of the measure with a 'gold standard'. This includes concurrent validity (correlation with a criterion measure of the same construct completed at the same time) and predictive validity (ability to predict expected future criterion).
- Construct validity – whether the results from a measure correspond to what would be predicted by the theoretical model on which the measure is based. This is further divided into convergent validity (correlation with other measures of the concept) and discriminant validity (not correlating with unrelated variables).

Once the measure has been chosen the next question to ask is what magnitude of difference on that measure is clinically relevant. A difference between scores may be statistically significant but may not be meaningful for clinicians and patients. Clinical significance has been defined as "the practical or applied value or importance of the effect of an intervention – that is, whether the intervention makes a real (e.g. genuine, palpable, practical, noticeable) difference in everyday life to the clients or to others with whom the clients interact" (Kazdin, 1999, p. 332). We, therefore, need to know what magnitude of change on an assessment score equates to a meaningful impact on functioning, behaviours, and well-being (Biddle, Fox, Boutcher, & Faulkner, 2000). In addition to reporting statistically significant differences, the magnitude of a clinically important effect for the outcome measures should be pre-defined (Stevinson, Lawlor, & Fox, 2004) when undertaking evaluation studies.

Administration Considerations - How Are You Going to Complete the Measure?

The practical arrangements for completing outcomes and the setting in which the intervention is evaluated will also influence the choice of measure. The constraining factors and available resources may vary for research and clinical purposes. In research studies, one source of bias when completing outcome measures is whether the assessor was 'blind', that is, whether the assessor knew which treatment the patient received. This is particularly pertinent in randomised controlled trials for evaluating interventions. For example, in a meta-analysis of exercise interventions for depression the outcome assessor was blind in only one of the 14 studies reviewed (Lawlor & Hopker, 2001). In a research context, if an independent assessor is unavailable then a self-report measure may be preferred where the respondent can complete it independently. However, self-report measures as the primary outcome may be susceptible to patient expectation bias (Mather et al., 2002). Within both clinical and research contexts the choice of measure may in part be determined by who it will be administered by. Some measures, particularly anxiety and depression scales completed as part of a clinical interview, require the assessor to have received training in conducting and interpreting these assessments.

The timing and location of follow up assessments is also relevant. Where follow up assessments are completed after patients have been discharged from the exercise intervention (or have completed it as part of a research evaluation) it is not always feasible to administer them face-to-face. It is often more pragmatic to send outcome questionnaires by post and where this approach is taken it is important that the questionnaires are appropriate for self-completion and do not place a great burden on the patient. The limitation with using postal outcomes is that people may not respond or may return incomplete responses. If multiple follow up points are planned then the measure should be appropriate for repeated administration (i.e., performance is not affected by "practice effect") and not too time-consuming.

The language(s) in which a measure has been published will inevitably influence whether it is used in particular countries. Most scales have been developed in British-English or American-English and so to be used in other languages, a translated version which has been evaluated is needed. However, mere translation of a standardised test is not appropriate when the norms for this test have been developed in one specific population/context, different from the index patient or research participant. In such cases, the test has to be restandardised/revalidated.

Assessing People with Illness Conditions and Disability –
Who Are You Completing the Measure with?

It is also necessary to consider who the measure was designed to be used with. Many psychological outcome measures have been developed for and evaluated with physically healthy people, yet are used with people who have physical or mental health problems. What is often disregarded is that the reliability and validity properties and cut-off scores (where relevant) apply to the population in which these were evaluated and do not necessarily generalise to patient populations.

People with physical illness or disability may have difficulty completing self-report measures. For example, lengthy questionnaires would be inappropriate for patients with cognitive impairments such as difficulties with attention, memory and concentration, or for those with motor problems or fatigue. Also, responses to somatic items may be confounded by the physical symptoms of a condition and not necessarily reflect a change in outcome following the intervention.

INTERNATIONAL CLASSIFICATION OF FUNCTION

In rehabilitation contexts, it is usually not sufficient to examine whether discrete organs or systems or group of muscles are working properly, but to understand the totality of that experience (which defies the Cartesian dualism, described earlier). The International Classification of Function (ICF) (World Health Organisation, WHO, 2001) is important in this respect, and provides a useful framework for selecting appropriate outcome measures (Heinemann, 2005; Jette & Haley, 2005; Mermis, 2005; Wade, 2003). The ICF serves as the international standard to describe and measure health and disability and classifies health in terms of various domains: the body, the individual, and the social sphere (WHO, 2001). These domains can be loosely mapped onto the notions of impairment, activity limitations, and participation restrictions; thereby embracing a biopsychosocial approach to health and disability (Lincoln & Nair, 2008). This distinction helps identify the level at which the outcome of an intervention is assessed.

Psychological outcomes for rehabilitation programmes have tended to focus on discrete (such as mood) or more global functions (such as quality of life), which are consonant with the possible aims of rehabilitation (Roberts, 2006). While psychological outcomes at an impairment level may be useful for a specific function, such outcomes at a participation restriction level may be useful for a global account of an individual's lived experience. Both these extremes are difficult constructs to measure from a psychological perspective (particularly in the affective and conative domains). Furthermore, there is evidence to suggest that impairments lead to no activity limitations, and vice versa; and activity limitations need not hamper participation (World Health Organisation, 2001). Therefore, the measures evaluated in this chapter will be mainly limited to those that fall within the remit of activity limitation and participation restriction, with special reference to quality of life and mood (for an overview of cognitive outcome measures in rehabilitation, see Lincoln & Nair, 2008).

QUALITY OF LIFE

Quality of life (QoL) is a notoriously difficult construct to measure due to the elusiveness of a precise operational definition. Generally, QoL is considered a conscious judgement (or appraisal) of satisfaction with one's life (Pavot & Diener, 1993). This being a generic construct, is often divided into more circumscribed aspects of QoL, such as "health-related" QoL (HRQL). While this distilled approach to QoL measurement helps to better contain the focus of the intervention (and assessment), it still remains a macro-construct that encompasses multiple outcomes. These cover a range of generic or condition-specific health status, well-being, adjustment and coping, and activities of daily living (ADL). In fact, Rejeski, Brawley and Shumaker (1996) delineate six types of HRQL measures related to physical activity: global indices of HRQL, physical functions, physical symptoms, emotional functions, social functions, and cognitive functions. Levasseur, Desrosiers, and St-Cyr Tribble (2008) hazard a definition of QoL: "the sum of cognitive and emotional reactions that an individual experiences associated with his/her achievements in the context of his/her culture and values, taking into account his/her goals, expectations, standards, and concerns" (p.2). This definition, they argue, includes the WHO-QoL Group definition and also includes the individual's reactions. Carr, Gibson, and Robinson (2001) suggest that HRQL is the gap between an individual's expectations of health and his/her experience of it. However, the perception of QoL is dynamic and varies between and within individuals over time. This lack of stability of this construct is related to its poor correlation with health/clinical conditions (the "disability paradox"). Carr et al. (2001) conclude that most existing measures do not take into consideration the individual's expectations, and cannot distinguish between "changes in the experience of disease and changes in expectations of health" (p1240).

QoL measures can be differentiated on the basis of various domains, one being, whether they are based on a theoretical framework of QoL, or are atheoretical. Measures which are based on theoretical models include the Patient Generated Index (Ruta, Garratt, Leng, Russell, & MacDonald, 1994), the Repertory Grid (Thunedborg, Allerup, Bech, & Joyce, 1993), and the World Health Organization's Quality Of Life profile (WHOQOL-100; 100 items) and the WHOQOL-BREF (26 items; WHOQOL Group, 1994). Another domain on which they differ is whether they are standardised or individualised measures. Carr and Higginson (Carr & Higginson, 2001) categorise the Schedule for the Evaluation of Individualised Quality Of Life (SEIQOL; Bernheim, 1999), the Patient Generated Index (PGI; Skevington, 1999), and the Disease Repercussion Profile (DRP; Chambers, 1982) as individualised measures. Standardised measures include the Subjective Quality of Life Profile (SQLP; Dazord, Leizorovicz, Gerin, & Boissel, 1994) and the WHOQOL-100 and BREF (WHOQOL Group, 1994) [please refer to Carr and Higginson (2001) for a review of these measures].

Carr and Higginson (2001) note that many widely used measures are not patient-centred, because of the way in which items were generated, the way in which they are scored and weighted (if at all), and the restrictions that questionnaires pose on patient's choice of answers. They recommend the use of individualised measures as opposed to measures that impose standardised models of QoL and have preselected domains.

Another distinguishing feature of QoL measures is related to who measures the construct. In some instances, for example, in evaluating QoL of an exercise intervention for someone who has had a stroke or a traumatic brain injury, which has left the individual with cognitive deficits or communication difficulties, proxy measures or proxies may need to be used. The use of proxies, however, immediately raises the question of how, if ever, a proxy can know and evaluate the *quality* of another's life. Any such evaluation will be coloured by the assessor's own beliefs, relationship with the patient, experience as a caregiver, caregiver burden and distress, etc. Nevertheless, there is evidence to suggest that a moderate degree of agreement exists between patient and proxy, particularly for the more observable domains of QoL (Dorman, Waddell, Slattery, Dennis, & Sandercock, 1997), but less so for subjective (ibid.) and psychosocial aspects of QoL (Sneeuw et al., 1998). Addington-Hall and Kalra (2001) conclude their essay "Who should measure quality of life" by suggesting that in the event of a discrepancy between a patient's and clinician's assessment of QoL, the patient should have the final word.

The problems associated with the construct of QoL and its measurement does not invalidate the potential uses of such a construct. Carr and Higginson (2001) identify it as an important factor in monitoring change or responses to treatment. However, to minimise some of the problems mentioned earlier, they suggest using QoL as an adjunctive measure, and moving away from the use of broad, multidimensional QoL measures, as these may be "less effective, accurate, and responsive than measures of specific patient outcomes in situations where treatment is aimed at achieving a particular outcome" (p1297), for example, improving adjustment or alleviating anxiety or depression.

Some of the more frequently employed QoL/HRQL measures used as outcome measures in exercise interventions are discussed below. As this is not an exhaustive description of these measures, the reader is encouraged to read the technical manuals of these tools before they are considered for use.

Sickness Impact Profile (SIP; Bergner, Bobbitt, Carter, and Gilson, 1981; Bergner et al., 1976; Gilson et al., 1975)

The SIP is one of the most widely recognised generic health status instruments. It is a 136-item, self- or interviewer-administered, behaviourally-based, health status questionnaire. Everyday activities are examined in two overall domains (physical and psychosocial), which comprise 12 categories in total. The physical categories include ambulation, mobility, body care and movement, and the psychosocial categories include sleep and rest, eating, work, home management, recreation and pastimes, ambulation, mobility, body care and movement, social interaction, alertness behaviour, emotional behaviour, and communication. The items are checked yes or no, endorsing items that describe themselves and their health; and 12 categories, two domains, and an overall score can be computed. It takes approximately 20-30 minutes to complete, and has been translated and validated in several languages. Test-retest reliability and internal consistency, and validity have been reported by Bergner et al. (1981). Two problems of the SIP are its length and the unavailability of a minimal clinically important change score. However, a 68-item shorter version (SIP 68) has been evaluated by Nanda, McLendon, Andersen, and Armbrecht (Nanda, McLendon, Andresen, & Armbrecht, 2003). It was compared to scales of instrumental activities of daily living and ADL, and the Short Form 36 Health Survey (SF-36) for convergent validity. Moderate correlations were observed with the SF-36 and high correlations with the original SIP. Reliability of proxy responses ranged between 0.26 and 0.85. An even shorter, 30-item, version has been developed and evaluated to assess quality of life after stroke (van Straten et al., 1997), which was deemed to be a clinimetrically sound measure. The SIP has been used as an outcome measure to evaluate aerobic training for people with multiple sclerosis (Petajan et al., 1996) and exercise rehabilitation for people with chronic obstructive pulmonary disease (COPD) (Emery, Schein, Hauck, & MacIntyre, 1998).

Short Form-36 Health Survey (SF-36; Ware, Snow, Kosinski, and Gandek, 1993)

The SF-36 is a multi-purpose, generic, health survey that assesses health concepts that are not specific to age, disease, or treatment group. The 36 items cover eight health concepts: bodily pain, physical functioning, role limitations due to physical problems, mental health, vitality, social functioning, role limitations due to emotional problems, and general health. Both dichotomous (yes/no) and polytomous (a scale) response categories are present. Summative scores are transformed to a zero to 100 scale, with higher scores representing better health, for each concept. The SF-36 can be self-administered or conducted by an interviewer. Reliability and validity studies have been conducted in various populations and settings, with adequate results. It has also been used to tap change over time in various diagnostic groups. A shorter version, the SF-12 (Ware, Kosinski, & Keller, 1996) is also available, which provides brief physical and mental health summary measures. However, compared to the SF-36, the shorter version is less robust when it comes to precision of measurements. Although the SF-36 has been used to tap change over time in various diagnostic groups, it is important to note that there is little evidence to suggest that the SF-36 is sensitive to detect change (Dixon, Heaton, Long, & Warburton, 1994). In fact, Biddle (2000) advises against the over-reliance of the SF-36 in studies of HRQL and suggests that more specific measures are used. Nevertheless, physical exercise programmes for patients with stroke (Lai et al., 2006), tai chi for treating knee osteoarthritis (Wang et al., 2008) and for people with traumatic brain injury (Gemmell & Leathem, 2006), graded exercise for people with chronic fatigue syndrome (Fulcher & White, 1997), have all used versions of the SF-36 to evaluate HRQL as an outcome measure.

Nottingham Health Profile (NHP; Hunt, 1986)

The NHP is a generic health-related quality of life measure used to evaluate perceived distress across various populations. It has two parts: Part I consists of

38 yes/no items in six dimensions: pain, physical mobility, emotional reactions, energy, social isolation and sleep; and Part II has seven general yes/no questions related to problems of daily living. The two parts may be used independently. Part I is scored using weighted values which provides a range of possible scores from zero (no problems at all) to 100 (presence of all problems within a dimension). The scores are presented as a profile, rather than an overall score. It can be self-administered or by the clinician/researcher, and can be completed in 5-10 minutes. It has been translated to various languages and is used extensively as a clinical and research instrument. The NHP scale can also adequately measure changes in perceived health following different interventions. The NHP and SF-36 have been compared and contrasted by researchers in various health conditions, and most researchers conclude that they are both reliable and valid measures of QoL. The efficacy of exercise interventions has been evaluated using the NHP for patients with clinical signs of congestive heart failure (Cider et al., 1997), and as an outcome measure to determine the efficacy of musculoskeletal physiotherapy exercise for chronic low back disorder (Goldby, Moore, Doust, & Trew, 2006).

EQ-5D (EuroQoL Group, 2008)

The EQ-5D is a standardised instrument that measures health outcome, and is used to measure QoL for a wide range of health conditions and interventions. It has five items (3 response options per domain), and visual analogue scale (0-100, with 100 being the best health state). Five domains are assessed: mobility, self-care, usual activity, pain, anxiety and depression; and scores are weighted on the five domains. A profile is obtained on the basis of these scores, and a weighted health index, based on norms derived from general population samples, can be calculated. Population norms are available for a number of countries. The EQ-5D can be self-administered or administered by a proxy, and compliments the SF-36, NHP, and SIP. Adequate test-retest reliability and internal consistency have been reported. However, there is evidence that patients reporting health problems on the EQ-5D have significantly lower mean scores on the SF-36 and SF-12 (Hurst, Kind, Ruta, Hunter, & Stubbings, 1997). The EQ-5D is also used to calculate change scores in the evaluation of interventions. The strengths of the EQ-5D are its worldwide use and its use in clinical, research, and economic evaluation of healthcare (by calculating Quality-adjusted life years, QALYs). It has been translated into various languages. A youth version is currently being developed (EuroQol Group, 2008). The EQ-5D has been used to evaluate tai chi for treating knee osteoarthritis (Wang et al., 2008), and a high intensity exercise programme for patients with rheumatoid arthritis (van den Hout et al., 2005).

Mood

The most frequently assessed psychological outcomes of mood following exercise interventions are depression and anxiety. While depression and anxiety are sometimes formally assessed for selecting people for an intervention (or research study) by using diagnostic interviews or screening tools, outcome is normally assessed using questionnaires. There are a multitude of measures available for this purpose, and a lack of consistency in their use between different health conditions. For example, in a systematic review (Sjosten & Kivela, 2006) of 13 studies evaluating the effects of physical exercise on depressive symptoms in older adults, five different depression measures were used. Therefore, only examples of commonly used mood measures in exercise interventions have been described here.

Some psychological outcomes, particularly anxiety and depression, can be assessed on a continuum (severity) or as a diagnosis (presence/absence). A diagnosis may be obtained using a cut-off on a measure or using specific criteria following a clinical interview. In some cases diagnostic criteria may be used for selecting patients and then a questionnaire is used to evaluate outcome in terms of improvement in severity rather than remission. Studies reporting the effects of exercise on depression have been criticised for providing insufficient detail about the psychiatric diagnosis of participants using standard criteria (Dimeo, Bauer, Varahram, Proest, & Halter, 2001). The lack of agreement between researchers regarding the criteria for defining depression has impeded our understanding of the relationship between physical activity and depression (Mutrie, 2000).

For trials evaluating exercise interventions for depression, Lawlor and Hopker (2001) have recommended the use of a dichotomous outcome (i.e. the likelihood of being depressed following the intervention) suggesting that this is more important in clinical terms. However, Callaghan (2004) has argued that depression may not be easily dichotomised and it is relevant to assess severity. Participants with a high score on a depression scale may not necessarily be clinically depressed. Also, an individual may be judged to have changed to a clinically significant degree on but did not change on the categorical criterion (Kazdin, 1999). The use of a continuous outcome measure enables growth curve analysis and inspection of the trajectory of scores over time which can be informative (e.g. Blumenthal et al., 1999).

Beck Depression Inventory (BDI; Beck and Steer, 1987)

The BDI is a 21-item measure of depressive symptoms and can be completed with an interviewer or self-administered. Reliability and validity have been widely evaluated and established (for a review see Beck, Epstein, Brown, & Steer, 1988). The BDI is commonly used with psychiatric and healthy samples and was used as an outcome in 10 out of 14 randomised controlled trials in a meta-analysis evaluating exercise for the management of depression (Lawlor & Hopker, 2001). One reason for its selection is to allow comparisons with results of drug trials (Singh, Clements, & Singh, 2001). The BDI has been updated to the BDI-II (Beck, Steer, & Brown, 1996) to be concordant with DSM-IV criteria for depression, although the original version still is still used. The BDI includes somatic symptoms of depression (e.g. sleep disturbance, appetite changes and tiredness) which can also reflect the symptoms of a health condition. However, scores can be separated in somatic and cognitive subscales. For example, Gowans, Dehueck, Voss, Silaj, and Abbey (2004) used the BDI as an outcome following land-based and water-based aerobic exercise for people with fibromyalgia because the cognitive/affective score is not confounded by somatic symptoms of the condition and was able to detect improvement in mood.

Examples of use of the BDI in assessing mood at outcome following exercise treatments include those people with chronic low back pain (Koldas Dogan, Sonel Tur, Kurtais, & Atay, 2008), fibromyalgia (Busch, Barber, Overend, Peloso, & Schachter, 2007; Gowans et al., 2004; Redondo et al., 2004) and older adults (Blumenthal et al., 1999; Singh et al., 2001). Although a measure of depression, the BDI was grouped under the heading of 'health related quality of life' outcome measures when reviewing exercise interventions for people with coronary heart disease (Jolliffe et al., 2001). This relates to the previous discussion of the overarching nature of QoL construct, which for some people includes mood.

Center for Epidemiological Studies Depression Scale (CES-D; Radloff, 1977)

The CES-D is a 20-item self-report questionnaire measuring the level of depressive symptoms in the past week and was designed for use in the general population. In addition to the total score subscale scores can be obtained for psychological symptoms, somatic symptoms, interpersonal problems and well-being. The CES-D correlated with clinicians' ratings and existing depression measures, in a sample including older adults (Radloff, 1977). The scale has mostly been widely used in community and epidemiology research rather than as part of clinical practice. Within exercise intervention it has been included as an outcome for people with ankylosing spondylitis (Lee, Kim, Chung, & Lee, 2008), COPD (Emery et al., 1998), rheumatoid arthritis (Wang et al., 2005), osteoarthritis (Wang et al., 2008), in addition to older adults (Penninx et al., 2002).

Visual Analog Mood Scales (VAMS; Stern, 1997)

Patients who have a neurological illness or injury, for example traumatic brain injury or stroke, may have communication impairments (such as aphasia) and/or cognitive impairments, including difficulties with memory, attention and concentration. Most self-report psychological outcome measures require intact communication and cognitive abilities, and therefore can be inappropriate for use with people who have such impairments. Visual analogue scales are an alternative format for obtaining self-reports. The VAMS were developed to assess mood states in patients with neurological impairments. They consist of eight unipolar scales: Afraid, Confused, Sad, Angry, Energetic, Tired, Happy, and Tense. Each item consists of a 'neutral' cartoon face with verbal label at the top of the page and a 100mm vertical line connecting it to the mood face and verbal label at the bottom of the page. The patient is asked to mark on the vertical line how they are currently feeling. Concurrent validity with self-reported mood has been found with healthy adults (Nyenhuis, Stern, Yamamoto, Luchetta, & Arruda, 1997; Stern, Arruda, Hooper, Wolfner, & Morey, 1997) and patients with stroke (Arruda, Stern, & Somerville, 1999; Bennett, Thomas, Austen, Morris, & Lincoln, 2006). Normative data has been reported for healthy adults, older adults, and psychiatric patients (Nyenhuis et al., 1997; Stern et al., 1997). The VAMS have been used as one of the outcome measures for evaluating the benefits of tai chi for people who have had a traumatic brain injury (Gemmell & Leathem, 2006). Further evaluation of the ability of the VAMS to detect change following exercise interventions is required.

Geriatric Depression Scale (GDS; Yesavage et al., 1983)

The GDS was designed specifically for use with older people and excludes somatic symptoms of depression. There are 30-item (Yesavage et al., 1983) and 15-item (Sheikh & Yesavage, 1986) versions with each question having a yes/no answer format. In functionally impaired, cognitively intact older adults living in the community, the GDS (15 items) correlated with measures of depression and was able to discriminate between depressed and non-depressed patients (Friedman, Heisel, & Delavan, 2005). The GDS is widely used with older people (Almeida & Almeida, 1999; Shah et al., 1997) and has been included as an outcome measure to evaluate exercise programmes with patients with stroke (Lai et al., 2006) and older adults (Mather et al., 2002; Tsang, Fung, Chan, Lee, & Chan, 2006).

Hamilton Rating Scale for Depression (HRSD; Hamilton, 1967)

The HRSD is a 17-item, interviewer-rated depression measure covering cognitive, behavioural, and somatic components of depression. As completion of the scale requires a trained clinician it is unsuitable for large-scale or community-based studies (Potts, Daniels, Burnam, & Wells, 1990). One of the reasons for using the scale has been to enable comparison with findings from the international depression literature (Mather et al., 2002). The scale has been found to have good diagnostic accuracy in adults over 65 years (Mottram, Wilson, & Copeland, 2000). Clinical criteria for evaluating the response to therapeutic intervention used in antidepressant studies has been defined as a reduction of $\geq 50\%$ or a score of ≤ 10 on the HRSD (Dimeo et al., 2001). However, where patients were those who had responded poorly to initial antidepressant treatment, a reduction in HRSD scores of $\geq 30\%$ has been considered to be clinically relevant (Mather et al., 2002). Examples of use in exercise intervention studies are with inpatients and outpatients with major depression (Dimeo et al., 2001) and older adults (Blumenthal et al., 1999; Mather et al., 2002).

State-Trait Anxiety Inventory (STAI; Spielberger, Gorusch, Lushene, Vagg, and Jacobs, 1983)

The STAI has 40 items, 20 measuring state anxiety and 20 measuring trait anxiety. It has been used widely with medical and psychiatric populations. Responses to each item are a four-point scale rating agreement with the statement. The state version of the STAI has been found to be sensitive to change following exercise intervention (Gowans, DeHueck, & Abbey, 2002). The state STAI has been used as an outcome measure for exercise interventions for older adults

(Blumenthal et al., 1999) and people with COPD (Emery et al., 1998) and fibromyalgia (Gowans et al., 2004).

Beck Anxiety Inventory (BAI; Beck and Steer, 1993)

The BAI is a 21-item scale measuring the severity of self-reported anxiety and was developed to discriminate anxiety from depression. Discriminant validity was supported by the finding that the BAI was correlated moderately with a clinician's rating of anxiety but only mildly with a rating of depression and so the scale may be advantageous to the STAI (Beck et al., 1988). Although, as stated in the manual (Beck & Steer, 1993), the scale was developed with psychiatric outpatients, and therefore, should be used cautiously with other clinical groups. It has been used as an outcome measure for a physical exercise based programme for patients with fibromyalgia (Redondo et al., 2004).

Hospital Anxiety and Depression Scale
(HADS; Zigmond and Snaith, 1983)

The HADS is a 14-item scale with seven items relating to depression and seven to anxiety, and separate scores are obtained for each subscale. The scale was designed to exclude somatic symptoms of psychological distress for use with nonpsychiatric medical patients in hospital settings. The HADS is advantageous as it provides information on the severity of both anxiety and depression using a single instrument. A review of over 200 studies concluded that the HADS is a reliable and valid scale for the assessment of anxiety and depression in medical patients and is sensitive to change following intervention (Herrmann, 1997). In addition, the total score has been used as a global measure of psychological distress with patients with cancer (Smith et al., 2002), cardiac patients (S. B. Roberts, Bonnici, Mackinnon, & Worcester, 2001) and stroke patients (Aben, Verhey, Lousberg, Lodder, & Honig, 2002). The HADS has been used to evaluate exercise interventions in a range of medical conditions, including back pain (Chatzitheodorou, Kabitsis, Malliou, & Mougios, 2007), traumatic brain injury (Bateman et al., 2001) and chronic fatigue syndrome (Fulcher & White, 1997; Powell, Bentall, Nye, & Edwards, 2001; Wallman, Morton, Goodman, Grove, & Guilfoyle, 2004).

General Health Questionnaire
(GHQ; Goldberg and Williams, 1988)

The GHQ is a widely used screening instrument for detecting psychiatric morbidity. There are versions which contain 12, 20, 28, 30, and 60 items. Patients are asked to compare their current state to their usual state and the scale can be completed by interview or self-report. Reliability and validity are reported in the manual (Goldberg & Williams, 1988). The GHQ includes psychosomatic items and so may also be measuring physical health status (Bowling, 1995). Although developed as a screening measure, the GHQ-12 has been used to assess outcome following exercise interventions in brain injury (Blake & Batson, in press), with older adults (Tsang et al., 2006) and people with chronic low back pain (Koldas Dogan et al., 2008).

Profile of Mood States
(POMS; McNair, Lorr, and Droppleman, 1971, 1992)

The POMS measures affective states by asking patients to rate agreement with 65 monopolar adjectives which make up six dimensions: tension-anxiety, depression-dejection, anger-hostility, vigour-activity, fatigue-inertia, and confusion-bewilderment. It is popular with psychologists for assessing mood change in experimental studies (Bowling, 1995). However, it has been criticised for only including one positive mood dimension and its use as a primary outcome measure of mood for exercise interventions has been questioned (Scully, Kremer, Meade, Graham, & Dudgeon, 1998). The POMS has been used extensively in physical activity research (Biddle, 2000) and was used by Petajan et al. (1996) to evaluate aerobic training in patients with multiple sclerosis.

CONCLUSION

The assessment of psychological outcomes is an essential aspect of evaluating exercise interventions, as it can serve as both global and specific measures of activity limitations and participation restrictions. However, the construct can be over-inclusive, and thereby problematic, due to the lack of a ubiquitous definition of the term. Therefore, clinicians and researchers should operationally define the notion of psychological outcome (and what facets of it they are measuring) at the outset. This approach will serve to identify the relevant outcome measures to be used, which will further guide the selection of a generic or specific measure.

Aspects to consider when selecting a psychological outcome measure include the psychometric properties, administration considerations, and interpretability of findings. There is a plethora of psychological outcome measures (generic or disease-specific) available, and the challenge lies in selecting the appropriate ones. While in clinical practice, idiographic, bespoke measures can be informative in that setting, for research purposes, the inclusion of (appropriate) standardised measures is useful. Heterogeneity in outcome measures can preclude the pooling of results for meta-analysis (Rietberg, Brooks, Uitdehaag, & Kwakkel, 2005), which presents difficulties when comparing outcomes across studies, and reduces the interpretability of findings.

Clinicians and researchers are encouraged to continue to employ psychological outcome measures in evaluating exercise interventions. However, a thorough understanding of the patient, the illness condition or disability, and the characteristics of the measures used, will enhance the evidence-base of the effectiveness of the intervention, and ensure that it is patient-centred.

REFERENCES

Aben, I., Verhey, F., Lousberg, R., Lodder, J., & Honig, A. (2002). Validity of the Beck Depression Inventory, Hospital Anxiety and Depression Scale, SCL-90, and Hamilton Depression Rating Scale as screening instruments for depression in stroke patients. *Psychosomatics, 43*, 386-393.

Addington-Hall, J., & Kalra, L. (2001). Who should measure quality of life? *BMJ, 322*, 1417-1420.

Almeida, O. P., & Almeida, S. A. (1999). Short versions of the Geriatric Depression Scale: A study of their validity for the diagnosis of a major depressive episode according to ICD-10 and DSM-IV. *International Journal of Geriatric Psychiatry, 14*, 858-865.

Arruda, J. E., Stern, R. A., & Somerville, J. A. (1999). Measurement of mood states in stroke patients: Validation of the Visual Analog Mood Scales. *Archives of Physical Medicine and Rehabilitation, 80*, 676-680.

Bateman, A., Culpan, F. J., Pickering, A. D., Powell, J. H., Scott, O. M., & Greenwood, R. J. (2001). The effect of aerobic training on rehabilitation outcomes after recent severe brain injury: a randomized controlled evaluation. *Archives of Physical Medicine & Rehabilitation, 82*, 174-182.

Beck, A. T., Epstein, N., Brown, G., & Steer, R. A. (1988). An inventory for measuring clinical anxiety: psychometric properties. *Journal of Consulting & Clinical Psychology, 56*, 893-897.

Beck, A. T., & Steer, R. A. (1987). *Beck Depression Inventory Manual*. San Antonio, TX: The Psychological Corporation.

Beck, A. T., & Steer, R. A. (1993). *Beck Anxiety Inventory Manual*. San Antonio, TX: Psychological Corporation.

Beck, A. T., Steer, R. A., & Brown, G. K. (1996). *Beck Depression Inventory Manual-2nd Edition*. San Antonio, TX: The Psychological Corporation.

Bennett, H. E., Thomas, S. A., Austen, R., Morris, A. M. S., & Lincoln, N. B. (2006). Validation of screening measures for assessing mood in stroke patients. *British Journal of Clinical Psychology, 45*, 367-376.

Bergner, M., Bobbitt, R. A., Carter, W. B., & Gilson, B. S. (1981). The Sickness Impact Profile: development and final revision of a health status measure. *Medical Care, 19*, 787-805.

Bergner, M., Bobbitt, R. A., Kressel, S., Pollard, W. E., Gilson, B. S., & Morris, J. R. (1976). The sickness impact profile: conceptual formulation and methodology for the development of a health status measure. *International Journal of Health Services, 6*, 393-415.

Bernheim, J. L. (1999). How to get serious answers to the serious question: "How have you been?": subjective quality of life (QOL) as an individual experiential emergent construct. *Bioethics, 13*, 272-287.

Biddle, S. J. H. (2000). Emotion, mood and physical activity. In S. J. H. Biddle, K. R. Fox & S. H. Boutcher (Eds.), *Physical activity and psychological well-being* (pp. 63-87). London: Routledge.

Biddle, S. J. H., Fox, K. R., Boutcher, S. H., & Faulkner, G. E. (2000). The way forward for physical activity and the promotion of psychological well-being. In S. J. H. Biddle, K. R. Fox & S. H. Boutcher (Eds.), *Physical activity and psychological well-being* (pp. 154-168). London: Routledge.

Blake, H., & Batson, M. (In Press) Exercise intervention in brain injury: a pilot randomised study of Tai Chi Qigong. *Clinical Rehabilitation*.

Blumenthal, J. A., Babyak, M. A., Moore, K. A., Craighead, W. E., Herman, S., Khatri, P., et al. (1999). Effects of exercise training on older patients with major depression. *Archives of Internal Medicine, 159*, 2349-2356.

Bowling, A. (1995). *Measuring Disease*. Buckingham: Open University Press.

Bowling, A. (1997). *Measuring Health. A review of quality of life measurement scales*. Buckingham: Open University Press.

Busch, A. J., Barber, K. A., Overend, T. J., Peloso, P. M., & Schachter, C. L. (2007). Exercise for treating fibromyalgia syndrome. *Cochrane Database of Systematic Reviews*(4), CD003786.

Callaghan, P. (2004). Exercise: a neglected intervention in mental health care? *Journal of Psychiatric & Mental Health Nursing, 11*, 476-483.

Carr, A. J., Gibson, B., & Robinson, P. G. (2001). Measuring quality of life: Is quality of life determined by expectations or experience? *BMJ, 322*, 1240-1243.

Carr, A. J., & Higginson, I. J. (2001). Are quality of life measures patient centred? *BMJ, 322*, 1357-1360.

Chambers, L. W. (1982). *The McMaster Health Index Questionnaire.* Hamilton, Ontario: McMaster University.

Chatzitheodorou, D., Kabitsis, C., Malliou, P., & Mougios, V. (2007). A pilot study of the effects of high-intensity aerobic exercise versus passive interventions on pain, disability, psychological strain, and serum cortisol concentrations in people with chronic low back pain. *Physical Therapy, 87*, 304-312.

Cider, A., Tygesson, H., Hedberg, M., Seligman, L., Wennerblom, B., & Sunnerhagen, K. S. (1997). Peripheral muscle training in patients with clinical signs of heart failure. *Scandinavian Journal of Rehabilitation Medicine, 29*, 121-127.

Dazord, A., Leizorovicz, A., Gerin, P., & Boissel, J. P. (1994). Quality of life of patients during treatment of type I diabetes. Importance of a questionnaire focused on the subjective quality of life. *Diabete et Metabolisme, 20*, 465-472.

Dimeo, F., Bauer, M., Varahram, I., Proest, G., & Halter, U. (2001). Benefits from aerobic exercise in patients with major depression: a pilot study. *British Journal of Sports Medicine, 35*, 114-117.

Dixon, P., Heaton, J., Long, A., & Warburton, A. (1994). Reviewing and applying the SF-36. *Outcomes Briefings, 4*, 3-25.

Dorman, P. J., Waddell, F., Slattery, J., Dennis, M., & Sandercock, P. (1997). Are proxy assessments of health status after stroke with the EuroQol questionnaire feasible, accurate, and unbiased? *Stroke, 28*, 1883-1887.

Emery, C. F., Schein, R. L., Hauck, E. R., & MacIntyre, N. R. (1998). Psychological and cognitive outcomes of a randomized trial of exercise among patients with chronic obstructive pulmonary disease. *Health Psychology, 17*, 232-240.

EuroQol Group (2008) *What is EQ-5D?* Retrieved [24.10.08], from http://www.euroqol.org/

Fox, K. R., Boutcher, S. H., Faulkner, G. E., & Biddle, S. J. H. (2000). The case for exercise in the promotion of mental health and psychological well-being. In S. J. H. Biddle, K. R. Fox & S. H. Boutcher (Eds.), *Physical activity and psychological well-being* (pp. 1-9). London: Routledge.

Friedman, B., Heisel, M. J., & Delavan, R. L. (2005). Psychometric properties of the 15-item geriatric depression scale in functionally impaired, cognitively intact, community-dwelling elderly primary care patients. *Journal of the American Geriatrics Society, 53*, 1570-1576.

Fulcher, K. Y., & White, P. D. (1997). Randomised controlled trial of graded exercise in patients with the chronic fatigue syndrome. *BMJ, 314*, 1647-1652.

Gemmell, C., & Leathem, J. M. (2006). A study investigating the effects of Tai Chi Chuan: individuals with traumatic brain injury compared to controls. *Brain Injury, 20*, 151-156.

Gilson, B. S., Gilson, J. S., Bergner, M., Bobbit, R. A., Kressel, S., Pollard, W. E., et al. (1975). The sickness impact profile. Development of an outcome measure of health care. *American Journal of Public Health, 65*, 1304-1310.

Goldberg, D., & Williams, P. (1988). *A user's guide to the General Health Questionnaire*. Windsor: Nfer-Nelson.

Goldby, L. J., Moore, A. P., Doust, J., & Trew, M. E. (2006). A randomized controlled trial investigating the efficiency of musculoskeletal physiotherapy on chronic low back disorder. *Spine, 31*, 1083-1093.

Gowans, S. E., DeHueck, A., & Abbey, S. E. (2002). Measuring exercise-induced mood changes in fibromyalgia: a comparison of several measures. *Arthritis & Rheumatism, 47*, 603-609.

Gowans, S. E., Dehueck, A., Voss, S., Silaj, A., & Abbey, S. E. (2004). Six-month and one-year followup of 23 weeks of aerobic exercise for individuals with fibromyalgia. *Arthritis & Rheumatism, 51*, 890-898.

Hamilton, M. (1967). Development of a rating scale for primary depressive illness. *British Journal of Social & Clinical Psychology, 6*, 278-296.

Heinemann, A. W. (2005). Putting outcome measurement in context: a rehabilitation psychology perspective. *Rehabilitation Psychology, 50*, 6-14.

Herrmann, C. (1997). International experiences with the Hospital Anxiety and Depression Scale-A review of validation data and clinical results. *Journal of Psychosomatic Research, 42*, 17-41.

Huitt, W. (2001). The mind. *Educational Psychology Interactive.* Valdosta, GA: Valdosta State University. Retrieved [26.10.08], from http://chiron.valdosta.edu/whuitt/col/summary/mind.html

Hunt, S. M., (1986). *Measuring Health Status*. London: Croom Helm.

Hurst, N. P., Kind, P., Ruta, D., Hunter, M., & Stubbings, A. (1997). Measuring health-related quality of life in rheumatoid arthritis: validity, responsiveness and reliability of EuroQol (EQ-5D). *British Journal of Rheumatology, 36*, 551-559.

Jette, A. M., & Haley, S. M. (2005). Contemporary measurement techniques for rehabilitation outcomes assessment. *Journal of Rehabilitation Medicine, 37*, 339-345.

Jolliffe, J. A., Rees, K., Taylor, R. S., Thompson, D., Oldridge, N., & Ebrahim, S. (2001). Exercise-based rehabilitation for coronary heart disease. *Cochrane Database of Systematic Reviews*(1), CD001800.

Kazdin, A. E. (1999). The meanings and measurement of clinical significance. *Journal of Consulting & Clinical Psychology, 67*, 332-339.

Koldas Dogan, S., Sonel Tur, B., Kurtais, Y., & Atay, M. B. (2008). Comparison of three different approaches in the treatment of chronic low back pain. *Clinical Rheumatology, 27*, 873-881.

Lai, S. M., Studenski, S., Richards, L., Perera, S., Reker, D., Rigler, S., et al. (2006). Therapeutic exercise and depressive symptoms after stroke. *Journal of the American Geriatrics Society, 54*, 240-247.

Lawlor, D. A., & Hopker, S. W. (2001). The effectiveness of exercise as an intervention in the management of depression: systematic review and meta-regression analysis of randomised controlled trials. *BMJ, 322*, 763-767.

Lee, E.-N., Kim, Y.-H., Chung, W. T., & Lee, M. S. (2008). Tai Chi for disease activity and flexibility in patients with ankylosing spondylitis--a controlled clinical trial. *eCAM, nem048.*

Levasseur, M., Desrosiers, J., & St-Cyr Tribble, D. (2008). Do quality of life, participation and environment of older adults differ according to level of activity? *Health & Quality of Life Outcomes, 6*, 30.

Lincoln, N., & Nair, R. D. (2008). Outcome measurement in cognitive neurorehabilitation. In D. T. Stuss, G. Wincour & I. H. Robertson (Eds.), *Cognitive Neurorehabilitation* (pp. 91-105). Cambridge: Cambridge University Press.

Mather, A. S., Rodriguez, C., Guthrie, M. F., McHarg, A. M., Reid, I. C., & McMurdo, M. E. (2002). Effects of exercise on depressive symptoms in older adults with poorly responsive depressive disorder: randomised controlled trial. *British Journal of Psychiatry, 180*, 411-415.

McNair, D. M., Lorr, M., & Droppleman, L. F. (1971). *Manual for the Profile of Mood States.* San Diego, CA: Educational and Industrial Testing Services.

McNair, D. M., Lorr, M., & Droppleman, L. F. (1992). *EdITS Manual for the Profile of Mood States (POMS)*. San Diego, CA: EdITS/Educational and Industrial Testing Service.

Mermis, B. J. (2005). Developing a taxonomy for rehabilitation outcome measurement. *Rehabilitation Psychology, 50*, 15-23.

Mottram, P., Wilson, K., & Copeland, J. (2000). Validation of the Hamilton Depression Rating Scale and Montgommery and Asberg Rating Scales in terms of AGECAT depression cases. *International Journal of Geriatric Psychiatry, 15*, 1113-1119.

Mutrie, N. (2000). The relationship between physical activity and clinically defined depression. In S. J. H. Biddle, K. R. Fox & S. H. Boutcher (Eds.), *Physical activity and psychological well-being* (pp. 46-62). London: Routledge.

Nanda, U., McLendon, P. M., Andresen, E. M., & Armbrecht, E. (2003). The SIP68: an abbreviated sickness impact profile for disability outcomes research. *Quality of Life Research, 12*, 583-595.

Nunnally, J. C. (1978). *Psychometric Theory*. New York: McGraw-Hill Book Company.

Nyenhuis, D. L., Stern, R. A., Yamamoto, C., Luchetta, T., & Arruda, J. E. (1997). Standardization and validation of the Visual Analog Mood Scales. *The Clinical Neuropsychologist, 11*, 407-415.

Pavot, W., & Diener, E. (1993). Review of the Satisfaction With Life Scale. *Psychological Assessment, 5*, 164-172.

Penninx, B. W., Rejeski, W. J., Pandya, J., Miller, M. E., Di Bari, M., Applegate, W. B., et al. (2002). Exercise and depressive symptoms: a comparison of aerobic and resistance exercise effects on emotional and physical function in older persons with high and low depressive symptomatology. *Journals of Gerontology B Psychological Sciences & Social Sciences, 57*, P124-132.

Petajan, J. H., Gappmaier, E., White, A. T., Spencer, M. K., Mino, L., & Hicks, R. W. (1996). Impact of aerobic training on fitness and quality of life in multiple sclerosis. *Annals of Neurology, 39*, 432-441.

Potts, M. K., Daniels, M., Burnam, M. A., & Wells, K. B. (1990). A structured interview version of the Hamilton Depression Rating Scale: evidence of reliability and versatility of administration. *Journal of Psychiatric Research, 24*, 335-350.

Powell, P., Bentall, R. P., Nye, F. J., & Edwards, R. H. (2001). Randomised controlled trial of patient education to encourage graded exercise in chronic fatigue syndrome. *BMJ, 322*, 387-390.

Radloff, L. S. (1977). The CES-D Scale: a self-report depression scale for research in the general population. *Applied Psychological Measurement, 1,* 385-401.

Redondo, J. R., Justo, C. M., Moraleda, F. V., Velayos, Y. G., Puche, J. J., Zubero, J. R., et al. (2004). Long-term efficacy of therapy in patients with fibromyalgia: a physical exercise-based program and a cognitive-behavioral approach. *Arthritis & Rheumatism, 51,* 184-192.

Rejeski, W. J., Brawley, C. J., & Shumaker, S. A. (1996). Physical activity and health-related quality of life. *Exercise & Sports Sciences Reviews, 24,* 71-108.

Rietberg, M. B., Brooks, D., Uitdehaag, B. M., & Kwakkel, G. (2005). Exercise therapy for multiple sclerosis. *Cochrane Database of Systematic Reviews*(1), CD003980.

Roberts, G. (2006). *Enabling Recovery: The Principles and Practice of Rehabilitation Psychiatry.* London: RCPsych Publications.

Roberts, S. B., Bonnici, D. M., Mackinnon, A. J., & Worcester, M. C. (2001). Psychometric evaluation of the Hospital Anxiety and Depression Scale (HADS) among female cardiac patients. *British Journal of Health Psychology, 6,* 373-383.

Ruta, D. A., Garratt, A. M., Leng, M., Russell, I. T., & MacDonald, L. M. (1994). A new approach to the measurement of quality of life. The Patient-Generated Index. *Medical Care, 32,* 1109-1126.

Scully, D., Kremer, J., Meade, M. M., Graham, R., & Dudgeon, K. (1998). Physical exercise and psychological well being: a critical review. *British Journal of Sports Medicine, 32,* 111-120.

Shah, A., Herbert, R., Lewis, S., Mahendran, R., Platt, J., & Bhattacharyya, B. (1997). Screening for depression among acutely ill geriatric inpatients with a short Geriatric Depression Scale. *Age & Ageing, 26,* 217-221.

Sheikh, J. I., & Yesavage, J. A. (1986). Geriatric Depression Scale: Recent evidence and development of a shorter version. *Clinical Gerontology, 5,* 165-173.

Singh, N. A., Clements, K. M., & Singh, M. A. (2001). The efficacy of exercise as a long-term antidepressant in elderly subjects: a randomized, controlled trial. *Journals of Gerontology A Biological Sciences & Medical Sciences, 56,* M497-504.

Sjosten, N., & Kivela, S. L. (2006). The effects of physical exercise on depressive symptoms among the aged: a systematic review. *International Journal of Geriatric Psychiatry, 21,* 410-418.

Skevington, S. M. (1999). Measuring quality of life in Britain: Introducing the WHOQOL-100. *Journal of Psychosomatic Research, 47,* 449-459.

Smith, A. B., Selby, P. J., Velikova, G., Stark, D., Wright, E. P., Gould, A., et al. (2002). Factor analysis of the Hospital Anxiety and Depression Scale from a large cancer population. *Psychology and Psychotherapy: Theory, Research and Practice, 75*, 165-176.

Sneeuw, K. C., Aaronson, N. K., Sprangers, M. A., Detmar, S. B., Wever, L. D., & Schornagel, J. H. (1998). Comparison of patient and proxy EORTC QLQ-C30 ratings in assessing the quality of life of cancer patients. *Journal of Clinical Epidemiology, 51*, 617-631.

Spielberger, C. D., Gorusch, R. L., Lushene, R., Vagg, P. R., & Jacobs, G. A. (1983). *Manual for the State-trait Anxiety Inventoru.* Paolo Alto, CA: Consulting Psychologists Press.

Stern, R. A. (1997). *Visual Analog Mood Scales Professional Manual.* Odessa, FL: Psychological Assessment Resources Inc.

Stern, R. A., Arruda, J. E., Hooper, C. R., Wolfner, G. D., & Morey, C. E. (1997). Visual analogue mood scales to measure internal mood state in neurologically impaired patients: description and initial validity evidence. *Aphasiology, 11*, 59-71.

Stevens, S. S. (1946). On the theory of scales of measurement. *Science, 103*, 677-680.

Stevinson, C., Lawlor, D. A., & Fox, K. R. (2004). Exercise interventions for cancer patients: systematic review of controlled trials. *Cancer Causes & Control, 15*, 1035-1056.

Thunedborg, K., Allerup, P., Bech, P., & Joyce, C. R. (1993). Development of the Repertory Grid for measurement of individual quality of life in clinical trials. *International Journal of Methods in Psychiatric Research, 3*, 45-56.

Trochim, W. (2006). Levels of measurement. Research Methods Knowledge Base. Retrieved 23.10.08, from http://www.socialresearchmethods.net/kb/measlevl.php

Tsang, H. W., Fung, K. M., Chan, A. S., Lee, G., & Chan, F. (2006). Effect of a qigong exercise programme on elderly with depression. *International Journal of Geriatric Psychiatry, 21*, 890-897.

van den Hout, W. B., de Jong, Z., Munneke, M., Hazes, J. M., Breedveld, F. C., & Vliet Vlieland, T. P. (2005). Cost-utility and cost-effectiveness analyses of a long-term, high-intensity exercise program compared with conventional physical therapy in patients with rheumatoid arthritis. *Arthritis & Rheumatism, 53*, 39-47.

van Straten, A., de Haan, R. J., Limburg, M., Schuling, J., Bossuyt, P. M., & van den Bos, G. A. (1997). A stroke-adapted 30-item version of the Sickness Impact Profile to assess quality of life (SA-SIP30). *Stroke, 28*, 2155-2161.

Wade, D. T. (2003). Outcome measures for clinical rehabilitation trials: impairment, function, quality of life, or value? *American Journal of Physical Medicine & Rehabilitation, 82*(10 Suppl), S26-31.

Wallman, K. E., Morton, A. R., Goodman, C., Grove, R., & Guilfoyle, A. M. (2004). Randomised controlled trial of graded exercise in chronic fatigue syndrome. *Medical Journal of Australia, 180*, 444-448.

Wang, C., Roubenoff, R., Lau, J., Kalish, R., Schmid, C. H., Tighiouart, H., et al. (2005). Effect of Tai Chi in adults with rheumatoid arthritis. *Rheumatology, 44*, 685-687.

Wang, C., Schmid, C. H., Hibberd, P. L., Kalish, R., Roubenoff, R., Rones, R., et al. (2008). Tai Chi for treating knee osteoarthritis: designing a long-term follow up randomized controlled trial. *BMC Musculoskeletal Disordorders, 9*, 108.

Ware, J., Jr., Kosinski, M., & Keller, S. D. (1996). A 12-Item Short-Form Health Survey: construction of scales and preliminary tests of reliability and validity. *Medical Care, 34*, 220-233.

Ware, J. E., Snow, K. K., Kosinski, M., & Gandek, B. (1993). *SF-36 Health Survey: Manual and Interpretation Guide*. Boston, MA: The Health Institute, New England Medical Center.

WHOQOL Group (1994) The development of the WHO quality of life assessment instruments (the WHOQOL). In: Orley, J., & Kuyken, W. (Eds). *Quality of life assessment: international perspectives* (pp.41-57). Berlin: Springer-Verlag.

World Health Organisation (2001). *International Classification of Functioning, Disability and Health*. Geneva, Switzerland: WHO.

Yesavage, J. A., Brink, T. L., Rose, T. L., Lum, O., Huang, V., Adey, M., et al. (1983). Development and validation of a geriatric depression screening scale: A preliminary report. *Journal of Psychiatric Research, 17*, 37-49.

Zigmond, A. S., & Snaith, R. P. (1983). The Hospital Anxiety and Depression Scale. *Acta Psychiatrica Scandinavica, 67*, 361-370.

AUTHOR BIOGRAPHIES

Paula Banbury; B.Sc. (Hons), M.Sc., RGN
Nottingham Back & Pain Team, Nottingham University NHS Trust,
Mobility Centre, City Campus, Hucknall Road, Nottingham NG5 1PJ, UK.
Tel:+44 115 9936626; Fax:+44 115 9936627
Paula.banbury@nuh.nhs.uk

Paula is a Clinical Nurse Specialist who has worked with the Nottingham Back and Pain Team, UK, for 8 years. Prior to this she worked in the Pain Team at the Queen's Medical Centre and completed an Msc in Health Policy and Organisation at the University of Nottingham in 1997. Paula enjoys teaching nursing students and local support groups about long term pain and is a member of the British Pain Society.

Dr Pamela Bartlo; PT, DPT, CCS
D'Youville College - Physical Therapy Department
320 Porter Ave, Buffalo, NY 14201, USA
Tel: 716-829-8390; Fax: 716-829-7680
e-mail: bartlop@dyc.edu

Pamela is a licensed Physical Therapist and a Board Certified Specialist in Cardiovascular and Pulmonary Rehabilitation. She is currently on faculty at D'Youville College in Buffalo, New York, USA. She also serves as the Director of the Transitional Doctorate of Physical Therapy at the college. Her areas of clinical expertise are in cardiovascular and pulmonary rehabilitation, as well as adult neurological rehabilitation. Pamela's research concentrates on knowledge levels of cardiovascular disease risk factors, supervised exercise for people with Type 2 Diabetes, and exercise programming for adults with developmental disabilities attending day habilitation.

Dr Holly Blake; B.A.(Hons), Ph.D., CPsychol.
Faculty of Medicine and Health Sciences, University of Nottingham,
Queen's Medical Centre, Nottingham, NG7 2UH, UK.
Tel: +44 (0)115 8231049; Fax: +44 (0)115 8230999
Email: Holly.Blake@nottingham.ac.uk

Holly is a Chartered Health Psychologist & Lecturer in the Faculty of Medicine and Health Sciences at the University of Nottingham, UK. She is a qualified health and lifestyle trainer, and has many years of experience in a healthcare setting, with diverse research interests focused on rehabilitation and psychosocial outcomes for people with chronic disease, complex service evaluation, workplace and community exercise intervention delivery and outcomes, workplace health programmes, health technologies, and physical activity interventions for people with long-term conditions.

Dr Helen Dawes; Ph.D M.Med.Sci MCSP
Reader, Movement Science Group, School of Life Sciences, Oxford Brookes University, Associate Research Fellow, Dept. of Clinical Neurology, University of Oxford, UK
Tel:+44(0)1865 483293; Fax:+44(0)1865 483242
Email: hdawes@brookes.ac.uk

Helen is a physiotherapist and British Association of Sport and Exercise Science research accredited physiologist in the UK. She is a Reader in Movement Science with current activities extending from exercise prescription for neurological populations in the university clinical exercise unit, to training of health and fitness professionals through to research activities. Her research extends from underlying neuroscience to service delivery, evaluating factors affecting optimal human performance in health and disease with a focus on optimising mobility and physical activity in neurological populations.

Professor Amanda Griffiths, Ph.D M.Sc PGCE CPsychol AcSS AFBPsS
Institute of Work, Health and Organisations, University of Nottingham,
International House, Jubilee Campus, Nottingham, NG8 1BB, UK.
Tel: +44 (0)115 8466637; fax: +44 (0)115 8466625
Email: Amanda.Griffiths@nottingham.ac.uk

Amanda is Professor of Occupational Health Psychology in the Institute of Work, Health & Organisations at the University of Nottingham, UK. She is a Chartered Occupational Psychologist and a Chartered Health Psychologist. Her research explores how working life can be more satisfying, healthy and productive, how people can best manage long-term health conditions, and thus how to minimise work incapacity due to ill health. It involves identifying optimum management strategies for an ageing and diverse workforce.

Dr Martin Hagger Ph.D CPsychol
Personality, Social Psychology, and Health Research Group, School of
Psychology, University of Nottingham, Nottingham, NG7 2RD, UK.
Tel: +44(0)115 8467929; Fax: +44(0)115 9515324
Email: martin.hagger@nottingham.ac.uk

Martin Hagger is Reader in Social and Health Psychology in the School of Psychology, University of Nottingham, UK, with diverse research interests in the areas of health and social psychology. His main focus is the social processes involved in people's 'self-regulation' and motivation of health behaviour, applying social cognitive and motivational models to change diverse health behaviours such as physical activity, dieting, binge drinking, and coping with illness. He is editor-in-chief of Health Psychology Review and the Psychology of Sport and Exercise, co-editor of Psychology and Health, associate editor of Stress and Health, and member of the editorial boards of British Journal of Health Psychology, Journal of Behavioral Medicine, Psychology, Health, and Medicine, and International Review of Sport and Exercise Psychology.

Charlotte Hilton, B.Sc (Hons)
School of Science and Technology, Nottingham Trent University, NG11 8NS, UK.
Tel: +44 (0) 115 8486601
Email: charlotte.hilton@ntu.ac.uk

Charlotte has many years experience working within in-patient and community mental health settings and more recently in a public health environment. Charlotte has been involved in the design, delivery and evaluation of exercise referral schemes and physical activity care pathways within primary care settings. Charlotte's research interests include the holistic evaluation of exercise initiatives aimed at adult chronic ill health improvement, family focussed health improvement initiatives and the integration of motivational interviewing into diverse behaviour change settings. Charlotte is also a member of the Motivational Interviewing Network of Trainers (MINT).

Elizabeth Johnson
Nottingham Back & Pain Team, Nottingham University Hospitals NHS Trust, Mobility Centre, City Campus, Hucknall Road, Nottingham, NG5 1PJ, UK.
Tel:+44 115 9936626; Fax:+44 115 9936627
Email: lizdavid.bicycle@btinternet.com

Liz qualified as a physiotherapist in 1980 and worked with the Nottingham Back and Pain Team at the Nottingham University Hospitals NHS Trust, UK. Following the biopsychosocial model, and using Cognitive Behavioural therapy techniques in a group setting, the Nottingham Back and Pain team teach self management skills for coping with long term pain. Although now retired, she worked within the team for many years, predominantly with musculoskeletal conditions and chronic pain.

Alec Knight, B.Sc. (Hons.), M.Sc.
Research Associate, Institute of Work, Health & Organisations, University of Nottingham, International House, Jubilee Campus, Nottingham, NG8 1BB, UK.
Tel: +44 (0)115 8232213; Fax: +44 (0)115 8466625
e-mail: alec.knight@nottingham.ac.uk

Alec is a Research Associate at the Institute of Work, Health and Organisations at the University of Nottingham, UK. He has been involved in research projects relating to occupational health and organisational psychology funded by the Economic and Social Research Council, the National Institute of Health Research, the European Agency for Safety and Health at Work, and Help The Aged. He is also in the final stages of his doctoral studies, which have focused on prejudice and discrimination against older workers.

Sumaira Malik, B.Sc (Hons), M.Sc.
Institute of Work, Health & Organisations, University of Nottingham,
International House, Jubilee Campus, Nottingham, NG8 1BB, UK.
Tel: +44 (0)115 846 6929; Fax: +44 (0)115 846 6625
Email: lwxsm5@nottingham.ac.uk

Sumaira is a doctoral candidate at the Institute of Work, Health and Organisations and a researcher in the Division of Nursing at the University of Nottingham, UK. She has a background in health psychology and is currently completing her thesis on the use and impact of online support communities for infertility. Her current research interests include physical activity and health, physical activity interventions, exercise in depressed populations, online support, e-health, and health and illness behaviours.

Alison McKeown
Clinical Psychologist in Training, Clinical Psychology Unit, Department of Psychology, University of Sheffield, Sheffield S10 2TN, UK.
Tel: +44 (0) 114 222 2000; Fax: +44 (0) 114 276 6515
Email: pcp06acm@sheffield.ac.uk

Alison is a clinical psychologist in training at the University of Sheffield, UK. She has an interest in the processes and mechanisms of individual change, and the factors that influence these processes, particularly in relation to psychological health and ill health.

Phoenix Mo, BSc (Hons)
Institute of Work, Health & Organisations, University of Nottingham, International House, Jubilee Campus, Nottingham, NG8 1BB, UK.
Tel: +44 (0)115 846 6929; Fax: +44 (0)115 846 6625
Email: lwxsm5@exmail.nottingham.ac.uk

Phoenix is a doctoral candidate in Health Psychology at the Institute for Work, Health and Organisations and a researcher in the Division of Nursing at University of Nottingham, UK. She completed her undergraduate degree in Psychology at the University of Hong Kong, and a masters degree in Health Psychology at the University of Nottingham. She is currently undertaking a PhD examining how HIV+ individuals use online support groups to cope with their diseases, and the effect of online support on disease management and quality of life. Her research interests include online support, physical activity and health, exercise in depressed populations, illness behaviours, and stigma among social minorities.

Dr Shirley Thomas, BSc (Hons), Ph.D., CPsychol
Institute of Work, Health & Organisations, University of Nottingham, International House, Jubilee Campus, Nottingham, NG8 1BB, UK.
Tel: +44 (0) 115 8467484; Fax: +44 (0) 115 8466625
Email: Shirley.Thomas@nottingham.ac.uk

Shirley is a Chartered Health Psychologist and Lecturer in Rehabilitation Psychology in the Institute of Work, Health & Organisations at the University of Nottingham, UK. Her research interests focuses on mood problems after stroke and she is currently conducting an evaluation of psychological treatments for low mood in stroke patients with aphasia. Her research interests also include the psychological aspects of disability and rehabilitation, mood and physical activity, and mental health and ageing.

Dr Roshan das Nair, BA, MSc, MPhil (Clinical Psychology), PhD, CPsychol
Institute of Work, Health & Organisations, University of Nottingham, International House, Jubilee Campus, Nottingham NG8 1BB, UK.
Tel: 0115 8468314; Fax: 0115 8466625
Email: roshan.nair@nottingham.ac.uk

Roshan is a Chartered Consultant Psychologist in HIV and Sexual Health at the Department of Clinical Psychology and Neuropsychology of the Nottingham University Hospitals NHS Trust, and Research Tutor on the Trent Doctorate in Clinical Psychology at The University of Nottingham, UK. He has an interest in health outcome measures and has recently completed a RCT of memory rehabilitation following brain damage, and a Rasch Analysis of the Nottingham Activities of Daily Living scale.

Caroline Neal, B.A.(Hons),B.Sc.(Hons)
Nottingham Back & Pain Team, Nottingham University Hospitals NHS Trust, Mobility Centre, City Campus, Hucknall Road, Nottingham, NG5 1PJ, UK.
Tel:+44 115 9936626; Fax:+44 115 9936627
Email:Caroline.Neal@nuh.nhs.uk

Caroline is an Occupational Therapist with the Nottingham Back and Pain Team, UK. Caroline worked in forensic mental health before joining the Nottingham Back and Pain Team in 2002. This team assess and treat long term non-malignant muskuloskeletal pain. Following the biopsychosocial model, and using Cognitive Behavioural therapy techniques in a group setting, the Nottingham Back and Pain team teach self management skills for coping with long term pain. She is also currently training to be a Cognitive Behavioural Psychotherapist at the University of Birmingham, UK.

Dr Frances M Wise, MBBS PhD(Melb) FAFRM(RACP)
Cardiac Rehabilitation Unit, Caulfield Hospital, 260 Kooyong Road
Caulfield VIC 3162, Australia.
Tel: +61 3 9076 6264; Fax: +61 3 9076 6220
Email: f.wise@cgmc.org.au

Frances is a Senior Rehabilitation Physician in the Cardiac Rehabilitation Unit at Caulfield Hospital, Melbourne, Australia. She has completed a PhD in Rehabilitation Medicine and has worked for many years as a clinician in the rehabilitation sector, as well as more recently in program evaluation. Her research interests include exercise in heart disease, behavioural change in cardiac rehabilitation, depression in heart disease, and psychosocial outcomes in stroke.

INDEX

A

absolute zero, 316
academics, viii, 274
accessibility, 27
accidents, 20, 68, 132, 156
accounting, 19, 183, 251, 253
accuracy, 9, 57, 58, 147, 329
achievement, 18, 221, 284
activation, 84, 105
acute, 1, 19, 20, 46, 67, 80, 84, 90, 95, 103,
    115, 127, 128, 129, 141, 164, 185, 190,
    199, 205, 207, 208, 230, 232, 264, 267, 278
acute stress, 267
Adams, 77, 90
adaptation, 94, 215
addiction, 222
Addison's disease, 257
adipose, 29, 209
adipose tissue, 29, 209
adjustment, 137, 141, 187, 231, 259, 321, 323
administration, 316, 319, 332, 337
administrative, 121
adolescence, 285
adolescent female, 308
adolescents, 57, 94, 97, 255, 257, 259, 285,
    286, 310
adult, 6, 24, 45, 75, 151, 172, 272, 286, 292,
    306, 341, 344
adult population, 6, 286, 293

adulthood, 285, 286
adverse event, 68, 198
aerobics, 75, 286
aetiology, 33, 79, 102, 283
affective disorder, 311
affective states, 331
age, x, 4, 11, 34, 35, 36, 64, 67, 73, 76, 89,
    121, 128, 133, 192, 199, 206, 229, 238,
    242, 257, 262, 263, 272, 276, 292, 302,
    316, 324
ageing, 18, 31, 39, 268, 343, 346
ageing population, 18
agents, 187
agility, 44, 132
aging, 89, 94
aid, 4, 184, 267, 298
air, 33, 175, 177
airways, 33
alcohol, 7, 19, 23, 32, 187
alcohol consumption, 23, 32
alcohol dependence, 7
alertness, 323
alpha, 317
altered state, 132
alternative, ix, xi, 27, 35, 118, 131, 136, 138,
    148, 165, 169, 215, 220, 279, 282, 283,
    295, 299, 302, 328
alternatives, 258
alters, 79
Alzheimer's disease, 24, 44
ambiguity, 243

ambivalence, 8
American Heart Association, 41, 69, 88, 156, 159, 171, 178, 179, 201, 202, 204, 206, 207, 209
American Psychiatric Association, 280, 303
amines, 309
Amsterdam, 179, 204, 209
analgesia, 113, 124
aneurysm, 25
anger, 331
angina, 137, 161, 188, 189, 190, 193, 195, 200, 207, 271
animal models, 135, 149
animals, 133
ankylosing spondylitis, 269, 328, 336
antecedents, 231, 238, 260, 300
anterior cruciate, 256
antibiotics, 200
antidepressant, xi, 35, 279, 281, 282, 283, 284, 288, 289, 293, 294, 295, 296, 297, 299, 303, 304, 309, 310, 311, 329, 338
antidepressant medication, xi, 35, 279, 281, 282, 288, 289, 295, 296, 297, 303
antidepressants, 285, 287, 295, 302, 304, 309
antioxidant, 96
antitumor, 43
anxiety disorder, 136
aortic regurgitation, 209
aortic stenosis, 137, 161, 199
apathy, 133
aphasia, 217, 328, 346
appetite, 136, 327
appraisals, 232, 254
apraxia, 132
aptitude, 252
argument, viii, 17, 24, 36, 106
arousal, 248
arrest, 214
arrhythmia, 195, 271
arrhythmias, 161, 199
arterioles, 162
artery, 23, 27, 42, 46, 67, 96, 162, 174, 184, 188, 190, 205, 207, 208, 209
arthritis, vii, 3, 32, 134, 172, 174, 194

assessment, 27, 105, 119, 121, 124, 125, 140, 149, 151, 168, 171, 181, 191, 192, 214, 271, 293, 294, 297, 301, 316, 318, 321, 322, 330, 331, 336, 340
assumptions, 316
asthma, 18, 218, 236, 271, 301
asymptomatic, 68, 156
ataxia, 132
Athens, 259
atherosclerosis, 44, 190, 205
athletes, x, 104, 130, 212, 215, 229, 230, 231, 235, 236, 237, 238, 239, 250, 252, 254, 256, 257
ATP, 164, 181
atrial fibrillation, 161
atrophy, 54, 80, 164
attitudes, 12, 14, 20, 23, 40, 58, 59, 109, 213, 218, 299, 303
attribution, 222
Australia, 14, 16, 156, 183, 184, 185, 192, 207, 214, 340, 347
autonomic nervous system, 156
autonomy, 137, 142, 243
autoregressive model, 236, 257
availability, 2, 301
avoidance, 103, 110, 114, 115, 126, 127, 129, 235
awareness, 9, 52, 58, 60, 62, 119, 133, 142, 143, 145, 147, 218
axon, 79
axons, 79

B

back, vii, 3, 104, 105, 106, 107, 108, 109, 113, 119, 120, 121, 122, 124, 126, 128, 129, 197, 263, 264, 269, 270, 276, 325, 330, 335
back pain, vii, 3, 47, 103, 104, 105, 106, 107, 108, 109, 113, 114, 121, 125, 126, 127, 128, 129, 130, 257, 269, 270, 277, 327, 330, 331, 334, 336
bad day, 220
barrier, 63, 65, 121, 122, 310

barriers, vii, viii, ix, 3, 4, 11, 22, 24, 46, 51, 58, 59, 60, 61, 64, 72, 80, 81, 94, 97, 99, 102, 108, 111, 118, 119, 120, 123, 125, 141, 148, 221, 263, 281, 299, 300, 303
basal ganglia, 73
basketball, 230
battery, 315
BDI, 327
BDNF, 80, 135
Beck Depression Inventory, 287, 289, 290, 291, 293, 294, 327, 332, 333
behavior, 92, 96, 98, 258, 304
behaviours, 2, 21, 23, 110, 114, 115, 118, 119, 147, 150, 185, 222, 231, 235, 252, 253, 282, 284, 318, 343, 345, 346
Belgium, 10
belief systems, 221
beliefs, ix, x, 12, 14, 33, 58, 101, 103, 108, 109, 110, 114, 115, 119, 124, 126, 127, 130, 187, 218, 221, 222, 223, 230, 231, 232, 234, 235, 249, 270, 304, 322
beneficial effect, 42, 139, 189, 213, 214, 221, 265, 268, 269, 272, 293
Best Practice, 204
beta-blockers, 192
bias, 119, 319
binding, 258
binge drinking, 343
biological markers, 2
biopsychosocial model, viii, 33, 101, 103, 105, 109, 110, 120, 123, 124, 125, 344, 347
bipolar, 266
bipolar disorder, 266
bleeding, 67, 213
blindness, 18
blood, 10, 19, 22, 25, 26, 28, 39, 41, 43, 67, 70, 84, 139, 157, 159, 160, 162, 173, 175, 177, 180, 181, 189, 191, 193, 195, 196, 199, 200, 203, 204, 208, 268, 301
blood clot, 67
blood flow, 67, 157, 160, 181, 189
blood pressure, 10, 25, 39, 41, 70, 139, 159, 173, 175, 177, 180, 189, 191, 193, 195, 196, 198, 203, 208
blood supply, 67
blood vessels, 160
BMA, 18
BMI, 8, 172, 174, 176
body composition, 139, 141, 147, 149, 203, 209
body image, 11, 218
body mass, 29, 39, 47
body mass index, 8, 29, 47
body size, 42, 218
body weight, 29, 32, 49, 97, 189
bone density, 22, 31, 43, 44, 46, 89
bone loss, 31, 35, 38
bone mass, 31, 44
bone mass density, 32
borderline, 208
boredom, 223
borrowing, 120
Boston, 340
bradykinesia, 74
brain damage, 132, 347
brainstem, 79
breast cancer, 34, 35, 42, 43, 44, 48
breathing, 104, 143, 146, 165, 271, 284
breathlessness, 27, 34
Britain, 145, 262, 263, 265, 266, 338
broad spectrum, 133
bronchitis, 33, 272
bursitis, 242
bypass, 174, 184, 188, 190, 200, 205
bypass graft, 174

C

CAD, 162
calcium, 32
caloric intake, 187
Canada, 136, 225
cancer, vii, 4, 18, 23, 24, 34, 35, 36, 37, 38, 41, 42, 44, 45, 46, 213, 214, 330, 339
capillary, 163, 164
cardiac arrest, 200
cardiac arrhythmia, 195
cardiac function, 179
cardiac output, 22, 160, 189
cardiac risk, 201

cardiac risk factors, 201
cardiomyopathy, 198
cardiopulmonary, 93
cardiovascular disease, ix, 18, 22, 25, 26, 30, 34, 42, 44, 45, 68, 84, 104, 134, 181, 183, 185, 189, 206, 207, 342
cardiovascular function, 196, 201
cardiovascular risk, 29, 89
cardiovascular system, ix, 54, 68, 155, 164, 166, 167, 169, 171
caregiver, 148, 322
caregivers, 148
cartilage, 242
case study, ix, 14, 93, 104, 116, 118, 120, 121, 122, 124, 131, 144
cataract, 176
cataract surgery, 176
causal attribution, 231
causal relationship, 10
causality, 255, 305
CDA, 99
CDC, 259
cell, 135
cell death, 135
Centers for Disease Control, 209, 259, 277
central nervous system, viii, 51, 78
central obesity, 208
cerebellum, 79
cerebral hemisphere, 67
cerebrovascular, 67, 68, 69, 70, 72, 73, 156, 280
cerebrovascular accident, 68, 156
cerebrovascular disease, 70, 72, 280
cerebrum, 79
cervical screening, 234, 257
CES, 286, 327, 338
CFA, 240, 242, 243, 248
CFI, 240, 243, 248
changing population, 18
chemicals, 119, 283
chemotherapy, 34, 38
chest, 195, 196
CHF, ix, 155, 156, 157, 158, 160, 161, 162, 163, 164, 165, 166, 167, 168, 169, 170, 171, 172, 174, 176, 177, 178, 179

childhood, 36, 285
children, 20, 62, 120, 255, 307
cholesterol, 19, 75, 88, 189
chronic disease, 2, 6, 11, 20, 22, 36, 55, 134, 214, 303, 308, 342
chronic diseases, 6, 20, 36, 55, 308
chronic fatigue syndrome, 130, 236, 256, 257, 324, 330, 335, 337, 340
chronic illness, 19, 36, 146, 216, 221, 231, 235, 239, 249, 257, 258
chronic obstructive pulmonary disease, 18, 36, 43, 45, 48, 272, 275, 277, 324, 334
chronic pain, 23, 25, 36, 126, 127, 128, 129, 224, 344
chronic renal failure, 26
chronic stress, 266, 267
CINAHL, 138
circulation, 268
citizens, 24
classes, 140, 144, 158, 167, 170, 188, 219, 296
classification, 55, 85, 106, 158
clients, 8, 66, 137, 254, 301, 318
clinical depression, 275, 286, 290, 293, 304, 305, 308, 310
clinical presentation, 33, 102, 106, 129
clinical trial, 26, 39, 40, 89, 127, 290, 305, 311, 336, 339
clinical trials, 26, 39, 40, 89, 290, 339
clinically significant, 106, 163, 164, 167, 295, 326
CNS, 79
Co, 84
coaches, 122, 252, 253
coagulation, 207
Cochrane, 27, 43, 45, 47, 48, 80, 94, 95, 126, 127, 128, 146, 151, 170, 181, 208, 285, 307, 334, 336, 338
Cochrane Database of Systematic Reviews, 45, 94, 128, 151, 208, 307, 334, 336, 338
codes, 59
cognition, 52, 69, 239, 255, 256, 315
cognitive abilities, 145, 328
cognitive deficit, 132, 322
cognitive deficits, 132, 322

cognitive dissonance, 221
cognitive function, 24, 44, 80, 90, 133, 141,
    145, 149, 153, 267, 321
cognitive impairment, ix, 131, 147, 221, 320,
    328
cognitive process, 237
cognitive processing, 237
cognitive representations, vii, 4, 254
cognitive tasks, 69
cognitive therapy, 289, 306
cohort, 90, 95, 152, 307
collaboration, 23
colleges, 1
colon, 34
colon cancer, 34
colorectal cancer, 42
common symptoms, 280
communication, 8, 122, 124, 132, 217, 322,
    323, 328
communication strategies, 217
communities, 13, 345
community service, 185
co-morbidities, 27, 168
comorbidity, 273
compensation, 110
competency, 97
competition, 223
competitive sport, 212
compliance, 29, 32, 215, 260, 278
complications, 3, 23, 30, 32, 37, 143, 196,
    198, 205, 209, 213
components, ix, 54, 56, 66, 81, 123, 125, 139,
    146, 183, 202, 231, 234, 236, 241, 249,
    317, 318, 329
composition, 139
concentrates, 134, 341
concentration, 132, 133, 146, 320, 328
conceptual model, 80, 154
concordance, 125, 185, 317
concrete, 298
conditioning, viii, 17, 59, 83, 106, 137, 138,
    145, 149, 151, 153, 216
conduction, 79
Confederation of British Industry, 262

confidence, ix, 20, 81, 131, 170, 185, 216,
    218, 243, 270, 284
confidence interval, 170, 243
confidence intervals, 170, 243
confinement, 221
confirmatory factor analysis, 234, 250, 257,
    258
confusion, 132, 331
congenital heart disease, 198
congestive heart failure, 178, 179, 180, 181,
    200, 325
consciousness, 132
consensus, 7, 65, 136, 154, 272, 280
consent, 238
construct validity, x, 229, 242, 250
construction, 340
consumption, 23, 32, 139, 157, 161
control condition, 291, 293
control group, 106, 140, 141, 143, 166, 286,
    287, 288, 289, 290, 291, 292, 293, 294,
    295, 296, 297
controlled research, 7, 9
controlled trials, 8, 30, 39, 43, 47, 77, 129,
    180, 203, 208, 286, 287, 296, 307, 319,
    327, 336, 339
COPD, vii, 4, 33, 39, 45, 48, 324, 328, 330
Copenhagen, 89
Coping, 239, 244, 246, 251, 257, 277
coping strategies, vii, x, 3, 4, 33, 43, 124, 125,
    229, 235, 236, 238, 249, 252, 253, 254, 256
coping strategy, 237, 251
coronary angioplasty, 176, 184, 203, 205, 206
coronary artery bypass graft, 188, 190
coronary artery disease, 23, 27, 42, 46, 162,
    184, 190, 205, 208, 209
coronary heart disease, vii, 4, 18, 26, 27, 30,
    36, 43, 47, 55, 68, 99, 111, 129, 130, 183,
    202, 203, 208, 213, 235, 327, 336
correlation, 317, 318, 321
correlations, 237, 245, 248, 317, 323
corticobasal degeneration, 96
corticospinal, 97
corticosterone, 135
cortisol, 92, 334
cost benefits, 271

cost-effective, 148, 149, 339
costs, 62, 128, 139, 262, 264, 265, 266, 269,
    281, 300
counseling, 65, 71, 288
covering, 329
C-reactive protein, 206
credit, xi, 261, 274
criticism, 218
cross-sectional, 265, 285, 292
cultural factors, 316
culture, 110, 225, 321
customers, 264
cycles, 71
cycling, 7, 10, 11, 31, 36, 56, 133, 140, 141,
    194, 217, 220
cytokine, 80

D

daily living, 67, 68, 71, 78, 82, 94, 108, 132,
    142, 151, 158, 190, 321, 323, 325
Dallas, 202
danger, 258
data analysis, 99
data collection, 147, 255
data set, 13
database, 210
DBP, 160
death, ix, 22, 26, 30, 34, 66, 68, 118, 132,
    135, 156, 183, 189, 204
deaths, 52, 156, 166, 183, 192, 280
decay, 236
decisions, 221
Deep Brain Stimulation, 74
defense, 135
defibrillator, 201
deficits, 3, 132, 139, 149, 152, 216, 283, 322
definition, 48, 102, 212, 282, 311, 321, 331
delayed gratification, 224
delivery, 8, 12, 20, 30, 53, 54, 56, 60, 65, 71,
    72, 73, 77, 78, 82, 149, 263, 342, 344
Delphi, 136
Delphi technique, 136
dementia, 52
demographics, 18, 316

demyelination, 79
denial, 235
density, 22, 31, 43, 44, 46, 89, 111, 163, 164,
    189, 190
dentate gyrus, 44
Department of Health and Human Services,
    22, 48, 192, 209
depressed, 25, 134, 136, 280, 284, 285, 286,
    289, 290, 292, 293, 294, 297, 299, 300,
    301, 302, 307, 308, 310, 326, 329, 345, 346
depressive disorder, 298, 306, 308, 336
Depressive disorders, 292
depressive symptomatology, 281, 289, 292,
    294, 297, 309, 337
depressive symptoms, xi, 35, 38, 279, 281,
    283, 285, 286, 287, 288, 289, 290, 292,
    293, 296, 297, 298, 299, 302, 305, 308,
    309, 310, 326, 327, 336, 337, 338
detection, 9, 272
developed countries, 19, 184, 266, 271
developed nations, ix, 183
developmental change, 257
developmental disabilities, 342
diabetes, vii, 4, 6, 18, 22, 29, 34, 36, 37, 38,
    39, 40, 41, 42, 43, 46, 47, 48, 55, 75, 84,
    89, 111, 134, 161, 203, 204, 213, 219, 236,
    301, 334
diabetes mellitus, 42, 43, 47
diabetic neuropathy, 201
diabetic retinopathy, 199
Diagnostic and Statistical Manual of Mental
    Disorders, 293
diagnostic criteria, 268, 293, 326
diastolic blood pressure, 160
diet, 20, 23, 29, 39, 46, 49
dietary, 29, 42, 187, 190
dieting, 343
diets, 208
differentiation, 234
difficult goals, 221
dilation, 207
directionality, 236
disabilities, 23, 24, 46, 58, 59, 60, 61, 62, 83,
    94, 95, 132, 133, 136, 138, 140, 143, 145,
    153, 190, 218

disabled, 59, 113, 203
discomfort, 158, 220, 221
discounting, 117
discourse, 114
discrimination, 345
discs, 112
disease activity, 32, 336
disease progression, 24, 75, 162, 163, 164, 167, 172, 177
diseases, viii, 18, 21, 33, 34, 51, 53, 86, 132, 134
dislocation, 242
disorder, 31, 73, 79, 306, 308, 314, 325, 335, 336
dissatisfaction, 125
distortions, 117
distraction, 111, 283
distress, 110, 114, 322, 324, 330
diuretic, 172, 174, 176
diversity, viii, 2, 17, 37, 220
dizziness, 193, 199, 221, 282
dopamine, 73, 74, 283
dorsi, 197
dose-response relationship, 299
draft, 255
drinking, 343
dropout rates, 299
drowning, 132
drowsiness, 282
drug therapy, 187
drug treatment, 74, 187, 281
drugs, 299
DSM, 288, 290, 292, 293, 327, 332
DSM-II, 288, 290
DSM-III, 288, 290
DSM-IV, 293, 327, 332
dualism, 314, 320
duality, 110
durability, 315
duration, 2, 18, 30, 31, 32, 55, 56, 57, 58, 66, 68, 72, 73, 78, 110, 145, 160, 162, 168, 171, 186, 187, 191, 194, 195, 196, 215, 220, 224, 238, 282, 292, 296, 297, 309
duties, 121, 270
dyspnea, 34, 178

dysthymia, 293

E

ears, 75, 242
eating, 35, 280, 323
ecological, 267
Economic and Social Research Council, 275, 345
Education, 15, 39, 43, 84, 91, 187, 226
e-health, 345
elderly, 52, 56, 60, 62, 72, 85, 208, 248, 267, 293, 294, 296, 297, 303, 307, 308, 310, 311, 335, 338, 339
elderly population, 52, 62, 85, 297
elders, 309, 310
e-mail, 155, 341, 344
embolism, 161, 199
emotion, 133, 236, 239, 242, 244, 245, 248, 250, 254, 257
emotion regulation, 254
emotional distress, 266, 304
emotional experience, 33, 102
emotional health, 191
emotional reactions, 321, 325
emotional responses, 117, 231, 232, 237, 239, 255
emotional well-being, 310
emotions, x, 114, 229, 235, 237, 249, 250, 251, 253, 254, 257
emphysema, 33, 272
employees, viii, 4, 263, 264, 265, 266, 268, 269, 270, 272, 273
employers, xi, 261, 262, 263, 265, 266, 267, 270, 273, 274
employment, 25, 262, 263, 265, 267, 269, 271, 272
empowered, 20, 253
encouragement, 4, 25, 36, 284
endocarditis, 161, 199
endocrine, 52
endocrine disorders, 52
endorphins, 119, 216, 283
endothelium, 189
end-stage renal disease, 236

endurance, 26, 29, 53, 54, 56, 64, 66, 70, 76, 81, 85, 86, 92, 137, 138, 139, 141, 142, 162, 163, 164, 171, 174, 179, 181, 188, 196, 197, 216, 292
energy, 4, 27, 29, 35, 38, 79, 109, 136, 152, 187, 188, 201, 264, 280, 282, 291, 300, 325
engagement, viii, 11, 13, 51, 64, 65, 132, 133, 144, 145, 264, 295, 300
England, 6, 10, 14, 19, 40
enrollment, 202
environment, 12, 14, 27, 33, 62, 63, 122, 133, 141, 220, 273, 336, 344
environmental factors, 58, 60, 74, 75, 79, 169
environmental influences, 63
epidemic, 38
epidemiologic studies, 34, 44
epidemiology, 259, 328
epilepsy, 18, 52, 137, 218
equating, 52
equilibrium, 74
ethnic minority, 154
EU, 259
euphoria, 283
Europe, 19, 37, 132, 183, 184, 268, 277
European Commission, 184, 204
European Union, 184, 227, 230
evening, 195
evidence-based policy, 273
evolution, viii, 83, 101
excitability, 78
exercise participation, 3, 4, 53, 58, 81, 140, 148, 213, 218, 300
exercise performance, 104, 162, 179, 188, 300
exercisers, 134, 294
exertion, 28, 34, 57, 158, 161, 166, 170, 173, 175, 177, 178, 193, 198, 203
experimental design, 130
expertise, 61, 123, 224, 341
exposure, 79, 126, 130, 132
external validity, 267, 270
extraction, 189
extraneous variable, 236

F

facial expression, 74
facilitators, viii, 46, 51, 61, 64, 87, 94
factor analysis, 232, 234, 250, 256, 257, 258
failure, 27, 38, 48, 117, 179, 273
family, 58, 63, 110, 119, 122, 148, 154, 263, 265, 344
family members, 122, 154
family support, 58
fat, 35, 43, 196, 208
fatigue, ix, 27, 32, 34, 53, 76, 79, 80, 81, 87, 91, 92, 93, 98, 119, 130, 131, 132, 136, 139, 157, 165, 173, 191, 221, 236, 256, 257, 320, 324, 330, 331, 335, 337, 340
fats, 29
fax, 343
fear, 23, 76, 110, 112, 114, 115, 126, 127, 129, 130, 136, 141, 217, 221, 270
fears, 33, 106, 196, 218, 258
February, 40, 150
feedback, 39, 300
feelings, ix, 35, 59, 101, 115, 116, 118, 119, 136, 137, 147, 212, 218, 220, 223, 280, 281, 284, 300
females, 76, 156, 280, 308
fever, 161, 199
fibrillation, 161
fibrinolysis, 189
fibromyalgia, 126, 128, 327, 330, 334, 335, 338
Finland, 214, 307
flexibility, 32, 36, 53, 56, 66, 137, 138, 141, 143, 144, 145, 146, 236, 282, 290, 297, 336
flight, 172
flow, 28, 33, 67, 157, 160, 181, 189, 207
focus group, 12, 77, 87
focusing, 4, 133, 144, 145, 165, 269, 280, 286
food, 153, 204
football, 230
Ford, 30, 41, 230, 243, 256
forensic, 347
forgetfulness, 282
forgetting, 135
Fox, 314, 318, 333, 335, 337, 339

fracture, 31
fractures, 32, 70, 201, 242
fragility, 31
France, 156
frustration, 142
functional changes, 67, 163
funding, 7
fusion, 54

G

gait, 28, 44, 47, 69, 71, 74, 75, 77, 88, 91, 96,
    98, 134, 149, 152, 173, 292
games, 216, 217, 218
ganglia, 73
gas, 180
gas exchange, 180
gender, 64, 76, 242, 304, 316
gender differences, 304
General Health Questionnaire, 143, 331, 335
general practitioner, 18, 19, 62, 231, 296, 301,
    310
general practitioners, 62, 231, 301
generalizability, 12
generalized anxiety disorder, 306
genetic disorders, 52
Geneva, 48, 99, 181, 210, 340
geriatric, 310, 335, 338, 340
GHQ, 331
globus, 74
glucose, 46, 196
glycosylated, 30
goal setting, 270
goals, 10, 46, 123, 185, 187, 221, 222, 284,
    321
gold, 318
gold standard, 318
government, 19, 20, 83, 137, 145, 213, 214,
    262, 285
government policy, 137
GPs, 214, 262, 301
grafts, 188, 190
grief, 231, 256
group membership, 223
group work, 77

groups, 1, 3, 10, 23, 35, 60, 62, 66, 70, 77,
    106, 107, 134, 143, 169, 171, 194, 198,
    213, 218, 269, 270, 271, 287, 288, 289,
    290, 291, 294, 296, 324, 330, 341, 346
growth, 85, 99, 135, 212, 326
growth factor, 85, 99, 135
growth factors, 99, 135
guidance, xi, 7, 20, 70, 105, 137, 141, 224,
    298, 313
guidelines, 3, 6, 8, 9, 10, 11, 12, 22, 28, 37,
    41, 42, 44, 59, 68, 69, 72, 103, 126, 159,
    172, 186, 187, 191, 195, 200, 207, 298

H

HADS, 330, 338
haemoglobin, 30
haemostasis, 204
hamstring, 197
handicapped, 174
hands, 107, 248, 249
harm, 82, 103, 113, 115, 223, 274
harmful effects, 104
hazards, 3
HDL, 43
head and neck cancer, 236, 258
head injuries, 152
head injury, 132, 142
head trauma, 153
headache, 52, 129
healing, 112, 135
Health and Human Services, 189, 209
health care, xi, 2, 12, 19, 23, 33, 111, 158,
    179, 187, 204, 226, 230, 261, 262, 273,
    280, 281, 285, 298, 299, 300, 302, 303,
    304, 310, 315, 316, 325, 334, 335, 342
health care professionals, 281, 285, 298, 300,
    302
health education, 293, 296, 297
health effects, 29, 213
health problems, 1, 18, 22, 24, 36, 37, 70, 110,
    134, 218, 263, 266, 271, 272, 273, 281,
    302, 314, 320, 325
health psychology, 345
health services, 263, 264, 270

health status, 32, 35, 134, 283, 321, 323, 333, 334
hearing, 132
hearing loss, 132
heart disease, ix, 18, 22, 26, 27, 36, 37, 68, 156, 180, 183, 184, 206, 235, 327, 347
heart failure, vii, ix, 4, 18, 25, 27, 36, 38, 39, 40, 44, 45, 47, 155, 156, 159, 178, 179, 180, 181, 184, 188, 200, 206, 208, 209, 271, 325, 334
heart rate (HR), ix, 56, 57, 104, 155, 157, 173, 175, 177, 181, 191, 192, 193, 195, 198, 201, 284
heat, 82, 88, 165
heating, 82
height, 139
helplessness, 300
hemiparesis, 90, 93
hemodynamic, 179
hemodynamics, 178, 181
hemostatic, 207
heterogeneity, 159, 298, 303
heterogeneous, 106
high blood cholesterol, 19
high blood pressure, 19, 22, 25, 301
high risk, 4, 68, 198, 200, 298
high-density lipoprotein, 189, 190
higher quality, 72
high-frequency, 291
high-level, 19
hip, 9, 31, 111, 127
hippocampal, 80
histology, 165
HIV, 18, 346
HIV/AIDS, 18
hockey, 230
holistic, 270, 315, 344
homogeneity, 317
Hong Kong, 346
hopelessness, 35, 266, 280, 300
hormone, 34, 135
hormones, 99, 308
hospital, 19, 20, 27, 36, 56, 132, 139, 141, 146, 147, 172, 174, 176, 186, 188, 190, 201, 205, 216, 230, 330

hospital care, 36
hospitality, 268
hospitalization, 235
hostility, 331
House, 144, 343, 344, 345, 346
household, 158, 174, 191, 217
household tasks, 158, 191
HPA, 283
HPA axis, 283
human, 3, 52, 54, 72, 97, 218, 342
Human Kinetics, 83, 86, 128, 152, 153, 202, 205, 277
human subjects, 97
humans, 208
Huntington's disease, 257
husband, 119, 172
hyperactivity, 189, 283
hypercholesterolemia, 172, 174
hypertension, 6, 18, 23, 25, 26, 36, 45, 67, 89, 111, 180, 187, 189, 199, 203, 208, 271
hypertrophic cardiomyopathy, 201
hypotension, 199
hypothesis, 78, 82, 231, 235, 237, 240, 242, 243, 247, 248, 249, 251, 252, 255, 283, 284, 306

I

IASP, 33, 43, 102, 127
ICD, 332
identification, 153
identity, x, 69, 117, 220, 223, 229, 232, 235, 236, 237, 238, 239, 242, 243, 248, 249, 250, 252, 253
IDS, 289
Illinois, 151
images, 118, 212
immune function, 80
immune response, 79
immune system, 22
immunological, 52
impairments, 18, 23, 28, 53, 61, 67, 69, 75, 87, 91, 132, 133, 139, 141, 143, 145, 152, 156, 253, 281, 321, 328
implantable cardioverter defibrillators, 206

implementation, 7, 56, 196, 274
impulsive, 133, 216
in situ, 323
in transition, 76
in vivo, 126, 130
inactive, 7, 30, 34, 299
incarceration, 221
incentive, 18
incidence, 18, 30, 34, 38, 46, 95, 136, 214,
    230, 268
Incidents, 114
inclusion, 8, 20, 25, 159, 254, 267, 287, 332
income, 120, 121, 154
independence, viii, ix, 17, 23, 37, 131, 139,
    140, 144, 145, 146, 166, 190, 196, 217
indication, 57, 74, 83, 255
indicators, 72, 146
indices, 321
indirect effect, 253
induction, 217, 218
industry, 58, 212
ineffectiveness, 125
inertia, 331
infarction, 184, 188, 190, 271
infections, 132, 200, 271
infectious, 52
infertility, 345
inflammation, 55, 79, 85, 86, 96, 103
inflammatory disease, 32, 79
inflammatory response, 55
inflammatory responses, 55
inherited, 113
inhibitor, 172
initiation, 163, 167
injections, 73
innovation, 21, 40
inoculation, 268
insight, 84
insomnia, 282
inspection, 326
instability, 107
institutions, 1, 13
instruction, 143, 144
instructors, 8
instruments, 323, 332, 340

insulation, 79
insulin, 23, 26, 30, 39, 42, 43, 49, 111, 187,
    190
insulin resistance, 26, 30, 190
insulin sensitivity, 23, 39, 49
integration, 3, 4, 40, 63, 65, 71, 72, 73, 81,
    147, 344
integrity, 97
intentions, 212, 220, 303
interaction, 77, 221, 283, 284, 293, 296, 323
interactions, 176, 291
interdisciplinary, 102, 123, 124, 125, 130
internal consistency, 323, 325
internet, 46, 96
interval, 133, 292, 316
intervention strategies, 42, 272, 276
interview, 290, 297, 319, 326, 331, 337
interviews, 12, 239, 316, 326
intimidating, 218, 301
intracranial pressure, 132
intramuscular, 160
intrinsic, 119
intrinsic rewards, 119
Investigations, 109
investment, 6, 19, 97, 121, 270
Ireland, 260
irritability, 35, 133, 135, 280
irritable bowel syndrome, 259
ischaemia, 67, 189, 193, 200
ischaemic heart disease, 280
ischemia, 161
ischemic, 57, 67, 71, 97, 156
ischemic heart disease, 156
ischemic stroke, 71, 97
isolation, 59, 120, 125, 284, 325
Israel, 97

J

JAMA, 39, 42, 44, 84, 209
Japan, 154
Japanese, 209, 210
job satisfaction, 275
jobs, 121, 187
joining, 347

joint damage, 32
joints, 31, 104, 142, 213, 242, 268
Jordan, 311
judge, 274
jumping, 70, 117

K

killing, 183
kinematics, 88
King, 43, 214, 226
knee, 33, 43, 111, 122, 127, 253, 264, 269, 324, 326, 340
knees, 122, 172

L

labour, 187
lactate level, 157, 163
land, 151, 165, 327
language, 217, 316, 319
later life, 285, 299
Latino, 303
law, 219
laws, 59
learning, 20, 76, 77, 80, 135, 218
left ventricle, 167
left ventricular, ix, 155, 156, 157, 162, 163, 179, 180
leg, 67, 84, 178
leisure, 13, 42, 59, 67, 89, 120, 143, 144, 154, 184, 190, 212, 217, 218, 301
leisure time, 59, 67, 184
lesioning, 74
lesions, 42
levator, 174
levodopa, 92, 93
life experiences, 114
life span, 165
life style, 32
lifestyle changes, 7, 23, 29
life-threatening, 4, 190, 200
lifetime, 38, 141, 283, 285
lift, 196, 216

ligament, 242, 256
likelihood, 11, 13, 67, 68, 73, 148, 196, 240, 267, 299, 326
limitation, 33, 146, 158, 319, 321
limitations, viii, ix, 57, 60, 81, 101, 109, 110, 131, 133, 145, 171, 199, 268, 270, 273, 287, 293, 297, 298, 303, 320, 321, 324, 331
Lincoln, 148, 150, 320, 321, 328, 333, 336
links, 13, 24
Lipid, 187, 190, 210
lipids, 43
lipoproteins, 190
litigation, 110, 265
loading, 240, 242
lobbying, 262
local community, 144, 301
local government, 214
localised, 268
location, 67, 133, 319
locomotion, 74, 139
locus, 119
Locus of Control, 222, 226
logical reasoning, 133
London, 14, 15, 40, 86, 97, 106, 126, 129, 130, 180, 225, 227, 257, 259, 270, 275, 276, 277, 278, 308, 333, 335, 337, 338
long distance, 105
longitudinal studies, 134
long-term services, 68
Los Angeles, 259
losses, 220
Lovelock, 46, 95
low back pain, 47, 103, 104, 105, 106, 107, 108, 113, 114, 121, 125, 126, 127, 128, 129, 130, 257, 269, 277, 327, 331, 334, 336
low risk, 82, 167, 198
low-density, 190
low-income, 154
low-intensity, 201, 301
low-level, 178
LTC, 18, 19, 21, 23
lumbar, 105, 107, 108
lungs, 33
Luxembourg, 276
lymphedema, 44

M

machines, 61, 165, 197, 201
macular degeneration, 174
magazines, 212
mainstream, 212
maintenance, viii, 29, 31, 33, 34, 47, 51, 62,
    151, 163, 188, 215, 216, 217, 219, 298, 303
maintenance tasks, 217
major depression, 136, 280, 285, 289, 298,
    303, 304, 305, 311, 329, 333, 334
major depressive disorder, 298, 306
maladaptive, 115, 116, 235, 237, 254
malaise, 32
males, 73, 132, 156, 280
malignant, 109, 347
manipulation, 106
manual workers, 268
Marfan syndrome, 199
marketing, 302
Marx, 62, 85
Massachusetts, 48
mastery, 146, 223, 283, 284, 300
MDA, 43
meanings, 336
measurement, 2, 9, 57, 84, 92, 192, 315, 316,
    321, 322, 333, 335, 336, 337, 338, 339
media, 212
median, 238
mediation, 252, 255
mediators, 55, 304
medication, 33, 35, 53, 76, 125, 234, 248,
    256, 258, 281, 289, 295, 296, 302
medications, xi, 35, 57, 74, 136, 168, 172,
    174, 176, 185, 187, 279, 281, 288, 295,
    296, 303
meditation, 165, 288
MEDLINE, 138
memory, 44, 80, 132, 320, 328, 346
memory loss, 132
men, x, 6, 10, 22, 34, 43, 44, 46, 48, 67, 71,
    75, 95, 96, 130, 153, 183, 205, 209, 229,
    238, 280
mental ability, 316
mental disorder, 18, 275, 303, 306

mental illness, 266, 286, 305, 314
mental retardation, 96
mercury, 161, 173, 175, 177
messages, 13, 19, 231
MET, 162, 191
meta-analysis, 30, 39, 43, 45, 46, 47, 48, 67,
    84, 88, 90, 92, 93, 98, 129, 130, 159, 180,
    203, 208, 275, 287, 305, 310, 319, 327, 332
metabolic syndrome, 30
metabolism, 90, 157, 162, 164, 168, 196, 215
middle-aged, 10, 44, 286, 292
migraine, 33, 40
Minnesota, 172, 174, 176, 181
minorities, 346
minority, 94, 154
misconceptions, 187
mitochondrial, 164, 181
mitral, 205, 209
mitral regurgitation, 209
mitral valve, 205
mobility, 22, 28, 31, 53, 54, 55, 69, 70, 71, 76,
    78, 80, 87, 90, 95, 96, 140, 158, 172, 174,
    221, 251, 252, 264, 323, 325, 342
modalities, ix, 149, 183, 187, 196, 213, 215,
    288, 291, 303
modality, 53, 81, 194, 196, 290
modeling, 255, 257
models, 56, 57, 62, 85, 134, 135, 149, 231,
    240, 242, 243, 248, 255, 257, 258, 322, 343
moderate activity, 83, 267
momentum, 215
money, 126
monoamine, 283
mood change, 331, 335
mood disorder, 296
mood states, 80, 328, 332
morbidity, 1, 34, 47, 184, 190, 205, 230, 258,
    259, 281, 292, 331
morning, 195
mortality, 1, 2, 27, 30, 34, 41, 43, 46, 47, 48,
    69, 89, 95, 99, 156, 158, 162, 167, 172,
    184, 188, 190, 201, 205, 208, 280, 281, 292
MOS, 239, 242, 260
motion, 2, 9, 137, 142, 165, 173, 197, 283

motivation, 11, 13, 14, 23, 31, 63, 85, 115,
    119, 133, 212, 213, 215, 220, 221, 223,
    224, 231, 256, 260, 264, 299, 300, 301,
    303, 343
motives, 86
motor activity, 151
motor function, 84, 93, 134, 139
motor vehicle accident, 132
movement, 52, 54, 58, 91, 103, 106, 111, 112,
    115, 141, 143, 146, 163, 197, 270, 273,
    282, 323
multidisciplinary, 13, 42, 105, 106, 124, 129,
    205
multiple sclerosis, 47, 52, 57, 59, 66, 79, 83,
    84, 85, 86, 88, 89, 91, 92, 93, 94, 95, 96,
    97, 98, 99, 134, 153, 324, 331, 337, 338
muscle atrophy, 157, 164, 215
muscle contraction, 160
muscle mass, 70
muscle relaxation, 142
muscle spasms, 142
muscle strength, 22, 31, 32, 53, 56, 80, 84, 95,
    105, 163, 164, 178, 196, 213
muscle weakness, 112
muscles, ix, 31, 55, 56, 63, 77, 104, 107, 108,
    141, 155, 157, 160, 161, 162, 215, 242,
    268, 284, 320
muscular dystrophy, 86
musculoskeletal pain, 124, 128
mutuality, 314
myelin, 79
myocardial infarction, 27, 161, 172, 184, 188,
    190, 191, 199, 200, 202, 205, 206, 207,
    208, 210, 259, 271, 278
myocarditis, 161, 199
myocardium, 160
myopathy, 93, 181

N

National Health Interview Survey, 41
National Health Service, 20, 262
natural, 220, 273, 276
natural environment, 220
natural science, 273, 276

neck, 120, 121, 124, 128, 236, 258, 269, 270
negative attitudes, 58
negative experiences, 218
negotiating, 63
negotiation, 172
neoplastic, 52
nerve, 111
nerves, 79, 111, 112, 242, 268
nervous system, 52, 61, 73, 79
nervousness, 248
network, 119
neural function, 135
neurobiological, 154, 311
neurogenesis, 44, 135, 306
neurological condition, vii, viii, 3, 29, 51, 52,
    53, 55, 56, 57, 58, 59, 60, 61, 62, 63, 64,
    65, 66, 77, 78, 82, 83, 86, 87
neurological disease, 53, 60, 83, 84
neurological disorder, 18, 52, 54, 84
neurological rehabilitation, 341
neuromotor, 152
neuromuscular diseases, 86
neuronal degeneration, 79
neuronal survival, 79
neurons, 73
neuroplasticity, 80
neuroprotection, 80
neuroscience, 342
neurotransmitter, 73, 134
neurotransmitters, 283
neurotrophic, 79, 97, 135
New England, 42, 128, 202, 207, 340
New Jersey, 126, 180, 225, 226
New York, 85, 126, 130, 149, 158, 200, 226,
    227, 258, 304, 308, 337, 341
New Zealand, 11, 107, 129, 303, 304
Newton, 34, 35, 45, 205
NHP, 324, 325
NHS, 18, 21, 40, 101, 341, 344, 346, 347
NNFI, 240, 243, 248
non-exercisers, 134
non-insulin dependent diabetes, 43, 111
non-random, 135, 286
normal, 3, 34, 55, 56, 60, 62, 63, 103, 112,
    142, 157, 189, 195, 270, 280

norms, 319, 325
North America, 94, 202
Nottingham Health Profile, 324
nucleus, 74
nurse, 188
nurses, 235, 301
nursing, 74, 77, 138, 174, 186, 301, 306, 310, 341
nursing care, 74
nursing home, 306, 310
nutrients, 187

outpatient, 19, 47, 96, 106, 130, 176, 188, 196, 198, 202, 209
outpatients, 179, 329, 330
overload, 215
overtime, 281
overweight, 10, 19, 21, 47, 96
overweight adults, 96
oxidative, 84, 94, 139, 157
oxidative stress, 84
oxygen, 22, 26, 38, 104, 139, 157, 161, 162, 179, 188, 189, 190, 191, 192, 205, 282, 290
oxygen consumption, 139, 157, 161

O

obese, 10, 14, 47, 49
obesity, vii, 4, 6, 10, 18, 22, 23, 26, 29, 34, 36, 43, 46, 47, 110, 207, 208, 213, 214, 218, 268, 301
objectivity, 2
occupational, viii, xi, 4, 133, 232, 261, 263, 264, 268, 269, 270, 271, 272, 274, 345
occupational asthma, 272
occupational health, 263, 264, 270, 345
occupational therapy, 133
oedema, 165, 172, 176
Ohio, 179
old age, 292
older adults, 25, 42, 44, 69, 70, 94, 143, 203, 216, 292, 293, 294, 295, 296, 297, 304, 308, 310, 326, 327, 328, 329, 331, 336
older people, 38, 292, 295, 296, 297, 310, 328
oligodendrocytes, 79
Oncology, 41, 44, 45, 48
online, 345, 346
open heart surgery, 209
organ, 164
orientation, 97, 133
orthopaedic, 223
osteoarthritis, 111, 127, 172, 259, 324, 326, 328, 340
osteopenia, 42
osteoporosis, 22, 23, 31, 32, 34, 36, 38, 40, 43, 48
osteoporotic fractures, 32
outcome of interest, 315

P

pacemakers, 199, 201
pacing, 112, 113, 201
pain management, ix, 33, 101, 105, 106, 107, 115, 121, 123, 124, 125, 129, 130
palliative care, 306
paradigm shift, 46, 55, 94, 153
paradox, 321
paradoxical, 79
paralysis, 217
parameter, 157, 159, 170, 240, 242
parameter estimates, 240
paranoia, 286
parasympathetic, 157
parents, 217
paresis, 153
Parkinson's Disease (PD), viii, 3, 51, 52, 59, 66, 73, 74, 75, 84, 85, 87, 88, 92, 96
parkinsonism, 88, 91, 93
partnership, 301
passive, 109, 124, 232, 235, 334
path analysis, 236, 240, 248, 250
path model, 240, 241
pathology, 52, 54, 84, 105, 112, 273
pathways, 344
patient care, 315
pedometer, 9, 30, 31, 38, 39, 47, 57, 84
peers, 23, 300
perception, x, 40, 77, 111, 201, 218, 229, 231, 232, 234, 235, 236, 239, 240, 242, 248, 249, 250, 254, 257, 300, 321

perceptions, x, 3, 11, 114, 129, 218, 221, 229, 231, 232, 234, 235, 236, 237, 238, 239, 240, 249, 250, 251, 252, 253, 254, 255, 257, 258, 259, 283, 303
perceptions of control, 235
perfusion, 204
pericarditis, 161, 199
peripheral nerve, 79
permit, 255, 298
personal accounts, 316
personal control, x, 229, 232, 234, 235, 236, 239, 242, 243, 249, 250, 251, 252, 253, 254, 255
personal efficacy, 234
personal responsibility, 222, 243
personality, 133, 231, 304, 305
persons with disabilities, 46, 94
persuasion, 300
pharmacological, 36, 69, 288
pharmacological treatment, 36
pharmacotherapy, 304, 305
Philadelphia, 38, 128
philosophy, 20
Phoenix, vi, 279, 345, 346
phone, 294
phosphate, 258
physical education, 153
physical exercise, xi, 3, 22, 24, 32, 54, 85, 133, 134, 139, 145, 208, 216, 222, 261, 269, 274, 278, 292, 300, 308, 310, 324, 326, 330, 338
physical fitness, 40, 43, 71, 141, 147, 208
physical health, vii, 3, 21, 24, 184, 219, 262, 285, 299, 301, 331
physical therapy, 76, 80, 86, 91, 133, 134, 145, 339
physical well-being, 267, 278
Physicians, 68
physiology, 150
physiotherapists, 106, 153, 224, 231, 252
physiotherapy, 90, 94, 97, 99, 168, 174, 217, 325, 335
pilot study, 39, 44, 47, 85, 89, 91, 92, 150, 258, 304, 305, 307, 334
placebo, 288

planning, x, 13, 121, 132, 220, 229, 237, 238, 239, 242, 248, 249, 250, 251, 252, 253, 254, 314, 316
plaque, 27
plasticity, 135, 149, 150
Plato, 54
play, 13, 14, 19, 55, 80, 137, 220, 266, 272, 283
pleasure, 136
point like, 137
policy instruments, 37
policy makers, 9
polio, 83
polyarticular, 32
POMS, 331
pools, 212
poor, 2, 8, 12, 14, 18, 23, 29, 33, 63, 102, 121, 122, 132, 266, 321
poor health, 266
population group, 3, 297
ports, 230, 259
positive mood, 331
positive relation, 235, 237
positive relationship, 235
postmenopausal women, 42
postoperative, 200
post-stroke, 28, 45, 47, 93, 96, 97
post-traumatic stress, 136
post-traumatic stress disorder, 136
postural hypotension, 201
posture, 31, 74, 143, 146
poverty, 265
power, 53, 54, 56, 66, 138, 243, 249
prediction, 251
predictive validity, 318
predictors, 48, 97, 238, 310
preference, 77, 106, 107
prejudice, 345
premature death, 2, 30, 36, 55
press, 57, 59, 60, 61, 64, 70, 82, 87, 99, 130, 197, 331
pressure, 10, 19, 22, 25, 39, 41, 67, 70, 132, 139, 159, 160, 164, 173, 175, 177, 180, 189, 191, 193, 195, 196, 198, 199, 200, 203, 208, 215, 301

primary care, 7, 8, 11, 15, 148, 187, 304, 308, 335, 344
prisons, 1
privacy, 218
private sector, 265
probability, 295
problem-focused coping, 231, 235, 236, 249, 252, 255
problem-solving, 133
production, 80, 164, 181, 216
productivity, 266, 275
professions, 273
Profile of Mood States (POMS), 331, 336, 337
prognosis, viii, ix, 17, 23, 37, 38, 101, 120, 127, 133, 165, 205
prognostic factors, 129
program, 38, 39, 46, 47, 71, 86, 90, 93, 95, 97, 98, 139, 141, 150, 151, 153, 154, 163, 179, 205, 240, 257, 289, 307, 310, 338, 339, 347
programming, 152, 342
progressive supranuclear palsy, 96
promoter, 80
prophylactic, 216
prostate, 34
prostate cancer, 34
protection, 231, 260, 267
protocol, 9
protocols, 37
proxy, 322, 323, 325, 334, 339
psoriasis, 257
psychiatric diagnosis, 326
psychiatric illness, 136
psychiatric morbidity, 331
psychiatric patients, 328
psychological distress, 260, 330
psychological health, 1, 35, 137, 145, 146, 345
psychological phenomena, 314
psychological processes, 109
psychological states, 220, 266, 268
psychological well-being, 6, 42, 137, 190, 235, 266, 267, 278, 284, 307, 309, 333, 335, 337
psychologist, 345

psychology, 133, 256, 293, 335, 345
psychometric properties, xi, 313, 316, 332, 333
psychopathology, 111, 151
psychosocial factors, 23
psychosocial functioning, 267, 278
psychosocial variables, 127, 256
psychotherapy, xi, 35, 136, 279, 281, 282, 287, 288, 289, 297, 305, 306, 307, 308
public, vii, 6, 7, 10, 11, 13, 14, 20, 36, 40, 52, 61, 86, 137, 144, 153, 216, 218, 277, 280, 291, 298, 302, 344
public health, vii, 6, 7, 10, 13, 14, 36, 52, 86, 137, 144, 153, 277, 280, 291, 344
Public Health Service, 209
public service, 40
pulmonary embolism, 137
pulmonary hypertension, 161, 199
pulmonary rehabilitation, 34, 39, 341
pulse, 191, 195
punitive, 264

Q

QALYs, 325
QLQ-C30, 339
quality research, 2, 137, 273
questionnaire, 2, 87, 147, 181, 234, 239, 257, 316, 323, 326, 327, 334
questionnaires, 12, 57, 58, 144, 316, 319, 320, 322, 326

R

radiation, 35
rain, 80, 220
Rasch analysis, 316
rating scale, 316, 335
ratings, 58, 327, 339
reactivity, 9, 283
reading, 117, 133, 294
reality, 134, 273
reasoning, 117, 133
reciprocal cross, 238, 251

recognition, 1, 262, 271, 285
reconstruction, 256
recreation, 141, 223, 255, 258, 323
recreational, 206, 230, 238
recurrence, 34, 188, 258, 306
regional, 209
regression, 307, 336
regression analysis, 307, 336
regular, 26, 31, 35, 36, 46, 55, 61, 63, 69, 72,
     80, 94, 104, 111, 121, 122, 159, 162, 190,
     212, 213, 217, 219, 221, 265, 283, 299,
     300, 301, 305
regulation, 254, 256, 257, 258
regulations, 59
rehabilitation program, 1, 25, 34, 36, 42, 55,
     62, 64, 94, 133, 137, 138, 141, 145, 168,
     171, 184, 186, 192, 195, 205, 209, 214,
     231, 263, 264, 270, 276, 320
reinforcement, 119
relapse, 43, 53, 281, 285, 292, 295, 298, 311
relapses, 78
relationship, x, 26, 30, 54, 75, 80, 86, 89, 114,
     119, 134, 222, 230, 236, 242, 249, 251,
     253, 266, 267, 283, 291, 298, 299, 302,
     304, 322, 326, 337
relationships, 10, 113, 120, 164, 223, 231,
     235, 236, 237, 251, 256
relaxation, 31, 33, 40, 125, 133, 140, 142,
     143, 146, 221, 288, 290
relevance, vii, 4, 115, 142, 216, 222
reliability,92, 98, 152, 181, 234, 239, 240,
     257, 316, 317, 318, 320, 323, 324, 325,
     327, 331, 336, 337, 340
remediation, 133
remission, 54, 289, 292, 326
remodeling, 163, 167
remyelination, 79
renal disease, 236
renin, 162
renin-angiotensin system, 162
repair, 149
repetitions, 26, 169, 170, 171, 197, 198
replication, 270
Research and Development, 90, 96, 97
resentment, 120

residential, 141
residuals, 240, 243, 248
resistive, 87, 159
resolution, 78
resources, 13, 59, 62, 119, 127, 172, 187, 194,
     280, 299, 319
respiratory, xi, 43, 161, 170, 173, 175, 177,
     215, 261, 263, 266, 271
respiratory disorders, xi, 261, 263, 266, 271
respiratory rate, 170, 173, 175, 177
responsiveness, 336
restenosis, 207
retinal detachment, 201
retinopathy, 199, 201
retirement, 264, 272
retirement age, 272
rewards, 119
rheumatoid arthritis, 36, 39, 40, 41, 42, 47, 48,
     151, 213, 269, 326, 328, 336, 339, 340
rhythm, 132
rings, 158
risk assessment, 272
risk factors, 19, 21, 26, 28, 29, 36, 42, 68, 69,
     70, 95, 128, 136, 154, 168, 185, 187, 189,
     196, 199, 201, 203, 265, 342
risk profile, 190
risks, 3, 24, 37, 55, 116, 165, 166, 167, 172,
     191, 213, 214, 262
RMSEA, 240, 243, 248
robotic, 134
routines, 282
Royal Society, 311
RPE, 57, 173, 175, 177
rugby, 230, 253
Russia, 156

S

sadness, 35, 136, 280
safety, x, 3, 27, 96, 110, 115, 116, 156, 163,
     167, 183, 198, 205, 207, 217, 277
sample, 12, 42, 59, 60, 139, 140, 142, 143,
     147, 234, 238, 239, 240, 242, 258, 269,
     286, 287, 289, 290, 291, 292, 293, 294,
     295, 296, 297, 298, 327

sarcopenia, 34
Sartorius, 281, 309
satisfaction, 216, 275, 301, 321
saturated fat, 29
savings, 6
SBP, 160, 161
scar tissue, 112
scepticism, 213
scheduling, 223
schizophrenia, 18, 266, 286
Schmid, 340
school, 1, 106, 135, 218, 268
school work, 268
sclerosis, 52, 78, 79, 84, 85, 87, 93
scores, 191, 288, 291, 293, 294, 295, 297,
    316, 318, 320, 324, 325, 326, 327, 329, 330
SDH, 95
search, 138, 232
search terms, 138
seasonality, 215
Second World, 103, 105
Second World War, 103, 105
secretion, 283
sedentary, 1, 2, 4, 11, 12, 13, 22, 36, 68, 69,
    76, 121, 130, 134, 139, 145, 153
sedentary lifestyle, 1, 13, 22, 36, 68, 121, 134,
    145
seizures, 137
selecting, xi, 313, 316, 320, 326, 332
Self, 15, 19, 20, 91, 94, 143, 224, 225, 258,
    276, 277, 278, 300
self worth, 223
self-awareness, 142
self-care, 19, 20, 40, 150, 282, 325
self-concept, 310
self-confidence, 267
self-determination theory, 92
self-efficacy, 42, 60, 63, 69, 92, 96, 142, 196,
    220, 221, 231, 267, 283, 284, 299, 300, 314
self-esteem, 23, 133, 136, 142, 143, 144, 146,
    147, 216, 222, 223, 259, 266, 267, 300, 314
self-identity, 69
self-management, 43, 106, 121, 124, 185, 235
self-monitoring, 9
self-regulation, 254, 256, 257

self-report, x, 2, 9, 33, 34, 38, 75, 111, 134,
    144, 147, 229, 238, 239, 288, 297, 304,
    316, 319, 320, 327, 328, 330, 331, 338
self-reports, 328
sensation, 110, 220
sensations, 220, 221, 223
sensitivity, 23, 39, 49, 218, 219
sensors, 2
sequelae, 137, 190
sequencing, 132
series, 139, 239, 315
serotonin, 283
sertraline, 295, 304
serum, 97, 334
services, iv, viii, 13, 17, 18, 19, 24, 37, 40, 68,
    137, 145, 218, 264, 274, 301, 310
severity, 3, 7, 88, 95, 111, 133, 158, 161, 224,
    257, 260, 295, 310, 315, 316, 326, 330
shock, 132
shortness of breath, 33, 172, 174, 176
short-term, 8, 34, 70, 180, 268, 292, 299, 302
side effects, 35, 143, 187, 282, 304, 309
sign, 113, 174, 176, 177
signals, 73
signs, 79, 152, 193, 195, 325, 334
sinus, 199
sites, 238
Sjogren, 267, 278
skeletal muscle, ix, 22, 28, 155, 157, 161, 162,
    164, 181
skeleton, 38
skills, 7, 54, 59, 61, 123, 133, 142, 185, 344,
    347
sleep, 135, 136, 323, 325, 327
sleep disturbance, 327
smoking, 23, 32, 187
smoking cessation, 187
soccer, 230
social activities, 158
social benefits, 223
social care, viii, 1, 17, 18, 19, 20, 37, 45
social context, x, 147, 211
social environment, 133
social exclusion, 24, 262, 265
social factors, 109

social impairment, 133
social influence, 103, 109, 119, 120, 148, 304
social influences, 103, 109, 119, 120
social integration, 3, 147
social isolation, 120, 325
social participation, 28
social psychology, 231, 343
social skills, 133
social support, 69, 119, 122, 133, 137, 143, 147, 235, 299
sodium, 187
software, 255
somatic symptoms, 293, 327, 328, 330
spasticity, 28, 69, 84, 132, 138, 140
spatial memory, 44
specificity, 215
spectrum, 133
speech, 61, 132, 133, 217
speed, 28, 30, 53, 54, 56, 57, 66, 77, 97, 98
spinal cord, 28, 42, 67, 79, 213
spinal cord injury, 42, 213
spine, 31, 107, 118, 121, 126
spines, 108
sporadic, 11
sports, x, 32, 87, 128, 130, 206, 229, 230, 235, 238, 239, 243, 245, 248, 249, 250, 252, 253, 254, 255, 256, 258, 259, 260, 264
sprains, 242
stability, x, 108, 141, 230, 236, 237, 249, 250, 251, 254, 321
stable angina, 184, 189
stages, 74, 76, 77, 78, 80, 82, 108, 109, 156, 216, 219, 220, 272, 309, 315, 345
STAI, 329, 330
standards, 37, 126, 159, 179, 204, 273, 321
statin, 172, 174
statistics, 178, 243, 248, 259, 266, 280, 316
stenosis, 189
stent, 184, 200, 207
stiffness, 31, 105, 121
stigma, 281, 282, 310, 346
stomach, 195
strain, 148, 150, 334
strains, 242, 299
stratification, 165

stress, 63, 64, 76, 79, 84, 99, 119, 135, 142, 148, 149, 154, 158, 160, 164, 165, 169, 171, 187, 198, 203, 208, 215, 231, 242, 256, 260, 266, 267, 268, 275, 277, 283, 308
stress fracture, 242
stressors, 267
stretching, 59, 81, 84, 106, 120, 138, 143, 283, 290
striatum, 73, 88
stroke volume, 160
strokes, 214
structural equation model, 258
Structural Equation Modeling, 257, 258, 259
students, 238, 341
subacute, 90, 97
subcortical structures, 67
subgroups, 298
subjective, 105, 142, 267, 278, 316, 322, 333, 334
subjective well-being, 267
subjectivity, 103
subluxation, 242
substantia nigra, 73
suffering, 18, 87, 105, 118, 120, 135, 190, 234, 253, 281, 299, 301, 302
suicide, 25, 280
supervision, 2, 198
supply, 22
support services, 137
support staff, 254
Surgeon General, 48, 209
surgery, 27, 74, 126, 161, 184, 196, 200, 205, 209, 213, 235, 259
surgical intervention, 200
survival, ix, 34, 42, 79, 183, 189, 190
survival rate, 34, 189
surviving, 68
survivors, 28, 35, 41, 46, 48, 68, 88, 93, 96, 97, 99
Sweden, 214
swelling, 32
Switzerland, 340
symptom, 34, 35, 191, 232, 251, 288
symptomology, 303
syndrome, 43, 334

synthesis, 78, 82, 287
systemic sclerosis, 89
systolic blood pressure, 160, 193, 199, 200

T

T2DM, 29, 30, 31
tachycardia, 199, 200
targets, 56, 58, 65, 69, 236, 237, 263, 264
taxonomy, 337
TBI, ix, 131, 132, 133, 134, 135, 136, 137,
    138, 139, 142, 143, 144, 145, 146, 147,
    148, 149, 151
TCC, 142
teaching, 111, 122, 341
temperature, 316
temporal, 236, 237
tendon, 242
tendons, 242, 268
tension, 112, 136, 196, 331
test-retest reliability, 98, 325
Texas, 202
thalamus, 74
therapeutic approaches, 76
therapeutic interventions, 164
therapists, 137
therapy interventions, 80, 81, 89
thinking, 33, 72, 111, 115, 117, 118
thinking styles, 115, 117, 118
Thomson, 271, 278
threat, 232, 236, 251
threatening, 166, 231, 236
threats, x, 52, 229, 258
threshold, 66, 93, 162, 201, 217
threshold level, 66, 162
thrombophlebitis, 161, 200
TIA, vii, 3, 29, 57, 67, 68, 69, 70, 72, 83
time periods, 317
timing, 53, 76, 82, 319
tissue, 33, 102, 105
tobacco, 19
tolerance, ix, 27, 48, 80, 94, 155, 156, 161,
    162, 163, 164, 168, 174, 178, 179, 190,
    194, 201, 204, 209
total cholesterol, 75

total energy, 291
toxic, 52, 132
training programs, 97, 206, 208
trait anxiety, 329
trajectory, 265, 315, 326
transfer, 70, 173
transformation, 45
transient ischemic attack, 57, 67
transition, 215, 216, 219
transition period, 215
translation, 235, 319
transplant, 178, 184, 192, 206
transplant recipients, 178
transport, 10, 11, 13, 56, 58, 61, 62
transportation, 60, 104
transversus abdominis, 108
trauma, 47, 231
traumatic brain injuries, 52, 132, 150, 152
traumatic brain injury, 136, 137, 138, 146,
    149, 150, 151, 152, 153, 154, 322, 324,
    328, 330, 335
travel, 10, 11
tremor, 74
triggers, 113, 118
triglyceride, 39
triglycerides, 189, 190
tuberculosis, 280
tumours, 132
turbulent, xi, 261
turnover, 265
type 2 diabetes, 29, 34, 36, 38, 39, 40, 42, 46,
    48, 55, 75, 203, 204, 213
type 2 diabetes mellitus, 38, 39

U

undergraduate, 238, 293, 346
United Kingdom, 103, 121, 225, 230
United States, 153, 156, 230, 306
universities, 9
unstable angina, 199
upper respiratory tract, 271
urinary, 54
US Department of Health and Human
    Services, 192, 209

V

validation, 335, 337, 340
validity, x, xi, 9, 12, 115, 181, 229, 234, 239,
    240, 242, 250, 257, 267, 270, 313, 316,
    318, 320, 323, 324, 327, 328, 330, 331,
    332, 336, 339, 340
values, 240, 321, 325
variability, 157, 181
variables, 127, 236, 238, 240, 248, 249, 250,
    251, 252, 253, 255, 256, 267, 273, 278,
    304, 318
variance, 231, 242, 251
variation, 220, 265
Vascular disease, 156
vascular system, 160
vasoconstriction, 160, 162
vasodilatation, 189
vein, 223
ventilation, 178
ventricle, 167
ventricular arrhythmia, 137, 193
ventricular tachycardia, 200
venue, 77
versatility, 337
vessels, 160, 174
victims, 70
Victoria, 204
virtual reality, 134
visible, 218
vision, 20, 45, 132, 221
Visual Analogue Scale, 289
vitreous, 201
vocational rehabilitation, 263
volleyball, 260
vomiting, 282
vulnerability, 79, 221, 284

W

waiting times, 281
walking, 7, 10, 11, 28, 30, 31, 34, 36, 39, 41,
    44, 46, 47, 49, 57, 59, 66, 71, 73, 74, 80,
    84, 89, 90, 92, 93, 94, 96, 97, 98, 112, 120,
    133, 139, 158, 161, 165, 169, 187, 194,
    220, 243, 253, 282, 286, 287, 293
war, 105
warrants, 147, 289
water, 31, 46, 141, 142, 146, 165, 217, 327
weakness, 69, 77, 84, 112, 141
wealth, viii, 36, 37, 101, 212
wear, 112
websites, 52
weight control, 20, 37, 187, 189
weight gain, 29, 165, 172, 215
weight loss, 13, 29, 39, 46, 119, 207, 212
weight management, 11, 187
weight reduction, 29, 30
wheelchair, 117, 118
white matter, 79
wind, 220
winter, 264
workability, 25
workers, 234, 267, 269, 270, 272, 278, 345
workforce, 262, 268, 271, 343
working conditions, 263
working population, 267
workload, 195, 200
workplace, 121, 262, 266, 272, 276, 277, 342
World Health Organization (WHO), 18, 19,
    35, 37, 48, 52, 89, 99, 156, 181, 183, 184,
    185, 210, 280, 281, 311, 320, 321, 322, 340
worry, 248
wound infection, 200
writing, 73, 132

X

xenografts, 43

Y

yes/no, 324, 325, 328
yield, 30, 31, 286
young women, 290